Global Applications of Culturally Competent Health Care: Guidelines for Practice

Marilyn "Marty" Douglas
Dula Pacquiao • Larry Purnell
Editors

Global Applications of Culturally Competent Health Care: Guidelines for Practice

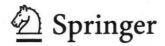 Springer

Editors
Marilyn "Marty" Douglas
School of Nursing
University of California San Francisco
Palo Alto
California
USA

Dula Pacquiao
School of Nursing
Rutgers University
Newark
New Jersey
USA

Larry Purnell
College of Health Sciences
University of Delaware
Sudlersville
Maryland
USA

ISBN 978-3-319-69331-6   ISBN 978-3-319-69332-3   (eBook)
https://doi.org/10.1007/978-3-319-69332-3

Library of Congress Control Number: 2018943678

Printed on acid-free paper

This Springer imprint is published by the registered company Springer International Publishing AG part of Springer Nature
The registered company address is: Gewerbestrasse 11, 6330 Cham, Switzerland

Preface

There are three areas that heighten the need for culturally competent care: globalization and its resultant increase in population and workforce diversity, global conflicts with consequent displacement of populations, and evidence of health inequities within the same country and across different countries globally. Today, global conflicts have forcibly displaced 65.6 million persons, creating an unprecedented 22.5 million refugees in the world (UNHCR 2018). An influx of this magnitude presents a challenge to nurses worldwide to provide care to persons who may have health beliefs and practices different from their own. In addition, these new groups of refugees and displaced persons augment the local and national racial and ethnic minority populations who are increasingly vulnerable to unequal access to health care and resultant poor health outcomes. This book was compiled as an effort to reduce the effects of social inequities on the health of these populations and to provide healthcare professionals with a resource for providing culturally competent care.

Health disparities are the differential consequences on the physical and mental well-being of population groups attributable to social inequalities. These inequities create cumulative disadvantages in human life conditions exposing certain groups to a greater number and intensity of health risks. Health is tied with the social conditions of life. Thus, health promotion should be grounded on the principles of social justice and protection of basic human rights supportive of health. While individual-based care and biomedical approaches to diseases are important, population health achievement is difficult without improving the conditions in which people are born, live, and work. This book attempts to demonstrate culturally competent care as a strategy to achieve health equity.

The Guidelines for Culturally Competent Health Care were developed by a task force convened by members of the Expert Panel on Global Nursing and Health of the American Academy of Nursing and also included members of the Transcultural Nursing Society. In preparing the guidelines, the task force members reviewed documents related to culturally competent health care from more than 50 publications and sources from around the world, including healthcare, governmental and nongovernmental organizations. Several versions of the guidelines were sent to global colleagues for peer review to assess global applicability. Eventually, the final version of the Guidelines was endorsed by the International Council of Nurses and distributed to its member national nursing organizations throughout the world. Nurses in these countries are now left to decide how to implement them.

The purpose of this book is to expand on previous work describing the Guidelines (Douglas et al. 2014) and to provide practical, clinical examples of how each of these guidelines can be integrated into practice by practitioners caring for diverse populations from around the world. This book will be useful for multidisciplinary healthcare students, clinicians, advanced practice nurses, administrators, educators, and those who provide community health or population-based care.

The first chapter provides the conceptual basis for culturally competent health care and presents a list of ten guidelines along with a few examples of implementation. Then a separate section is devoted to each guideline. Within each section is a chapter with an in-depth discussion of the guideline and its rationale, followed by three or more chapters with clinical case studies of examples of how the guideline was implemented in a particular cultural setting. All case studies follow a similar format and are written by international authors with clinical expertise and work experience in the culture being presented.

It is recognized that these guidelines must be adapted to each situation. Within each setting, there are cultural norms embedded in their respective social, economic, and political system in which they exist. Therefore, in conclusion, the guidelines and their accompanying case studies are intended to be examples of how culturally competent care can be delivered. They are not meant to be requirements for professional practice but rather to assist the practitioner, educator, administrator, or researcher in planning care for a culturally diverse population.

Palo Alto, CA, USA   Marilyn "Marty" Douglas
Newark, NJ, USA   Dula Pacquiao
Sudlersville, MD, USA   Larry Purnell

References

Douglas M, Rosenketter M, Pacquiao D, Clark Callister L, Hattar-Pollara M, Lauderdale J, Milsted J, Nardi D, Purnell L (2014) Guidelines for implementing culturally competent nursing care. J Transcult Nurs 25(2):109–221. https://doi.org/10.117/1043659614520998. Accessed 29 Oct 2017
United Nations High Commissioner for Refugees (UNHCR) Figure at a glance. Statistical yearbooks. http://www.unhcr.org/en-us/figures-at-a-glance.html. Accessed 9 Jan 2018

Acknowledgements

The Co-Editors wish to acknowledge and thank all of our professional colleagues around the world who have made this work possible. In particular, these include the members of the American Academy of Nursing Expert Panel on Global Nursing and Health's Task Force on Global Standards of Culturally Competent Care. This task force was comprised of the three co-editors of this book plus Lynn Clark Callister, PhD, RN, FAAN, Marianne Hattar-Pollara, PhD, RN, FAAN, Jana Lauderdale, PhD, RN, FAAN, Jeri Milstead, PhD, RN, FAAN, Deena Nardi, PhD, PMHCNS-BC, FAAN, Marlene Rosenkoetter, PhD, RN, CNS, FAAN, and Joan Uhl Pierce, PhD, RN, FAAN. This task force formulated the original Standards of Practice for Culturally Competent Care and published them as Guidelines for Practice, which form the basis of the structure and content for this book.

Special acknowledgement must be given to Joan Uhl Pierce, PhD, RN, FAAN, who was the first chair of the task force, and whose initiative was to enlist past presidents of the Transcultural Nursing Society as members of the Academy's task force on this topic.

In addition, we would like to specifically acknowledge Dr. Marianne Hattar-Pollara for her vision of expanding these Guidelines to book form. She was also instrumental in coordinating and participating in the key planning session for this book.

Finally, we wish to acknowledge the Transcultural Nursing Society (TCNS), in particular the Transcultural Nursing Scholars, who created the forum for common interest and commitment in promoting culturally competent practices in education, research, and practice. TCNS has its mission "to enhance the quality of culturally congruent, competent, and equitable care that results in improved health and well-being for people worldwide" and a vision "to provide nurses and other healthcare professionals with the knowledge base necessary to ensure cultural competence in practice, education, research, and administration."

Contents

1 Conceptual Framework for Culturally Competent Care   1
Dula Pacquiao

Part I   Guideline: Knowledge of Cultures

2 Knowledge of Cultures   31
Larry Purnell

**3 Case Study: Building Trust Among American
Indian/Alaska Native Communities—Respect
and Focus on Strengths**   43
Janet R. Katz and Darlene P. Hughes

**4 Case Study: An 85-Year-Old Immigrant from the Former
Soviet Union**   49
Lynn Clark Callister

**5 Case Study: Caring for Urban, American Indian,
Gay, or Lesbian Youth at Risk for Suicide**   53
Jana Lauderdale

Part II   Guideline: Education and Training

6 Education and Training in Culturally Competent Care   61
Larry Purnell

**7 Case Study: Traditional Health Beliefs of Arabic
Culture During Pregnancy**   77
Jehad O. Halabi

**8 Case Study: Perceived Cultural Discord and Possible
Discrimination Involving a Moroccan Truck Driver
in Italy**   85
Alessandro Stievano, Gennaro Rocco,
and Giordano Cotichelli

9   Case Study: A Multiracial Man Seeks Care in the
    Emergency Department   89
    Marianne R. Jeffreys

Part III   Guideline: Critical Reflection

10 Critical Reflection   97
    Larry Purnell

11 Case Study: Human Trafficking in Guatemala 113
    Joyceen S. Boyle

12 Case Study: A Young African American Woman
    with Lupus 119
    Donna Shambley-Ebron

13 Case Study: Intimate Partner Violence in Peru 125
    Roxanne Amerson

Part IV   Guideline: Cross Cultural Communication

14 Cross Cultural Communication: Verbal and Non-Verbal
    Communication, Interpretation and Translation 131
    Larry Purnell

15 Case Study: Korean Woman with Mastectomy Pain 143
    Sangmi Kim and Eun-Ok Im

16 Case Study: An 85-Year-Old Saudi Muslim Woman
    with Multiple Health Problems 149
    Sandra Lovering

17 Case Study: Communication, Language, and Care
    with a Person of Mexican Heritage with
    Type 2 Diabetes 155
    Rick Zoucha

18 Case Study: Stigmatization of a HIV+ Haitian Male 161
    Larry Purnell, Dula Pacquiao, and Marilyn "Marty" Douglas

Part V   Guideline: Culturally Congruent Practice

19 Integrating Culturally Competent Strategies
    into Health Care Practice 169
    Marilyn "Marty" Douglas

20 Case Study: Perinatal Care for a Filipina
    Immigrant 187
    Violeta Lopez

21 Case Study: Maternity Care for a Liberian Woman 193
    Jody R. Lori

**22 Case Study: Care of a Malay Muslim Woman
     in a Singaporean Hospital** 197
Antoinette Sabapathy and Asmah Binti Mohd Noor

**Part VI   Guideline: Cultural Competence in Health Care Systems
           and Organizations**

**23 Building an Organizational Environment of
     Cultural Competence** 203
Marilyn "Marty" Douglas

**24 Case Study: Culturally Competent Strategies Toward
     Living Well with Dementia on the Mediterranean Coast** 215
Manuel Lillo-Crespo and Jorge Riquelme-Galindo

**25 Case Study: Culturally Competent Healthcare Organizations
     for Arab Muslims** 221
Stephen R. Marrone

**26 Case Study: A Lebanese Immigrant Family
     Copes with a Terminal Diagnosis** 229
Anahid Kulwicki

Part VII   Guideline: Patient Advocacy and Empowerment

**27 Advocacy and Empowerment of Individuals, Families and
     Communities** 239
Dula Pacquiao

28 Case Study: Zapotec Woman with HIV in Oaxaca, Mexico ... 255
Carol Sue Holtz

**29 Case Study: Maternal and Child Health Promotion Issues
     for a Poor, Migrant Haitian Mother** 261
Joyce Hyatt

**30 Case Study: Caring for a Pakistani Male
     Who Has Sex with Other Men** 267
Rubab I. Qureshi

Part VIII   Guideline: Multicultural Workforce

31 Culturally Competent Multicultural Workforce 275
Dula Pacquiao

**32 Case Study: Internationally Educated Nurses
     Working in a Canadian Healthcare Setting** 287
Louise Racine

**33 Case Study: Recruitment of Philippine-Educated Nurses
     to the United States** 293
Leo Felix Jurado

**34 Case Study: Health Care for the Poor and
Underserved Populations in India** 299
Joanna Basuray Maxwell

Part IX   Guideline: Cross Cultural Leadership

35 Attributes of Cross-Cultural Leadership 307
Dula Pacquiao

**36 Case Study: Integrating Cultural Competence and
Health Equity in Nursing Education** 315
Susan W. Salmond

**37 Case Study: Cross-Cultural Leadership for Maternal
and Child Health Promotion in Sierra Leone** 323
Florence M. Dorwie

**38 Case Study: Nursing Organizational Approaches
to Population and Workforce Diversity** 329
Lucille A. Joel, Dula Pacquiao, and Victoria Navarro

Part X   Guideline: Evidence Based Practice and Research

**39 Designing Culturally Competent Interventions
Based on Evidence and Research** 339
Marilyn "Marty" Douglas

**40 Case Study: Domestic Violence of an Elderly Migrant
Woman in Turkey** 361
Gülbu Tanriverdi

**41 Case Study: Sources of Psychological Stress for a
Japanese Immigrant Wife** 369
Noriko Kuwano

**42 Case Study: Early Childbearing and Contraceptive
Use Among Rural Egyptian Teens** 375
Azza H. Ahmed

**43 Case Study: A Chinese Immigrant Seeks Health
Care in Australia** 381
Patricia M. Davidson, Adam Beaman,
and Michelle DiGiacomo

Contributors

Azza H. Ahmed, D.N.Sc., R.N., I.B.C.L.C. School of Nursing, Purdue University, West Lafayette, IN, USA

Roxanne Amerson, Ph.D., R.N., C.T.N.-A., C.N.E. School of Nursing, Clemson University, Greenville, SC, USA

Adam Beaman, M.P.H. School of Nursing, Johns Hopkins University, Baltimore, MD, USA

Joyceen S. Boyle, Ph.D., R.N., M.P.H., FAAN College of Nursing, University of Arizona, Tucson, AZ, USA

College of Nursing, Augusta State University, Augusta, GA, USA

Lynn Clark Callister, R.N., Ph.D., FAAN School of Nursing, Brigham Young University, Provo, UT, USA

Giordano Cotichelli, Ph.D., R.N. Faculty of Medicine, University of Ancona, Ancona, Italy

Patricia Davidson, Ph.D., Med., R.N., FAAN School of Nursing, Johns Hopkins University, Baltimore, MD, USA

Michele DiGiacomo, Ph.D. University of Technology Sydney, Sydney, NSW, Australia

Florence Maria Dorwie, D.N.P., R.N.C., A.P.N.-B.C. Sa Leone Health Pride, Inc., North Bergen, NJ, USA

New York Presbyterian Columbia University Medical Center, New York, NY, USA

Marilyn "Marty" Douglas, Ph.D., R.N., FAAN School of Nursing, University of California, San Francisco, San Francisco, CA, USA

Jehad O. Halabi, Ph.D., R.N., T.N.S. College of Nursing, King Saud bin Abdulaziz University of Health Sciences—National Guard, Al Ahsa, Kingdom of Saudi Arabia

Carol Sue Holtz, Ph.D., R.N. School of Nursing, Kennesaw State University, Kennesaw, GA, USA

Darlene P. Hughes, M.S.N., R.N. College of Nursing, Washington State University, Spokane, WA, USA

K Bay Air, Homer, AK, USA

Joyce Hyatt, Ph.D., D.N.P., C.N.M. Nurse Midwifery Program, School of Nursing, Rutgers University, Newark, NJ, USA

Eun-Ok Im, Ph.D., R.N., FAAN School of Nursing, Duke University, Durham, NC, USA

Marianne Jeffreys, Ed.D., R.N. Graduate College and College of Staten Island, The City University of New York (CUNY), New York, NY, USA

Lucille A. Joel, Ed.D., R.N., A.P.N., FAAN School of Nursing, Rutgers University, Newark, NJ, USA

Leo-Felix M. Jurado, Ph.D., R.N., A.P.N., FAAN Department of Nursing, William Paterson University, Wayne, NJ, USA

Janet R. Katz, Ph.D., R.N. College of Nursing, Washington State University, Spokane, WA, USA

Sangmi Kim, Ph.D., R.N. School of Nursing, Duke University, Durham, NC, USA

Anahid Kulwicki, Ph.D., R.N., FAAN School of Nursing, Byblos Campus, Lebanese American University, Byblos, Lebanon

Noriko Kuwano, Ph.D., R.N., M.W., P.H.N. International Nursing Department, Oita University of Nursing and Health Sciences, Oita, Japan

Jana Lauderdale, Ph.D., R.N., FAAN School of Nursing, Vanderbilt University, Nashville, TN, USA

Manuel Lillo-Crespo, Ph.D., M Anthro., M.S.N., R.N. Facultad Ciencias de la Salud, Department of Nursing, University of Alicante, Alicante, Spain

Clinica Vistahermosa Hospital, Alicante, Spain

Violeta Lopez, Ph.D., R.N., F.A.C.N., FAAN Nat Yong Loo Lin School of Medicine, Alice Lee Center for Nursing Studies, Clinical Research Center, National University of Singapore, Singapore, Singapore

Jody R. Lori, Ph.D., C.N.M., F.A.C.N.M., FAAN PAHO/WHO Collaborating Center, School of Nursing, University of Michigan, Ann Arbor, MI, USA

Sandra Lovering, R.N., B.S.N., M.B.S., D.H.Sc. King Faisal Specialist Hospital and Research Center, Jeddah, Kingdom of Saudi Arabia

Stephen Marrone, Ed.D., R.N., N.E.A., C.T.N.-A Harriet Rothkoft Heilbrunn School of Nursing, Long Island University of Nursing, Brooklyn, NY, USA

Joanna Basuray Maxwell, Ph.D., R.N. Department of Nursing, Multicultural Institute and Faculty Development, Towson University, Towson, MD, USA

Victoria Navarro, M.S.N., R.N. Joint Commission International, Oakbrook, IL, USA

Asmah Binti Mohd Noor, M.Sc., R.N., N.I.C.U. Nanyang Polytechnic, Singapore, Singapore

Dula Pacquiao, Ed.D., R.N., C.T.N.-A., T.N.S. School of Nursing, Rutgers University, Newark, NJ, USA

School of Nursing, University of Hawaii, Hilo, Hilo, HI, USA

Larry Purnell, Ph.D., R.N., FAAN School of Nursing, University of Delaware, Newark, DE, USA

Florida International University, Miami, FL, USA

Excelsior College, Albany, NY, USA

Rubab I. Qureshi, M.D., Ph.D. School of Nursing, Rutgers University, Newark, NJ, USA

Louise Racine, Ph.D., R.N., FAAN College of Nursing, University of Saskatchewan, Saskatoon, SK, Canada

Jorge Riquelme-Galindo, M.S.N., R.N. Department of Nursing, University of Alicante, Alicante, Spain

Gennaro Rocco, Ph.D., R.N., FAAN Centre of Excellence for Nursing Scholarship, Ipasvi Rome Nursing Board, Rome, Italy

Antoinette Sabapathy, R.N., S.C.M., C.N.M., W.H.N.P. Nursing Maternity Unit, Gleneagles Hospital, Singapore, Singapore

Susan W. Salmond, Ed.D., R.N., A.N.E.F., FAAN School of Nursing, Rutgers University, Newark, NJ, USA

Donna Shambley-Ebron, Ph.D., R.N., C.T.N.-A. College of Nursing, University of Cincinnati, Cincinnati, OH, USA

Alessandro Stievano, Ph.D., M.Sc.N., R.N. University of Rome, Rome, Italy

Center for Nursing Excellence, Ipasvi Rome Nursing Board, Rome, Italy

Gülbu Tanriverdi, Ph.D. Canakkale School of Health, Terzioglu Campus, Canakkale Onsekiz Mart University, Canakkale, Turkey

Rick Zoucha, Ph.D., P.M.H.C.N.S.-B.C., FAAN Joseph A. Lauritis Chair for Teaching and Technology, School of Nursing, Duquesne University, Pittsburgh, PA, USA

Conceptual Framework for Culturally Competent Care

Dula Pacquiao

Of all the forms of inequality, injustice in health care is the most shocking and inhumane.
Martin Luther King, Jr. (1966)

1.1 Introduction

Social determinants have been shown to have a greater negative impact on populations who experience cumulative disadvantages in society and manifested in poorer health status. Health promotion requires a broad understanding of the mechanisms by which social disadvantages create health inequities in vulnerable populations. Vulnerable groups are more likely to experience poverty, social exclusion, and limited access to social resources and privileges. Key to improving population health is through culturally competent practice to achieve health equity by promoting a culture of health and healthy communities (Lavizzo-Mourey 2015), grounded in the principles of social justice, human rights, and beneficence. Table 1.1 presents the Global Guidelines for Culturally Competent Health Care and sample applications of each. These guidelines articulate the ethical and moral principles of culturally competent care to achieve health equity for individuals, families, and populations.

D. Pacquiao, Ed.D., R.N., C.T.N.-A., T.N.S.
School of Nursing, Rutgers University,
Newark, NJ, USA

School of Nursing, University of Hawaii, Hilo,
Hilo, HI, USA

1.2 Social Determinants of Health

Social determinants of health are the conditions in which people are born, grow, live, work, and age (WHO 2015a) as well as the systems put in place to deal with illness (CDC 2015). These social circumstances are shaped by a wider set of economic, social, and political forces influencing the distribution of money, power, and resources. Social determinants of health are mostly responsible for health inequities among populations within a society and across the globe. They determine the extent to which a person or group possesses the physical, social, and personal resources to identify and achieve personal aspirations, satisfy needs, and cope with the environment (Raphael 2004). Social determinants of health pertain to the quantity and quality of a variety of resources that a society makes available to its members, such as, income, food, housing, employment, and health and social services.

Both individual- and group-level determinants have been identified (Diez-Roux 2004; Kaufman 2008). At the individual level, factors, such as race and ethnicity, gender, employment, social class, income, and experience with discrimination, are associated with health disparity. At the group level, social factors such as strength of social capital, social cohesion, collective efficacy,

© Springer International Publishing AG, part of Springer Nature 2018
M. Douglas et al. (eds.), *Global Applications of Culturally Competent Health Care: Guidelines for Practice*, https://doi.org/10.1007/978-3-319-69332-3_1

Table 1.1 Guidelines for the practice of culturally competent nursing care

Guideline	Description
Knowledge of cultures	Nurses shall gain an understanding of the perspectives, traditions, values, practices, and family systems of culturally diverse individuals, families, communities, and populations they care for, as well as knowledge of the complex variables that affect the achievement of health and well-being
Education and training in culturally competent care	Nurses shall be educationally prepared to provide culturally congruent healthcare. Knowledge and skills necessary for assuring that nursing care is culturally congruent shall be included in global healthcare agendas that mandate formal education and clinical training, as well as required ongoing, continuing education for all practicing nurses
Critical reflection	Nurses shall engage in critical reflection of their own values, beliefs, and cultural heritage in order to have an awareness of how these qualities and issues can impact culturally congruent nursing care
Cross-cultural communication	Nurses shall use culturally competent verbal and nonverbal communication skills to identify client's values, beliefs, practices, perceptions, and unique healthcare needs
Culturally competent practice	Nurses shall utilize cross-cultural knowledge and culturally sensitive skills in implementing culturally congruent nursing care
Cultural competence in healthcare systems and organizations	Healthcare organizations should provide the structure and resources necessary to evaluate and meet the cultural and language needs of their diverse clients
Patient advocacy and empowerment	Nurses shall recognize the effect of healthcare policies, delivery systems, and resources on their patient populations and shall empower and advocate for their patients as indicated. Nurses shall advocate for the inclusion of their patient's cultural beliefs and practices in all dimensions of their healthcare
Multicultural workforce	Nurses shall actively engage in the effort to ensure a multicultural workforce in healthcare settings. One measure to achieve a multicultural workforce is through strengthening of recruitment and retention effort in the hospital and academic setting
Cross-cultural leadership	Nurses shall have the ability to influence individuals, groups, and systems to achieve outcomes of culturally competent care for diverse populations. Nurses shall have the knowledge and skills to work with public and private organizations, professional associations, and communities to establish policies and guidelines for comprehensive implementation and evaluation of culturally competent care
Evidence-based practice and research	Nurses shall base their practice on interventions that have been systematically tested and shown to be the most effective for the culturally diverse populations that they serve. In areas where there is a lack of evidence of efficacy, nurse researchers shall investigate and test interventions that may be the most effective in reducing the disparities in health outcomes

Source: Douglas, M.K., Rosenkoetter, M., Pacquiao, D.F., Callister, L.C., Hattar-Pollara, M., Lauderdale, J, Milstead, J., Nardi, D., Purnell, L. (2014), Guidelines for Implementing Culturally Competent Nursing Care. *Journal of Transcultural Nursing* 25 (2):110. Reprinted with permission from Sage Publications, Inc.

and diversity of social networks influence quality of life and health outcomes (Burris et al. 2002). Sampson and Raudenbush (1999) observed that collective efficacy includes such informal mechanisms as behaviors, norms, and actions that residents of a given community use to achieve public order. Collective efficacy develops when members of the community have strong feelings of trust and solidarity for each other. When community members feel strongly bonded to each other, they cooperate to deter crime and share ownership of their neighborhood. Individual- and societal-level variables are intimately linked to produce health vulnerability.

1.2.1 Socioeconomic Status

Socioeconomic position is one's relative position as compared to others in society, which is determined by individual characteristics such as income, level of education, occupation, and employment (Babones 2010). Income, education, and occupation have all been shown to predict morbidity and mortality (Miranda et al. 2012; Seith and Kalof 2011; Williams et al. 2012). Poverty is a socioeconomic position that results from a combination of these individual characteristics, with consequent limitation to one's capacity for self-governance and subsequent dependence on society for survival. Dependence and lack of autonomy in turn foster marginalization of the affected group by mainstream society. Social marginalization excludes or limits access to institutional resources and privileges by certain individuals and groups, creating a cycle of poverty and social dependence.

Poverty is associated with a number of risk factors that affect morbidity, disability, and mortality. This association is observed globally, among the poorest and wealthiest countries alike. The poor face challenges in accessing adequate general healthcare and prenatal care. Wilkinson and Pickett (2010) found a strong correlation between the degree of income disparity within a society and health outcomes. Populations in countries with greater socioeconomic inequality experience poorer health outcomes than those living in societies with greater parity. For example, the proportion of the population reporting mental illness was much lower in Japan (9%), a country with a very small income gap as compared to 20% in countries with a greater degree of income inequality such as New Zealand, Australia, and the UK (Wilkinson and Pickett 2010).

In the USA, African Americans, American Indians and Alaskan Natives, and Hispanics are minority groups that are most greatly affected by poverty. Predominantly African American communities reside in neighborhoods with a poverty level greater than 40% (Iceland 2012). Neighborhoods with concentrated poverty and higher proportions of people of color are more likely to exhibit signs of material deprivation and economic disinvestment. Some individuals who are not poor but living in these neighborhoods are exposed to the same kind of challenges as poor residents.

According to the US Census (2016), the official poverty rate dropped slightly from 14.8% in 2014 to 13.5% in 2015; close to 43 million were living in poverty. The highest rates of poverty were among African Americans and American Indian and Alaskan Natives. Although African Americans represented only 13.3% of the US population, they bore a disproportionate burden of poverty with the highest rate between 24% (rural residents) and 33.8% (metro residents)—more than double the national average (USDA 2017). In 2015, children (18 years and younger) comprised 33.6% of the people living in poverty with a poverty rate of 19.7%. Nearly 32% of Black children and 28.9% of Hispanic children were in deep poverty compared to 11.4 for non-Hispanic Whites. Deep poverty is defined as income less than half the threshold (Institute for Research on Poverty 2016). White neighborhoods have twice as many social services as in predominantly African American and Latino neighborhoods despite their greater need for such services (Lin and Harris 2009). Hispanics were more likely than African Americans to enter poverty between 2009 and 2011 but were more likely than African Americans to get out of poverty. African Americans also spent longer periods of time in poverty with an average of 8.5 months compared to 6.5 months among Hispanics (Edwards 2014).

1.2.2   Environment

Chronic stress is experienced by residents of neighborhoods with concentrated poverty associated with high crimes, dilapidated infrastructure, and environmental hazards from toxic pollutants. In the USA, children who are poor and of African descent have a higher prevalence of asthma (25%) as compared to poor White (16%) and Hispanic children (13%) (Seith and Kalof 2011). Neighborhoods with concentrated poverty lack resources such as safe public spaces, transportation, affordable and healthy food venues, and quality schools and healthcare services.

Wilson (1996) noted that the high rate of joblessness has concentrated poverty, particularly in inner-city neighborhoods in the USA, as jobs requiring low education and skills moved to suburban communities along with the flight of White residents from urban areas. More recently there has been a steady shift in demand away from the less skilled toward the more skilled jobs in advanced economies, creating dramatic inequalities in wage and income between the more and the less skilled, as well as unemployment among the less skilled (Slaughter and Swagel 1997). These same changes in labor demands have caused widening income gaps in a number of developing countries as well as in advanced economies. In countries with relatively flexible wages set in decentralized labor markets, such as the USA and, increasingly, the UK, the decline in demand for less-skilled labor has translated into lower relative wages for these workers. Trade liberalization in Mexico in the mid-to-late 1980s led to increased relative wages of high-skilled workers but has not boosted the demand for unskilled labor nor raised unskilled wages. In fact, the demand for unskilled labor has declined, and their wages have fallen in some developing countries (Slaughter and Swagel 1997).

Pervasive joblessness undermines social organization and social capital of neighborhoods that could otherwise buffer the effects of poverty in these communities. According to Wilson (1996), the lack of role models from adults who are gainfully employed has contributed to the widespread degradation of work ethic in the young and the belief that education brings economic returns. African American communities in the northeast USA that were largely composed by freed slaves from the south have built strong social networks and connections that supported each other. According to Fullilove (2004), the urban gentrification movement dismantled this social network causing "root shock" especially among younger generations of African Americans who were separated from a stable network of social and emotional integration in racially divided communities.

Obesogenic environment refers to features of the living and working spaces that contribute to the development of obesity. In the USA, Drewnowski and Specter (2004) observed an association between poverty and obesity. As income decreases, the rate of obesity increases. Low-income families are more likely to consume poor-quality diets that include higher concentra-

tions of calories, sugar, refined grains, salt, and fat because these are less costly. These energy-dense foods are processed for longer shelf life and enhanced palatability but have low nutritional value and are a factor in causing obesity. Healthier foods such as fruits, vegetables, and lean sources of protein are often inaccessible, easily perishable, and beyond the means of those in poverty. Thus the poor are at risk for malnutrition, food insufficiency, and obesity with its associated health risks of diabetes, hypertension, and cardiovascular diseases. In 2011–2012, 8.4% of Americans between 2 and 5 years of age, 17.7% of those between 6 and 11 years, and 20.5% of the 12–19-year-old population were considered obese. The prevalence of obesity was highest for preschool-aged children between 2 and 4 years of age in households with incomes at or below the federal poverty threshold (CDC 2015).

In 2014, nearly 40% of the world's adult population was overweight and 13% were obese. At least 42 million children under the age of 5 were overweight or obese. The rate at which obesity is increasing among middle- and lower-income countries is 30% higher than those of higher-income countries (WHO 2015b). Obesity is steadily becoming a health crisis among the poor worldwide, more so than starvation. Income and gender differences in the rate of overweight and obesity are more pronounced among low-income and lower-middle-income countries. For example, in low-income countries, the rate of obesity among women is more than three times higher than that of men (7.3% and 2.2%, respectively). In lower-middle-income countries, obesity among women is twice that of men (10.4% vs. 5.1%).

Overall, African Americans have a higher rate of obesity, nearly 50% compared to the rate of obesity among Whites, Hispanics, and Asians (43%, 33%, and 11%, respectively). In addition, African Americans have higher rates of high blood pressure than Whites and nearly twice that of Mexican Americans (CDC 2014a). Income and education are correlated with obesity in women in the USA. Women with higher income and more years of education, particularly with college degrees, are less likely to be obese (CDC

2014b). Heart disease and obesity are risk factors for diabetes, another chronic health condition that disproportionately affects African Americans. African Americans are 70% more likely to be diagnosed with diabetes compared to Whites and are two times more likely to die from the disease. The prevalence of visual impairment is 20 per 100 adults with diabetes among African Americans as compared to 17 per 100 adults with diabetes among Whites (United States Department of Health and Human Services-Office of Minority Health [USDHHS-OMH], 2014).

1.2.3 Social Stratification

People do not get sick randomly but in relation to their living, social, political, and environmental circumstances (Bambas and Casas 2001). Socioeconomic and political structures create conditions resulting in wealth or poverty, job stability or instability, educational advancement or exclusion, acceptance or marginalization, and community progress or deprivation. Leading causes of death have been primarily attributed to lifestyle factors. However, lifestyle factors do not rest solely on individual choice but rather on life conditions and circumstances that contribute to unhealthy behaviors (WHO 2015b). Conventional explanations of poor health, such as lack of access to medical care and unhealthy lifestyles, only partially explain differences in health status (Marmot and Bell 2009). The seminal Whitehall I and II studies of British civil servants (Marmot et al. 1978, 1991) found a social gradient in health among Caucasians who were not poor and had equal access to health services. This social gradient existed for heart disease, some cancers, chronic lung disease, gastrointestinal disease, depression, suicide, sickness absence, back pain, and general feelings of ill health. Higher social position was associated with better health.

Social gradient is conditioned by the *status syndrome* (Marmot 2006). The lower individuals are in the social hierarchy, the less likely they are able to meet their needs for autonomy, social integration, and participation (Marmot 2006).

The Whitehall studies confirmed that access to healthcare services does not guarantee equity of health outcomes, suggesting that health status is more significantly shaped by life conditions. Despite universal access to healthcare services, differential health status was observed among thousands of White British civil servants. This suggests that programs and policies providing equal access and opportunity fall short in achieving equity of outcomes because of failure to consider the fundamental differences in the needs and statuses of population groups.

1.3 Vulnerable Populations

Vulnerable populations comprise groups of people who have systematically experienced greater social or economic obstacles to health that are historically linked to discrimination or exclusion. These factors may be based on their racial or ethnic group, religion, socioeconomic status, age, gender, gender identity or sexual orientation, and migration status. Other obstacles are associated with mental health, cognitive, sensory or physical disability, and geographic location of residence (USDHHS 2010). As a consequence, vulnerable populations experience multiple cumulative adversities in life with consequent predisposition to higher and multiple health risks (Frohlich and Potvin 2008). A group's vulnerability is linked with a particular society's social, cultural, and environmental inequalities that are differentially manifested in health inequity. Vulnerable populations may include the poor with limited literacy and education; victims of war, violence, enslavement, and sex trafficking; migrant workers and those without legal status; mentally ill and individuals with cognitive and physical disabilities; females in male-dominated societies; and victims of stigma and discrimination such as LGBTQ, HIV/AIDS infected, incarcerated, prostitutes, etc.

A common thread across vulnerable populations is poverty that can stem from lack of access to quality education, resources supporting achievement, and job opportunities. Poverty not only predisposes individuals to social discrimination and exclusion but also prevents access to basic services and opportunities that can improve their lives. The consequence of social discrimination and stigma is disempowerment and chronic underachievement, unemployment, and poverty. The poor experience the added burden of the "poverty penalty." According to Mendoza (2011) the five penalties of poverty are poor quality, higher prices, nonaccess, non-usage, and catastrophic spending burden. Those with the least financial means end up paying more in order to participate in the market economy as compared to those with more economic means. Because poor neighborhoods have less proximity to goods and services, residents have fewer options for competitive pricing of goods and services. When priced out of the market, the poor must prioritize their necessities of daily living, often forgoing services, preventive healthcare services, and healthier food. They lack the disposable income to take advantage of lower prices offered when purchasing larger quantities of goods and services, a situation that is compounded by their lack of storage space and transportation. Because of limited access to a variety of healthcare providers and services, the poor have less autonomy and choices in healthcare decisions, which in turn impact the effectiveness of healthcare, education, compliance, and outcomes. The poverty penalty contributes to the downward spiral of vulnerable populations and their health.

McEwen and associates (2015) have done seminal work distinguishing the effects of chronic, unmitigated stress from acute, episodic stress and its link to health. The chronic stress experienced with poverty, subordination, and discrimination produces allostatic load or "wear-and-tear" effects. Primarily mediated by neuroendocrine responses in three regions of the brain (hippocampus, amygdala, and prefrontal cortex), allostatic load triggers a cascade of mental, emotional, and physical effects. These include insomnia, depression, post-traumatic stress disorders, impaired cognitive ability, and engagement in high-risk behaviors such as tobacco, alcohol, and drug use. These behaviors further aggravate allostatic load effects. Physical effects are mediated by the hypothalamic-pituitary axis, resulting in sustained high levels of stress hormones that predispose one to the development of obesity, hypertension, immunosuppression, and impaired coping (McEwen et al. 2015).

Krieger (2011) has posited that individuals and groups embody their material and social world as evident in the differential patterning of disease exposure and susceptibility and ultimately mortality. Epidemiological data reflect the biological embodiment of social inequalities of individuals within the same family and population groups in communities across the globe. In other words, the cumulative impact of social adversities differentially experienced by humans across their life course shapes their health and well-being. The author emphasizes the role of social inequalities as the root cause of health inequities that condition the life chances and health trajectories of groups in society. Krieger argues that remedies should be focused on social change because of its greater impact on vulnerable individuals and groups, moving away from the individualistic paradigm that emphasizes self-responsibility for one's health. In other words, accountability for change rests heavily on society and the government. According to Krieger, the progress in decreasing smoking in the USA was largely facilitated by public policies mandating labeling of tobacco products as carcinogenic by the Surgeon General, legislation prohibiting targeted marketing of tobacco to minorities and youth, and legal measures compelling scientific and economic accountability of tobacco companies for their product and its health effects. While smoking cessation programs focusing on individual-level change are helpful, social policies have greater impact on population health because they address sociopolitical inequity.

1.4 Health Inequity

Health inequity is the disparity due to differences in social, economic, environmental, or healthcare resources. According to Whitehead (1992) health inequities are differences in health status that are unnecessary, avoidable, and considered unfair and unjust. Health inequity implies a need for collective moral obligation to correct unfair structure and practices that places an unequal burden of risks for poorer health among socially disadvantaged groups (Braverman 2014). Although evidence of health inequity exists in all societies, the gap between the privileged and vulnerable groups is mitigated by decreasing the impact of social inequalities that create the pathways to poor health.

Using data from the World Values Survey with over 15,000 respondents from 44 countries representing developed and developing nations in several continents, Babones (2010) found that individual indicators of socioeconomic status (income, education, and occupation) affect self-reported health status worldwide, independently and collectively. People of high income have more than 50% greater odds of reporting good health than those with low income, even when education and occupational class remained the same. Those with higher levels of education have more than 60% greater odds of reporting good health than people with lower educational achievement (Babones 2010). Selected examples of health disparities in some countries are presented.

1.4.1 Africa

1.4.1.1 North Africa and Middle East

Differences in health system size, structure, and financing occur in Middle Eastern countries. Public healthcare programs in the Arab countries provide comprehensive coverage of all levels of care, including prevention, ambulatory care, and inpatient services either completely free of charge or at a nominal fee (Kronfol 2012a). There are gaps in coverage such as nonprescription drugs, dental care, cosmetic surgery, and smoking cessation. Some countries prohibit fertility treatments and abortion based on religious and bioethical grounds. Dental services are limited even in countries that adopted social health insurance such as Lebanon. Many dentists practice in the private sector and cities, limiting access to dental services by rural and poor residents. Mental health services are frequently not available in public clinics. People with mental retardation, severe mental health problems, and low education as well as the elderly are most disadvantaged (Kronfol 2012b).

Rural residents in Middle Eastern countries and North Africa such as Sudan are more at risk of poverty and social exclusion. Geographic distance and lack of transportation pose barriers to access and utilization of preventive health services such as vaccination and antenatal services (Ibnouf et al. 2007). There is also concern about the safety, cost of transportation, and ease of boarding public buses. Most people walk or use private transportation to the clinics. The poor elderly and functionally impaired individuals are greatly disadvantaged. In many Muslim countries, a male guardian is needed to arrange for transport which further limits access because of the need to wait for this person to get off work, and many clinics are closed before he gets home from work (Kronfol 2012a).

In countries like Tunisia, Syria, and Egypt, gender significantly influences access and utilization of health services by women. In general, women prefer female physicians for reproductive health issues (Romdhane and Grenier 2009). Gender congruence and sensitivity of health providers affect service use by women (Kronfol 2012c). Although women are major healthcare users as well as providers, they are underrepresented in healthcare decision-making. Religion has an important influence on specific health practices such as male and female circumcision, the practice of medicine and litigation, the belief in fate and destiny, and other social determinants of health. There are legal, religious, medical, and social factors that serve to support or hinder women's access to safe abortion services in the 21 predominantly Muslim countries in the Middle East and North Africa, where 1 in 10 pregnancies ends in abortion (Hessini 2007; Kronfol 2012a). Gender-related issues include improving women's access to healthcare, education and literacy for girls and women, employment, and social protection for women and female genital mutilation (Kishk 2002).

Ethnic minorities in Arab countries experience discrimination in healthcare, public places, and public transport. Language barriers and differences in health beliefs and practices have been documented among Bedouins in a Beirut Hospital (Kronfol 2012a). Barriers are also related to nationality in the Gulf countries (e.g., Kuwait and United Arab Emirates) because separate healthcare facilities are reserved for nationals of the country, non-nationals, or expatriates. Facilities for nationals receive more government support. This differentiated care setting promotes segregation and unequal treatment of individuals and groups based on nationality (Kronfol 2012a).

1.4.1.2 Sub-Saharan Africa

According to Benatar (2013), in 2008, 54% of South Africans had an income below $3/day. While the top 10% earned 58% of annual national personal income, 70% of the population received a mere 16.9%. The Gini coefficient, a measure of income inequality, increased from 0.6 in 1995 to 0.679 in 2009. Infant mortality rates (IMR) have remained stable between 1990 and 2005 reflecting White and Black disparities—18 per 1000 live births among Whites as compared to 74 per 1000 live births among Black South Africans. IMR differed across geographical regions with 27/1000 live births in the Western Cape and 70/1000 live births in the Eastern Cape. Overall maternal mortality increased from 150/100,000 pregnancies in 1998 to 650/100,000 in 2007. Sub-Saharan Africa has endured disproportionately high prevalence of HIV/AIDs compared to other countries in the world. South Africa accounts for almost 17% of the world's population living with HIV/AIDS. The country has the largest antiretroviral treatment program in the world, yet only 40% of eligible adults are receiving treatment. The prevalence of HIV infection among those older than 19 years ranges from 16.1% in the Western Cape to 38.7% in KwaZulu-Natal (Benatar, Sullivan and Brown 2017).

UNESCO's EFA Global Monitoring Report (2015) noted that not a single country in sub-Saharan Africa has achieved gender parity in either primary or secondary education, with the poorest girls as most disadvantaged. In 2012, at least 19 countries around the world had fewer than 90 girls for every 100 boys in school; 15 of these countries were in sub-Saharan Africa. In the Central African Republic and Chad in 2012, the number of girls in secondary was half that of

boys. In Angola, the situation has actually worsened, from 76 girls per 100 boys in 1999 to 65 in 2012. The country with the greatest inequity in primary and lower secondary is Chad. In Guinea and Niger, approximately 70% of the poorest girls had never attended school compared with less than 20% of the richest boys. Gender disparities in secondary education have barely changed in sub-Saharan Africa since 1999, with approximately eight girls for every ten boys enrolled. In a few poor countries, such as Rwanda, new gender gaps at the expense of boys have emerged. In Lesotho, only 71 boys were enrolled for every 100 girls in 2012, a ratio unchanged since 1999 (UNESCO 2015).

Although gender gaps in youth literacy are narrowing, the report had predicted that fewer than seven out of every ten young women in sub-Saharan Africa were literate in 2015. Two-thirds of adults who lack basic literacy skills are women, a proportion unchanged since 2000. Half of adult women in sub-Saharan Africa cannot read or write. Gender-based school disparities that have been attributed to gender-based violence, child marriages, and secondary school dropout by pregnant girls remain a persistent barrier to girls' education. If existing laws mandating older age for females at marriage were enforced, this would result in an overall 39% increase in years of schooling in sub-Saharan Africa. Pregnancy has been identified as a key driver of dropout and exclusion among female secondary school students in sub-Saharan African countries, including Cameroon and South Africa. The prevalence of premarital sex before age 18 years, increased in 19 out of 27 countries in the region between 1994 and 2004 (UNESCO 2015).

1.4.2 Asia

1.4.2.1 China

As the most populous nation in the world, China's population as of January 1, 2017 was approximately 1.38 billion people, representing an increase of 0.53% (7.3 billion people) from 2016. China has a population density of 148 people per square kilometer. In 2016, the number of births exceeded the number of deaths by 7,315,733, but because of external migration, the population increased by only 41,254. The sex ratio of the total population was 1.051 (1051 males per 1000 females), which is higher than the global sex ratio (Countrymeters 2017a). Since the 1950s, the process of industrialization in China has shifted its economy from agriculture to manufacturing, which has significantly increased its energy consumption and created mass rural to urban migration. In 2011, the proportion of the population living in urban areas surpassed those living in rural areas for the first time, and an additional 200 million rural-to-urban migrants are anticipated during the next 10 years (Gong et al. 2012). Industrialization has led to serious environmental and ecological problems, both in urban and surrounding areas, including increased air and water pollution, local climate alteration, and a major reduction in natural vegetation and production (Fang et al. 2003). A major threat is the absence of continuous healthcare coverage for rural-to-urban migrants who are at risk of dual infectious disease burden from exposure to pathogens associated with rural poverty like parasitic worms in the soil and pathogens such as tuberculosis in crowded urban environments. Urbanization has led to changes in patterns of human activity, diet, and social structures with profound implications for noncommunicable diseases, e.g., diabetes, cardiovascular disease, cancer, and neuropsychiatric disorders. Urban residents have experienced an increase in the levels of cholesterol- related diseases (Lee 2004) and an overall decline in quality of life.

According to statistics from China's Ministry of Environmental Protection, cities in the Yangtze River Delta, Pearl River Delta, and Beijing-Tianjin-Hebei region suffer over 100 haze days every year, with particulate matter/PM2.5 concentration of two to four times above the World Health Organization guidelines, which can lead to systemic damage to human health (Pan et al. 2012). PM2.5 are small-sized particles in the air that can reach a large surface area of the respiratory system that carry a variety of toxic heavy metals, acid oxides, organic pollutants, and other chemicals, as well as microorganisms such as bacteria and viruses. Heavy metals and polycyclic aromatic hydrocarbons carried by PM2.5 can enter and deposit in human alveoli, causing inflammation and lung diseases, as well as enter the circulation and affect the normal functioning of the cardiovascular system. Exposure to PM2.5 can lead to significantly increased mortality from cardiovascular, cerebrovascular, and respiratory diseases, as well as greater cancer risks (Pan et al. 2012).

Air pollution in China is mainly caused by burning coal in factories and power plants and oil combustion by vehicles. During winter, homes are heated through a central heating system powered by coal burning; hence "smog" days are more frequent in winter seasons. Rohde and Muller (2015) have analyzed national reports on hourly air pollution from 1500 sites in China over 4 months including airborne particulate matter, sulfur dioxide, nitrogen dioxide, and ozone. Significant widespread air pollution is observed across Northern and Central China, not limited to major cities and geologic basins. Sources of pollution are widespread but are particularly intense in the northeast corridor from near Shanghai to north of Beijing. Rohde and Muller found that 92% of the Chinese population experienced more than 120 h of unhealthy air (based on US-EPA standard) and 38% experienced average concentrations that were unhealthy. The authors concluded that this level of exposure contributes to 1.6 million deaths/year (0.7–2.2 million deaths/year at 95% CI), roughly 17% of all deaths in China.

Wheat is the third largest crop and an essential contributor to food security in China and the world. Higher levels of air pollution in the North China Plain region during winter and spring, which correspond to the early growing phase of winter wheat, significantly reduce sun radiation and increase relative humidity, resulting in decreased photosynthetic rate, higher risks of fungal infection, and negative effects on wheat yields (Liu et al. 2016). Particulate matter such as cement dust, magnesium-lime dust, and carbon soot deposited on vegetation can inhibit plants' respiration and photosynthesis and cause chlorosis and death of leaf tissues because of the thick crust formation and alkaline toxicity from wet weather. The dust coating may also affect the normal action of pesticides and other agricultural chemicals. Accumulation of alkaline dusts in the soil can increase soil pH to levels adverse to crop growth (Last et al. 1985).

1.4.2.2 India

Being the second most populous country in the world, India's population as of January 1, 2017 was estimated at 1.33 billion representing an increase of 1.26% (16.6 million) from 2016. In 2016, the number of births exceeded the number of deaths by 17,154,513, but due to external migration, the population declined by 541,027. The sex ratio of the total population was 1.068 (1068 males per 1000 females) which is higher than the global sex ratio (Countrymeters 2017b). Forty-one percent of India's population is predicted to live in urban areas by 2030 (United Nations 2004). India's rapid urbanization comes with opportunities to make cities more livable and transform their economy, but this also comes with negative consequences by weakening an already inadequate social service infrastructure creating lack of basic services and pressure on resources. Cities have a transport crisis, road congestion, and pollution from noise, air, and waste. Public health concerns are associated with lack of quality housing, clean water, and sanitation.

In addition to urbanization, gender inequity is a significant social determinant of health of Indians. Being female is associated with lack of education, employment, health access, and autonomy. Studies indicate that Indians in urban areas and women in particular have poorer health outcomes than rural Indians and men, respectively. India has the largest number of people with diabetes than any other country, and the prevalence of diabetes among urban Indians rose from 2.1 to 12.1% from 1970 to 2003 (Ramachandran et al. 2003). The study by Mohan et al. (2016) using a cross-sectional sample of 6853 rural, poor urban, and middle-class urban women between 35 and 70 years old revealed that urban middle-class women have the highest levels of anthropometry, body mass index, cholesterol, waist-to-hip ratio, hypertension, and diabetes as compared to poor urban and rural Indian women. The study

also noted high occurrence of cardiovascular disease, stroke, and diabetes in middle-aged urban women. The higher rates of greater body mass index, waist-to-hip ratio, and cholesterol in urban middle-aged women may be attributed to greater caloric and fat intake and decrease in comparative physical activity. While some Hindus are vegetarian, saturated fat is derived from use of ghee (clarified butter), coconut milk, and cream in the food preparation. Middle-class urban women have the highest cardio-metabolic risks compared to poor urban and rural women (Mohan et al. 2016).

The rate of cardiovascular disease rates among individuals 30–60 years of age is 405 per 100,000 in India as compared to in Great Britain (180/100,000) and China (280/100,000) (Chauhan and Aeri 2013). Higher prevalence of cardiovascular disease is noted in urban than rural India. There has been a tenfold increase in the prevalence of coronary artery disease in urban India during the last 40 years, and rates have ranged between 1.6 and 7.4% in rural populations and 1 and 13.2% in urban populations (Gupta 2012).

The American College of Cardiology's Pinnacle India Quality Improvement Program (PIQIP) found that women had fewer patient medical encounters than men, including visiting a physician, hospital, or clinic for evaluation, testing, or treatment. Although women had a higher rate of noncommunicable diseases, they received less medication prescriptions than men (Kalra et al. 2016). Women are more at risk for hypertension, diabetes, and hyperlipidemia but receive less medical care than men. Sengupta and Jena (2009) found rural and urban women suffer from goiter, 1.93 and 3.62 times more than men, respectively. Urban women were observed to suffer more from asthma than their male counterparts.

In 2011, the Indian population over 65 years comprised 90 million and is predicted to exceed 227 million by 2050. Women are considered a disadvantaged group among the aging population. Although Indian women live longer than men, they consistently report poorer health, higher disabilities, lower cognitive function, and lower utilization of health services (Rao 2014).

Kakoli and Chaudhuri (2008) found wide health disparities between elderly men and women even after controlling for demographics, medical conditions, and known risk factors. However controlling for economic independence reduced the gaps significantly, suggesting that financial empowerment may be the key to improving health outcomes of elderly women.

The Longitudinal Aging Study conducted in the southern states of Karnataka and Kerala and two northern states of Rajasthan and Punjab found that elderly women have lower cognitive function than elderly men and the disparity was linked with gender discrimination evident in women having poorer education and less social engagements, both of which impact their health. Higher level of discrimination against women was observed in the two northern states (Population Reference Bureau 2012).

In India, gender bias is evident in all life stages of a woman—female infanticide, poor education facilities, dowry practices, stereotypical roles of women as homemakers, and discrimination against widows. Although dowry practices have been declared illegal, some families continue to expect payment by the bride's family to the groom's family before marriage. The burden of dowry payments has created a strong preference for sons and marginalization of females as a burden to their families. It is exceptionally hard for elderly women to have good health and quality of life. Although there are existing government initiatives for female children, they do not address the current generation of elderly women who continue to face discrimination, poverty, poor education, and poor health.

1.4.3 North America

1.4.3.1 United States

The USA is the only one among the most economically developed member countries of the Organization for Economic Co-operation and Development (OECD) that does not provide universal healthcare access to its citizens. Yet, it outspends all other members on healthcare. In 2012, the USA spent 16.9% of its GDP on healthcare, representing 7.5% points above the OECD average of 9.3%. Forty-eight percent of US healthcare is publicly financed, well below the average of 72% in OECD countries (OECD 2014a). The USA lags behind other developed countries and some less developed countries in many health outcomes (OECD 2014b). Health coverage for able adults below 65 years of age is generally acquired through employer-sponsored health insurance. An employer-sponsored system of access to care fosters inequity by favoring high wage earners with good benefits over low-income groups whose employers may not have the ability to provide optimal or any coverage for their employees.

At the end of 2014, more than seven of every ten uninsured individuals in the USA have at least one full-time worker in their family, and an additional 12% have a part-time worker in the family. Yet, for these families, employment does not translate to enough income to be able to purchase health insurance. While access to healthcare does not guarantee equity in health outcomes, lack of universal access perpetuates social and health inequity. Many gaps in coverage remain. While Medicare is available for adults 65 years and older, procurement of supplemental benefits depends on the financial capacity of the individual or his/her family. Medicaid and the State Children Health Insurance provide healthcare access to eligible indigent families and their children. However, because these costs are shared by each state with the federal government, funding is not the same across different regions. In addition, some healthcare practitioners do not accept patients with Medicaid, leaving these patients with even fewer options.

The Patient Protection and Affordable Care Act or the Affordable Care Act (ACA) was signed into law by President Obama on March 23, 2010, with a goal to provide access to health coverage to more than 40 million Americans. ACA aims to expand healthcare coverage to most US citizens and permanent residents by requiring most people to obtain or purchase health insurance (USDHHS 2015). To date, ACA has failed to reach its goal of expanding access to affordable health insurance for many Americans because of lack of political will to establish a universal system of healthcare that offers equity of access to quality healthcare for all.

Racial and ethnic minorities in the USA receive lower quality and intensity of healthcare compared with Whites across a wide range of preventive, diagnostic, and therapeutic services and disease states (Washington et al. 2008). The adjusted rate of preventable hospitalizations is higher among African Americans and Hispanics compared with the rate for non-Hispanic Whites (Moy et al. 2011). Among adults aged 65 years or more, racial and ethnic differences in influenza vaccination rates persist, with African Americans consistently having the lowest each year (Setse et al. 2011).

The Agency for Healthcare Research and Quality/AHRQ (2014) reported continuing evidence of suboptimal quality of care and access to health services among minority and low-income groups despite the ACA. Health disparities and access to care have shown no improvement for disadvantaged groups. The Centers for Disease Control and Prevention (CDC 2011) reported that despite progress over the past 20 years, racial/ethnic, economic, and other social disparities in health persist. Racial and ethnic minorities experience greater rates of poverty, unemployment, lack of health insurance, shorter life expectancy, and higher morbidity and mortality rates than White Americans, as shown in Table 1.2 (AHRQ 2014; CDC 2011).

In 2014, individuals below poverty level were at the highest risk of being uninsured. Over eight in ten of uninsured individuals were in low- or moderate-income families, with incomes below 400% of the poverty line, a requirement to receive subsidies for health insurance. While 45% of the uninsured were non-Hispanic Whites, people of color are at higher risk of being uninsured than non-Hispanic Whites. People of color make up 40% of the overall population but account for over half of the total uninsured population. The disparity in insurance coverage is especially high for Hispanics, who account for 19% of the total population but more than a third (34%) of the uninsured population. Hispanics and African

Table 1.2 Racial and ethnic health disparities in the USA

Health disparity	Most vulnerable/disadvantaged groups
Life expectancy from birth	African Americans
Mortality	
Cancer	African Americans
Complications of diabetes	African Americans
Coronary artery disease and stroke	African Americans
Homicide	African Americans
Motor vehicular deaths	American Indian and Alaskan Natives (AIANs)
Suicide	AIANs
Morbidity	
Childhood asthma	Puerto Ricans and African Americans
Diabetes	African Americans, AIANs
Human immunodeficiency virus (HIV)	African Americans, AIANs, males who have sex with men (MSM)
Hypertension and its complications	African Americans
Obesity	African Americans, Mexican-Americans
Infant mortality	African Americans
Low birth weight	African Americans
Extremely preterm birth	African Americans
Preterm birth	African Americans
Health behaviors	
Smoking	AIANs

Sources: Agency for Healthcare Research and Quality Advancing Excellence in Health Care (2014). *2014 National healthcare quality and disparities report.* Rockville, MD: USDHHS
Centers for Disease Control and Prevention. (2011). *Health disparities and inequalities report.* Atlanta, GA: Author

Americans have significantly higher uninsured rates (20.9% and 12.7%, respectively) than Whites (9.1%) (Kaiser Family Foundation 2015).

Health inequities occur along racial and ethnic lines. Differences in life expectancy between African and White American populations remain although the gap has narrowed. African Americans, on average, have a life expectancy of 4 years shorter than Whites (CDC 2014a).

African Americans comprise only 25% of the population living in poverty (Iceland 2012), but the effect of poverty is worsened by discrimination and marginalization. The mortality rate of infants born to Black women is 2.3 times higher than infants born to White women, and the maternal mortality rate for Black women is 3 times higher than that of White women (USDHHS, HRSA-MCHB 2013). Almost half of African American women (46%) are hypertensive compared to 30% of White women (CDC 2014c). African American women are victims of interpersonal violence at a rate of 7.8 per 1000 females aged 12 years and older as compared to White women and Latinas (6.2 and 4.0, respectively) (National Coalition on Black Civic Participation 2014).

1.4.3.2 Canada

Despite a universal healthcare system in Canada, low-income Canadians are less likely to see a specialist when needed, have more difficulty getting care on weekends or evenings, and are more likely to wait 5 days or more for an appointment with a physician. Canadians with below-average incomes are three times less likely to fill a prescription and 60% less able to get a needed test or treatment due to cost than above-average income earners (Mikkonen and Raphael 2010).

Men living in the wealthiest neighborhoods on average live more than 4 years longer than men in the poorest neighborhoods. In comparison, women in wealthiest neighborhoods live almost 2 years longer than women in the poorest neighborhoods. Those living in the most deprived neighborhoods had higher suicide and death rates. Adult-onset diabetes and heart attacks are far more common among low-income Canadians. Food insecurity is common in households led by lone mothers and aboriginal households. Food-insufficient households are more likely to report having diabetes, high blood pressure, and food allergies than households with sufficient food. Children in food-insecure households are more likely to experience a wide range of behavioral, emotional, and academic problems than children

living in food-secure households (Mikkonen and Raphael 2010).

Social exclusion is evident among recent immigrants and aboriginal populations in Canada. Recent immigrants have higher unemployment rates and lower labor force participation than Canadian-born workers. Compared to non-Aboriginal Canadians, First Nation Aboriginal people earn much less income, have twice the rate of unemployment, are more likely to live in crowded conditions, and are much less likely to graduate from high school. Aboriginal Canadians live the shortest lives and have higher rates of infant mortality, suicide, major depression, alcohol, and childhood sexual abuse than non-Aboriginal Canadians (Mikkonen and Raphael 2010).

1.4.3.3 Mexico

Mexico is considered most advanced of all the developing countries in the world. Since 2004, Mexico has extended healthcare coverage to 52 million previously unenrolled Mexicans through the *Seguro Popular*. Although some areas like Mexico City has an impressive number of tier one hospitals with top-notch medical advancements, many public hospitals are underfunded, lack medical technology, and offer limited services. Access to quality care is reserved for those who can pay for private hospital care (Izek 2016).

According to Guthrie and Fleck (2017), type 2 diabetes is the leading cause of death and disability in Mexico and has been declared a national health emergency. In 2013, the country has launched the National Strategy for the Prevention and Control of Overweight, Obesity and Diabetes through public health, medical care, and fiscal and regulatory policies. Mexico accounts for the most hospitalizations (many of them preventable) related to diabetes, among the 35 OECD countries. Many Mexicans are diagnosed with diabetes at a relatively early age with 3.25% of cases detected between 20 and 39 years, compared to the OECD average of 1.7% (Guthrie and Fleck 2017).

The rapid increase in obesity, diabetes, hypertension, and hypercholesterolemia in Mexico puts women of reproductive age at higher risk for preexisting hypertensive disorders and diabetes mellitus (WHO 2016). Socioeconomic disparities are evident in maternal mortality rates (MMR) from direct causes. MMR from direct maternal deaths has been declining between 2006 and 2013; the rate among women residing in the poorest municipalities decreased from 119.1 to 72.7 deaths per 100,000 live births as compared to the decline from 35.2 to 26.9 deaths per 100,000 live births among women in the wealthiest municipalities. Between 2008 and 2010 the poorest quintile had a statistically significant higher MMR from indirect causes than the wealthiest quintile (WHO 2016). Between 2000 and 2013, the number of stillbirths decreased from 9.2 to 7.2 per 1000 as compared to the 2015 worldwide average of 18.4 per 1000 births. Approximately 51% of stillbirths occurred intrapartum, with 40% occurring at 28 weeks' gestation or later, comparable to the global estimate of 33–46% for third-trimester stillbirths (Murguia-Peniche et al. 2016).

1.4.4 European Countries

Bask (2011) examined the accumulation of problems among welfare recipients by using two waves of data from annual surveys of living conditions in Sweden in 1994–1995 and 2002–2003. The analysis focused on such factors as chronic unemployment, economic problems, health problems, experiences of threat or violence, crowded housing, lack of a close friend, and sleeping problems. Being single (with or without children) and immigrant was associated with the most clusters of problems. Interestingly, education and economic factors were not significant, which was attributed by the author to the fact that Sweden is a welfare state with an ambitious universal social policy agenda involving redistributive activities and extensive spending on public welfare.

A study comparing all-White British civil servants with Whites and Blacks in the USA found that socioeconomic status was related to health (Adler et al. 2008). Subjective social status (SSS), that is, the perception of one's socioeconomic position, was also associated with health status. Occupation was a more important determinant of SSS among British civil servants compared to education and income among the US subjects. SSS was significantly related to overall health and depression in all groups and to hypertension in all groups except African American males. Socioeconomic factors did not predict SSS scores for Black Americans as well as they did for the British subjects and White Americans. Overall, relationships between SSS and health were stronger for the British and White US subjects than for African Americans, suggesting other factors, such as racial characteristics, influence their health.

Studies done in a number of countries showed that health disparities affect racial and ethnic minorities more than dominant groups in the same society. A longitudinal study of inpatient psychiatric admissions of adolescents in London found that young Blacks are nearly six times more likely than those in the White group to be admitted with psychosis, followed by "Other" (other ethnic groups and those with mixed ethnic background) and Asians. Young people with psychosis in the Black and Other groups were around three times more likely to experience formal detention on admission (Corrigall and Bhugra 2013). In Spain, Romanies (Gypsies), a marginalized group, were found to have greater prevalence of migraines compared to the general population. Romanies suffering from migraines had the worse self-reported health status and greater incidence of depression (Jimenez-Sanchez et al. 2013).

1.4.5 Latin America and Caribbean

In Latin and Caribbean countries, the poor tend to use fewer public resources than middle- and upper-income groups. Large patterns of health inequalities between socioeconomic groups, as well as between gender and ethnic groups, suggest a link between health outcomes and material and social living conditions. There is a growing impact of social determinants reflected by inequalities in health and overall well-being of the poor populations (Bambas and Casas 2001).

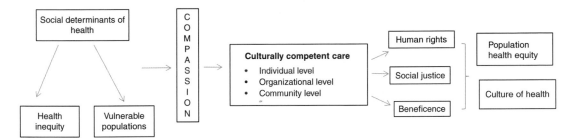

Fig. 1.1 Framework for culturally competent healthcare

1.5 Framework for Culturally Competent Healthcare

This section explains the key concepts undergirding the framework for culturally competent healthcare (see Fig. 1.1). The goal of culturally competent care is the achievement of health equity, particularly for vulnerable populations who are most affected by the social determinants that lead to health inequity. In order to achieve health equity, culturally competent care must be grounded in the principles of social justice and human rights.

1.5.1 Social Justice and Human Rights

Human rights are founded on the principle that all human beings have dignity and equal value. Article 25 of the Universal Declaration of Human Rights promulgated by the UN Assembly in 1948 emphasized the right of everyone to a standard of living adequate for the health and well-being for oneself and one's family, including food, clothing, housing, medical care, and necessary social services. UDHR also emphasized the right to security in the event of unemployment, sickness, disability, widowhood, old age, or other lack of livelihood in circumstances beyond his control (ICHRP 2012). These human rights are indivisible and must coexist as a collective in order to assure protection of an individual's dignity and well-being. The right to health is not possible without assuring economic, social, and cultural rights (UN 1948).

Assurance of health and well-being must take steps to address social determinants of health, which are multiple, complex, and interrelated. Human rights protection is critical particularly for individuals and groups who are vulnerable because of social exclusion, poverty, and other structural factors hindering their social mobility and autonomy. Health is intimately linked with such life realities as poverty, unemployment, educational opportunities, and living environments. Although human beings have universal rights, there is ample evidence that the privileged groups enjoy unfair advantages over the disempowered groups.

Social justice places the responsibility on society and its institutions to safeguard the health and well-being of the vulnerable while ensuring protection of the basic human rights of everyone. Achieving health equity, however, requires a moral obligation to redistribute resources to uplift those who do not have enough to live a decent life. Rawls (1971) first proposed a theory of justice with a set of principles governing the distribution of primary social goods, such as liberties, opportunities, income, and wealth. A just society according to Rawls is one that renders the most vulnerable less vulnerable.

Powers and Faden (2008) argue that injustice does not arise solely from the distribution of material goods and services but also in the allocation of non-distributive aspects of well-being. Victims of social subordination, discrimination, and stigma experience lack of respect, attachment, and autonomy that impact their well-being. The authors recommend that social justice needs to integrate the distributive and non-distributive aspects of justice. Indeed, improvement of health and well-being of vulnerable groups should address inequity in the allocation of material goods and services as well as prevent maldistribution of goodwill such as love, respect, compassion, and advocacy. Both are essential to becoming a fully participating member of society. These nonmaterial variables can make individuals either flourish or diminish their life chances in society (Powers and Faden 2008).

1.5.2   Cultural Competence

Several definitions and alternate terms exist in the literature on cultural competence. The definition by Cross et al. (1989) was adopted by the Office of Minority Health in developing the National Standards for Culturally and Linguistically Appropriate Services (CLAS) (USDHHS 2001). Cultural competence is defined as a set of congruent behaviors, attitudes, and policies that come together in a system, agency, or among professionals that enable them to work effectively in cross-cultural situations. Cross et al. used competence to indicate different levels of capacity at the individual, organizational, and system levels. At the system level, the needs of the community and society are addressed. Cultural competence initiatives have achieved some success at the individual care level, particularly in using linguistically congruent services, accommodation of different values and practices in healthcare, and education of health professionals. However, the evidence of lingering and widening health disparities among diverse groups demonstrate that culturally competent initiatives have not eliminated population health disparities.

1.5.2.1 Individual Level
Cultural competence is based on the requisite knowledge, attitudes, skills/behaviors, and practices that value and respect differences. At the individual level, knowledge pertains to a level of understanding of different cultural values, beliefs, and practices of individuals and families seeking care. Attitudes include respect, openness, sensitivity, self-awareness, and critical reflection. Skills include cross-cultural communication, cultural assessment, cultural conflict management, and accommodation of cultural differences.

1.5.2.2 Organizational Level
Organizational practices constitute development of infrastructure, leadership and management, and care delivery systems that promote culturally competent care. Healthcare organization initiatives may include (a) programs for training and development of multidisciplinary employees in culturally competent care; (b) offering services during hours and in locations convenient to patients who are unable to take time off work, have no private transportation, and need someone to look after their children when they go for their medical appointments; (c) providing trained interpreters and translators with expertise in common languages or dialects presented by patients; (d) offering menus and pastoral services that accommodate ethnic and religious differences of patients; and (e) providing adequate social services to address needs of patients and families.

1.5.2.3 Community Level
Community-level cultural competence is an area that needs development. This is a critical approach to address social determinants of health in vulnerable populations who have limited social capital. Bourdieu (1977) first defined social capital as the aggregate of actual or potential resources that are linked to a durable network of institutionalized memberships in a group and that provides and maintains material and symbolic gains for its members. While poor ethnic enclaves may offer emotional support and acceptance for their members, lack of economic and symbolic capital poses many constraints on their ability to be financially secure and influence the conditions in which they live. By contrast, individuals and communities with higher socioeconomic status and who are accepted as part of the dominant group have access to a social network that can enhance their socioeconomic position and power. Social and economic stratification in society is culturally reproduced, perpetuating vulnerability of some groups and privileged positions of others.

Culturally competent professionals and organizations are actively engaged with vulnerable communities. By forging multisectoral and multidisciplinary social networks in partnerships with the community, they promote broad awareness of the community's problems and compel power brokers to make changes on their behalf through policies and programs that can transform their lives. Social networks may be comprised of scientists, academicians, local politicians, bureaucrats, health professionals, advocates, and members of the community who can foster social connections built on mutual trust, reciprocity, and collective cooperation (Putnam 2000). Mutual trust and engagement are based on a common norm of conduct, shared goals, commitment, and understanding (Coleman 1990). The goal of community-level cultural competence is community empowerment and social change that are only possible with prolonged engagement and collaboration with the community. Sustainability of initiatives is enhanced by community champions who are trained and mentored to push for change and monitor the implementation and outcomes of change.

As shown in Tables 1.3 and 1.4, community-level strategies are distinct from individual- and organizational-level approaches. While individuals and organizations may have a plan of action, without acceptance and engagement by the community, these approaches will not be sustainable.

Successful partnerships and collaborations are built on a good understanding of the community and its people and prolonged engagement with them that is built on mutual trust and reciprocity. Partnership is a close cooperation between two or more parties having specified and joint rights and responsibilities and equal share of the risks as well as the rewards. Partners join forces in pursuit of a shared goal, commitment, rights, and obligations to participate and will be affected equally by the benefits and disadvantages arising from the partnership. Partnerships require mutual trust and respect for each other in order to create joint teamwork and coalitions and eliminate boundaries among them (Carnwell and Carson 2005).

By contrast, collaboration involves cooperation with less formalized set of responsibilities

Table 1.3 Examples of implementing guidelines for culturally competent nursing care

Caregivers	Healthcare organizations Leaders/managers
Guideline #1: Knowledge of cultures	
1. Participate in learning modules on the general principles of culturally competent care	1. Facilitate staff participation in classes on culturally competent care and knowledge of cultural groups served
2. Participate in learning modules on specific knowledge of the most common cultural groups served	2. Organize cultural awareness activities to promote cultural competence (such as, Heritage Days with culturally diverse speakers, media, ethnic food, etc.)
3. Identify the nurse's healthcare beliefs and values that may be different than those of the patient and family	3. Provide accessible resources for staff to learn about specific cultures and common language terms used by populations served
Guideline #2: Education and training	
1. Attend required orientation and annual in-service classes on cultural diversity	1. Provide orientation and annual in-service training in cultural competence for all levels of staff, including all management, professional, and nonprofessional staff in any department with patient contact
2. Attend continuing education classes or other learning experiences to maintain cross-cultural skills	2. Provide classes to increase staff's cultural knowledge about the ethnically diverse patients who receive health services in the facility
3. Mentor healthcare colleagues in culturally competent care	3. Provide classes to enhance nurses' skills in cross-cultural assessment and communication skills
4. Role model lifelong learning of cultural competence	4. Use a variety of modalities to teach cultural competency, such as workshops, conferences, online training, films, and immersion experiences
	5. Partner with transcultural experts to provide staff with continuing education courses, consultation, and practice skills for culturally competent care

(continued)

Table 1.3 (continued)

Caregivers	Healthcare organizations Leaders/managers
Guideline #3: Critical reflection	
1. Reflect on one's own cultural beliefs, values, and practices 2. Analyze patient care problems through the prism of critical reflection	1. Incorporate critical reflection into performance evaluations of staff 2. Promote critical reflection of staff through team meetings and case study discussions in which staff uses critical reflection 3. Host programs and workshops for staff that encourage critical reflection and self-awareness of cultural values and beliefs
Guideline #4: Cross-cultural communication	
1. Consider culturally specific variations in communication, such as, body language; eye contact; distance between speakers; voice volume, tone, intonation, and inflections; and willingness to share thoughts and feelings 2. Use pain scales in the preferred language of the patient or use "faces of pain" scale for those who do not speak language of caregivers 3. Develop skills in using interpreters and translators 4. Provide patients with discharge materials that are translated into their preferred language 5. Distribute educational materials in the patient's preferred language	1. Provide budget for translation of materials 2. Develop, produce, and/or distribute patient education materials in the languages of populations served 3. Coordinate a program to effectively use interpreters within the agency 4. Use symbols and pictograms in hospitals, clinics, and other healthcare organizations whenever possible
Guideline #5: Culturally competent practice	
1. Establish a trusting relation through open and sensitive communication, active listening, and respect of patient's cultural beliefs and practices 2. Conduct a cultural assessment that includes patient's preferences on the following: language, designated decision-maker, perception of causes of health and illness, and culturally defined treatment modalities 3. Incorporate cultural assessment information into plan of care 4. Demonstrate skill in cultural brokering, bridging, and negotiation in conflict situations	1. Develop policies that reflect local cultural beliefs, norms, and practices 2. Supervise staff to ensure that effective cross-cultural nursing practice is being delivered 3. Provide staff with adequate resources to deliver culturally competent practice 4. Evaluate effectiveness of culturally appropriate services 5. Revise policies related to culturally appropriate services as needed

Table 1.3 (continued)

Caregivers	Healthcare organizations Leaders/managers
Guideline #6: Culturally competent healthcare systems and organizations	
1. Participate on agency committees on cultural diversity 2. Participate in agency-sponsored cultural diversity events 3. Maintain annual cultural competency educational requirements	1. Develop systems to promote culturally competent care delivery 2. Ensure that mission and organizational policies reflect respect and values related to diversity and inclusivity 3. Assign a managerial-level task force to oversee diversity-related issues within the organization (93) 4. Establish an internal budget for the provision of culturally appropriate care, such as for the hiring of interpreters, producing multi-language patient education materials, adding signage in different languages, etc. (94) 5. Include cultural competence requirements in job descriptions, performance measures, and promotion criteria 6. Develop a data collection system to monitor demographic trends for the geographic area served by the agency (95) 7. Obtain patient satisfaction data to determine the appropriateness and effectiveness of services 8. Collaborate with other health agencies to share ideas and resources for meeting the needs of culturally diverse populations 9. Bring healthcare directly to the local ethnic population 10. Enlist community members to participate in the agency's program planning committees, for example, for smoking cessation or infant care programs
Guideline #7: Patient advocacy and empowerment	
1. Assist patients and families in accessing resources to resolve cultural differences in preferences for care 2. Help patients and their families communicate their care preferences to those who provide care	1. Implement an impartial mechanism that patients and families can use to address cultural preferences for care 2. Create a forum for nurses to examine respectful interactions with their patient populations
Guideline #8: Multicultural workforce	
1. Participate in mentoring culturally diverse staff 2. Volunteer to visit schools to speak with students about healthcare professions	1. Establish a priority of hiring bilingual/bicultural provider staff 2. Celebrate cultural differences through institutional special events 3. Establish policies for zero tolerance for discrimination by all care providers 4. Develop a mentoring network for support of culturally diverse staff 5. Send staff to schools with large ethnic student bodies to encourage students to choose healthcare professions
Guideline #9: Cross-cultural leadership	
1. Participate in community activities and/or organizational initiatives to promote delivery of culturally competent care 2. Participate in professional associations dedicated to the promotion of culturally competent healthcare	1. Participate in collaborative partnerships to facilitate participation and promote effective communication with the community of diverse consumers 2. Contribute to establishing systems for coordinating care between all levels of healthcare services, both internally and with the culturally diverse community at large 3. Provide support for staff participation in collaborative research and integration of best evidence in care specific to diverse patient populations

(continued)

Table 1.3 (continued)

Caregivers	Healthcare organizations Leaders/managers
Guideline #10: Evidence-based practice and research	
1. Participate in journal clubs to review the transcultural health literature 2. Participate in committees that monitor satisfaction of patients from diverse cultural backgrounds and assess efficacy of care given 3. Participate in agency committees to investigate a cross-cultural nursing problem that is unique to an area of practice 4. Implement research-based protocols regarding culturally competent care	1. Provide nursing staff with resources for improving library search and research critique skills of the staff 2. Establish journal clubs to review current literature about the most common cultural groups served to ensure evidence based practice 3. Develop advanced practice nurse (APN) consultants to facilitate implementation of evidence-based cross-cultural practice 4. Consult with local faculty for expertise in research process and study design 5. Collaborate with colleagues to establish a national agenda of priorities for transcultural nursing research 6. Develop interdisciplinary teams of researchers to collaborate on quality improvement projects or research studies and to apply for funding 7. Conduct research through networks with high proportions of patients from diverse populations 8. Collaborate with national and international colleagues to design and implement large scale intervention studies of cultural phenomena 9. Host workshops and conferences to disseminate evidence on effective approaches to culturally congruent nursing practice

Source: Douglas, M.K., Rosenkoetter, M., Pacquiao, D.F., Callister, L.C., Hattar-Pollara, M., Lauderdale, J, Milstead, J., Nardi, D., Purnell, L. (2014), Guidelines for Implementing Culturally Competent Nursing Care. *Journal of Transcultural Nursing* 25 (2):116–118. Reprinted with permission from Sage Publications, Inc.

Table 1.4 Community societal strategies

Perform community assessment
• Identify strengths and deficits of the community
• Collect demographic, SES (income, education, occupation), and crime statistics
• Describe characteristics of vulnerable population group applicable to specific community
• Document ethnohistory (racial and ethnic relationships, social hierarchy, internal and external migration)
• Graph morbidity and mortality patterns
• Ascertain resources for health-related initiatives
• Identify gatekeepers, stakeholders, and potential partners (academic, health, religious, politicians)
• Appreciate previous experience with community advocacy and activism
• Identify existing health resources and collaboratives
• Locate potential venues for community initiatives
• Recognize the impact of existing policies on health and SES (land use, zoning, sanitation, economic development, housing, funding of social programs)
Create partnerships and collaboratives within the community
• Seek common goals and objectives
• Promote long-term engagement and advocacy by members of collaboratives
• Promote immersion of partners in local community
• Develop plan of action
• Create a demand for safe and better places to live; responsive and equitable healthcare system and elimination of health disparities
• Strengthen vulnerable kids and families
• Delineate specific responsibilities of partners

Table 1.4 (continued)

• Seek funding sources
• Seek venues for community action
• Develop evaluation strategies and outcomes to be achieved
• Monitor implementation of planned action
• Monitor interconnections of policies and structures with community health
Build cognitive and social capital of vulnerable communities
• Establish trust and mutual goals with vulnerable groups
• Promote respectful communication and collective solidarity
• Promote awareness of collective problems, efforts to create change, and outcomes across groups
• Emphasize connections between social determinants and poor health
• Engage members of community by developing local champions
• Use bridging, mentoring, and modeling techniques
• Structure incentives for continued engagement and participation of community
• Facilitate access of community members to ongoing planning and implementation
• Engage community members to collect data and monitor progress of initiatives
• Increase awareness and participation of local community in planning, implementation, and evaluation
• Establish a system for ongoing feedback and resolution of conflicts
• Empower community members in data collection, communicating directly with stakeholders, and making decisions about their health
• Publicize impact of initiatives in community and broader society
• Give credit to community members and partners for achievements

or involvement than a formal partnership. A collaborative exists when several people pool their common interests, assets, and professional skills to promote broader interests for the community's benefit. Fundamentally, the relationship between collaborators is nonhierarchical, and shared power is based on knowledge and expertise, rather than role or title (Henneman et al. 1995). The defining attribute of collaboration is the sharing of expertise in a joint venture for an agreed purpose. While effective collaboration needs some of the same attributes of partnership such as team work, mutual trust and respect, and a highly connected network, there are, however, lower expectations of reciprocation and less sharing of risks and rewards than with a formal partnership. It is important to create and nurture both types of relationships to strengthen community capacity to obtain services, resources, and power for health achievement as shown in the following example. A health science center of a local university partnered with the city government to provide health services for the homeless in the city. Multidisciplinary faculty and students have exclusive access to the homeless in differ-

ent shelters run by the city while the city gains additional healthcare manpower and expertise to promote health of the homeless. The university also collaborated with the local hospital to refer patients for emergencies and laboratory tests, police department for security at the shelter during clinic hours, and nearby churches to offer parking for students and faculty.

Building healthy communities involves empowering communities with the cognitive and social capital to transform their own lives for health. Culturally competent strategies at this level must follow a specific process of community assessment before any partnership or collaboration begins. The process of identifying the problem, setting priorities, and selecting a plan of action and outcomes to be monitored must involve the community. The effectiveness of this process is built on mutual trust among the partners/collaborators and the community which develops from prolonged and committed engagement with the community. Health promotion for vulnerable communities must be informed by an in-depth knowledge of the community's strengths, the people (residents, gatekeepers, and stakeholders), shared values, and concerns.

Community strategies require collaborations and partnerships that cut across disciplines and sectors of the community.

1.5.3 Compassion

The antecedent to cultural competence at the community level is the compassionate understanding of the vulnerable (Pacquiao 2016). Compassion stems from both an empathic understanding and sympathetic connection with the suffering of the vulnerable. It evolves from the understanding of the plight of the disadvantaged and feeling their suffering. Compassion motivates one to engage in collaboratives and partnerships with vulnerable populations to advocate for beneficial changes in the lives of vulnerable populations. Compassion compels one to move from non-maleficent actions (preventing harm to others) to beneficent ones (making a difference for others) by engaging in multisectoral collaboration and partnerships with vulnerable communities to address social determinants of poor health. Culturally competent professionals develop partnerships with local communities and stakeholders to build neighborhood social capital and collective empowerment and efficacy in securing or changing social and economic policies in order to improve their lives. Culturally competent professionals understand that the agent accountable to make changes in the lives of vulnerable populations is beyond the purview of the individual but rather on society and the government.

1.5.4 Application of Levels of Cultural Competence

The following example occurred in the poorest district of a large city in Eastern USA with a large population of low-income African American residents with high prevalence of obesity, diabetes, asthma, cancer, and cardiovascular disease. The district has many abandoned homes, a dilapidated infrastructure, and high unemployment and crime rates. Fast-food venues and *bodegas* (small neighborhood stores) are prevalent in the neighborhood. The area is considered a food desert as many households have limited access to large grocery stores offering affordable and quality healthy foods. One of the city's municipal council members, an African American educator, is a resident of this district. Several generations in his family have remained in this same neighborhood. His family has a broad social network of influential African Americans who were former residents of the community but have remained engaged in the community. The council member is trusted by the community and emerged as the district's champion and advocate in the city council. The council convenes monthly town meetings for residents to share issues and concerns. His social network of community leaders, educators, politicians, scientists, and students are invited to these meetings.

The goal of one of the initiatives developed was to decrease obesity by improving access to healthy foods and safe places to exercise. Ongoing culturally competent strategies to improve the lives and well-being of residents include the following:

1.5.4.1 Individual Level
- Multidisciplinary healthcare staff and students in health professions, education, and social work conduct health promotion activities at senior centers, barber shops, schools, homeless shelters, and local churches.
  - Culturally congruent communication is practiced emphasizing respect for elders and people of lower SES and the use of low-literacy brochures and instructions.
  - African American healthcare practitioners are recruited to provide services, and community members serve as cultural mediators.
  - Women and religious leaders are encouraged to bring their partners, husbands, brothers, male friends, and sons to be screened. African American men tend not to participate in health screening. Close follow-up is done for men through women family members.
  - Assessment of weight, blood pressure, blood glucose, and level of physical activity.

- Counseling on age- and gender-appropriate BMI levels is done because of the widespread acceptance of larger body size in the community.
- Counseling on healthy food purchasing, reading labels, meal planning and preparation, and meal portion sizes emphasizing low cost and healthier options. Emphasis is placed on modifying ethnic menus to reduce salt, fat, and calories as well as increase fiber. Poor urban African American diets tend to have low fiber and high sodium, sugar, and fat content.
- Accessing food pantries in the area and referral to Meals on Wheels—a federally funded program that delivers meals to homebound individuals such as the elderly and disabled who are unable to purchase or prepare their own meals. Counseling is provided on how to obtain a variety of food products that are nutritious, low cost, and healthy.
- Providing age-appropriate exercise classes such as home exercises and group walks for clients in unsafe neighborhoods.

- Multidisciplinary healthcare staff and students in health professions operate the mobile clinic that goes into different neighborhoods to conduct health assessment, counseling, disease management, referral, and follow-up. Community members serve as volunteers to recruit, remind, and bring people to the venues where the van is located on specific days of the week.
- Home health nurses, nursing students, and a nurse practitioner conduct home visits for homebound residents unable to avail of the mobile van service.

1.5.4.2 Organizational Level
- Local primary schools partner with a nonprofit community organization (donates land, vegetable seeds, and soil) and a local university (performs soil analysis) to involve students in gardening in the school grounds. Soil analysis is important as the city is situated in ten superfund sites and toxic pollutants are found in most areas, making them unsuitable for growing edible foods unless the top soil is replaced.

- Partnership among local schools, police, and residents to ensure safe access of school children to the local park after school. Most parents keep their children at home because of high crimes.
- Local schools open their gyms for students after school hours in addition to providing tutoring as most students do not have adequate support at home and many parents are working. The majority of adults have high school education.
- A local medical school obtained a grant to bring local farmers to sell their produce monthly at the school. Farmers requested a safe place to sell, and the medical school located in the neighborhood was chosen as the venue because it is accessible to buses.
- The local community and county hospitals sponsor health fairs aimed at decreasing obesity, particularly during the summer months and traditional festivals celebrated by the local community.
- Local schools introduce students to fresh fruits and vegetables and provide demonstration on healthy food preparation. Because of lack of large grocery stores offering fresh and low-cost fruits and vegetables, young kids have limited exposure to them.
- The local community and county hospitals enlist community members to participate on hospital-wide committees that address chronic diseases and nutrition for clients in their catchment areas.

1.5.4.3 Community Level
- Collaboration between the police chief and the council member in addressing safety concerns of residents. To address complaints about delays in police response, residents were instructed to document the date and time they called, date and time of police response, person called at the police station, and the reason for the call. Trust in the police is critical to residents feeling safe in their neighborhood and motivate them to get out of their homes.
- The council created an advisory council comprised of local business owners to create jobs and offer healthy food choices and menus.

- The nonprofit community organization encourages the use of vacant lots by residents for community gardens. Residents can rent the lot for $1 annually for as long as the produce is consumed and shared with neighborhood residents. The organization offers technical assistance, seeds, and soil to renters. Preliminary observations noted increased interactions and connections among community members offering the potential for building social capital of the neighborhood.
- Residents were given an organizational chart of the city with appropriate contact details so they know the person or office to call for specific problems.
- The council conducts periodic walks with local residents in their neighborhood to ease safety concerns, improve social interactions among residents, and motivate them to get out and walk.
- Cameras were installed by the city on local streets in high-crime neighborhoods.

1.6 Health Equity

Elimination of health inequity and advocacy for vulnerable populations is central to culturally competent care. Social determinants of health are socially constructed institutionalized forces that create one's "place" in society, with some more privileged than others (Jenkins 2002). The social construction and reproduction of "place" is embodied in internalized habits of the vulnerable. Oscar Lewis (1966) has documented a sense of helplessness and fatalism among poor Mexicans and Puerto Ricans. This finding has been supported by later studies of poor Hispanics (Baer and Bustillo 1993; Poss and Jezewski 2002). Fatalism and helplessness are the antithesis of self-empowerment and self-reliance. Yet the same predispositions are found useful among the poor in coping with life conditions that are beyond their control (Leyva et al. 2014). Culturally competent strategies should be directed toward changing the life circumstances of poor Hispanics to dismantle the cycle of socially constructed "place" and habits of helplessness and fatalism. By simply valuing their cultural values and beliefs and doing little or nothing to change the status quo of their social circumstances, culturally competent strategies cannot achieve health equity because social determinants of their poor health are not being addressed.

Vulnerable populations are generally comprised of people who are viewed as different by mainstream society. Cultural competence is at the core of advocacy and beneficent acts for the vulnerable because it bridges differences and builds coalitions through mutual respect, reciprocity, and shared goals. To achieve health equity, cultural competence should primarily focus on health and its social determinants. Emphasis on health rather than disease moves cultural competence beyond individual disease-based care toward population health promotion that accounts for the social, economic, cultural, and political contexts of people's lives.

1.7 Culture of Health

A culture of health is a cohesive system of values, beliefs, and practices that support health throughout the life course and across different life contexts. As health is embedded in life conditions, culturally competent approaches should cut across different sectors and disciplines.

Health is achieved in homes, employment, schools, and communities. These are places healthy people inhabit. Building healthy communities requires four strategies: (a) making health a shared value; (b) fostering cross-sector collaboration to improve well-being; (c) creating healthier, more equitable communities; and (d) strengthening integration of health services and systems (Lavizzo-Mourey 2015).

1.8 Summary

Equity of health outcomes is achieved by addressing the fundamental conditions that predispose certain groups to poor health more than others. Health promotion should be grounded in understanding the social pathways to poor health that are rooted in the living and working conditions of people. Because social determinants of health have different trajectories for populations, healthcare should stop the cycle of vulnerability in certain groups. Health is achieved by preventing and mitigating existing social inequities that render vulnerable populations to suboptimal life chances in society. Thus, central to health promotion are the maintenance of safeguards to preserve basic human rights and the application of social justice to benefit those that need them the most. Cultural competence is a pathway to creating healthy communities, replete with healthy values, beliefs, and ways of life where health is a collective responsibility and not solely that of the individual alone. Healthy communities breed healthy individuals and families because everyone is socialized and have access to a healthful way of life. Healthy communities have built social capital for health with a widespread network of support and surveillance that ensures health for everyone.

References

Adler N, Singh-Manoux A, Schwartz J et al (2008) Social status and health: a comparison of British civil servants in Whitehall-II with European- and African-Americans in CARDIA. Soc Sci Med 66: 1034–1045

Agency for Healthcare Research and Quality Advancing Excellence in Health Care (2014) National healthcare quality and disparities report. USDHHS, Rockville

Babones S (2010) Income, education, and class gradients in health in global perspective. Health Sociol Rev 19(1):130–143

Baer RD, Bustillo M (1993) Susto and mal de ojo among Florida farmworkers. Emic and etic perspectives. Med Anthropol Q 7(1):90–100

Bambas A, Casas JA (2001) Assessing equity in health. Conceptual criteria. In: PAHO, equity and health: views from the Pan American Sanitary Bureau, Publication 8. Author, Washington DC, pp 12–21

Bask M (2011) Cumulative disadvantage and connections between welfare problems. Soc Indic Res 103:443–464

Benatar S (2013) Editorial: challenges of health disparities in South Africa. S Afr Med J 103(3):154–155. https://doi.org/10.7196/SAMJ.6622

Benatar S, Sullivan T, Brown A (2017) Why equity in health and in access to health care are elusive: insights from Canada and South Africa. Glob Public Health 4:1–25. https://doi.org/10.1080/17441692.2017.1407813

Bourdieu P (1977) Outline of a theory of practice. Cambridge Univ. Press, New York

Braverman P (2014) What are health disparities and health equity? We need to be clear. Public Health Rep 129(S2):5–8

Burris S, Kawachi I, Sarat A (2002) Integrating law and social epidemiology. J Law Med Ethics 30(4):510–521

Carnwell R, Carson A (2005) Understanding partnerships and collaboration. In: Canrwell R, Buchanan J (eds) Effective practice in health and social care. Open University Press, McGraw Hill, London, pp 1–19

CDC (2011, Jan 14) CDC health disparities and inequalities report—United States, 2011. MMWR 60(Suppl). https://www.cdc.gov/mmwr/pdf/other/su6001.pdf

CDC (2014a) Health, United States, 2013. http://www.cdc.gov/nchs/data/hus/hus13.pdf#018

CDC (2014b) Adult obesity facts. http://www.cdc.gov/obesity/data/adult.html

CDC (2014c) High blood pressure. http://www.cdc.gov/bloodpressure/facts.htm

CDC (2015) Prevalence of childhood obesity in the United States, 2011-2012. http://www.cdc.gov/obesity/data/childhood.html

Chauhan S, Aeri BT (2013) Prevalence of cardiovascular disease in India and its economic impact—a review. Int J Sci Res Publ 3(10):1–5

Coleman J (1990) The foundations of social theory. Harvard University Press, Cambridge

Corrigall R, Bhugra D (2013) The role of ethnicity and diagnosis in rates of adolescent psychiatric admission and compulsory detention: a longitudinal case-note study. J R Soc Med 106:190–195

Countrymeters (2017a) China population. (2017). http://www.countrymeters.info/en/China/

Countrymeters (2017b) India population. (2017). http://www.countrymeters.info/en/India/

Cross T, Bazron B, Dennis K et al (1989) Towards a culturally competent system of care, vol I. Georgetown University Child Development Center, CASSP Technical Assistance Center, Washington, DC

Diez-Roux AV (2004) The study of group-level factors in epidemiology: rethinking variables, study designs and analytical approaches. Epidemiol Rev 26(1):104–111

Drewnowski A, Specter S (2004) Poverty and obesity: the role of energy density and energy cost. Am J Clin Nutr 79:6–16

Edwards A (2014) Dynamics of economic well-being: poverty, 2009-2011. U.S. Department of Commerce, Economics and Statistics Administration, (Household Economics Studies: 70–137). http://www.census.gov/prod/2014pubs/p70-137.pdf

Fang JY, Piao S, Field CB, Pan Y, Guo QH, Zhou L, Peng C, Tao S (2003) Increasing net primary production in China from 1982 to 1999. Front Ecol Environ 1(6):293–297. https://doi.org/10.2307/3868089

Frohlich KL, Potvin L (2008) The inequality paradox: the population approach and vulnerable populations. Am J Public Health 98(2):216–220

Fullilove MT (2004) Root shock: how tearing up city neighborhoods hurts America and what we can do about it. One World/Ballantine Books, New York

Gong P, Liang S, Carlton EJ et al (2012) Urbanisation and health in China. Lancet 379(9818):843–852

Gupta R (2012) Regional variations in cardiovascular risk factors in India: India heart watch. World J Cardiol 4(4):112. https://doi.org/10.4330/wjc.v4.i4.112

Guthrie A, Fleck F (2017) Quality care is key to tackling Mexico's diabetes emergency. Bull World Health Organ 95:393–394. https://doi.org/10.2471/BLT.17.020617

Henneman EA, Lee JL, Cohen JI (1995) Collaboration: a concept analysis. J Adv Nurs 21:103–109

Hessini L (2007) Abortion and Islam: policies and practice in the Middle East and North Africa. Reprod Health Matters 15(29):75–84

Ibnouf AH, van den Borne HW, Maarse JA (2007) Utilization of antenatal care services by Sudanese women in their reproductive age. Saudi Med J 28(5): 737–743

Iceland J (2012) Poverty in America: a handbook. Berkeley: University of California Press

Institute for Research on Poverty, University of Wisconsin-Madison (2016) Who is poor? http://www.irp.wisc.edu/faqs/faq3.htm

International Council on Human Rights Policy (ICHRP) (2012) Article 25: Universal declaration of human rights. http://ichrp.org/en/article_25_udhr

Izek I (2016) Mexico City: disparities in healthcare. http://pulitzercenter.org/projects/neonatal-outcomes-developing-developed-world-without-breath

Jenkins R (2002) Pierre Bourdieu. Routledge, London

Jimenez-Sanchez S, Jimenez-Garcia R, Alonso-Blanco C et al (2013) Prevalence of migraine headaches in the Romany population in Spain: demographic, lifestyle and co-morbidity. J Transcult Nurs 24(1):6–13

Kaiser Family Foundation (2015) Key facts about the uninsured population. http://kff.org/uninsured/factsheet/key-facts-about-the-uninsured-population/

Kakoli R, Chaudhuri A (2008) Influence of SES, wealth and financial empowerment on gender differences in health and healthcare utilization in later life: evidence from India. Soc Sci Med 66(9):1951–1962

Kalra A, Pokharel Y, Glusenkamp N et al (2016) Gender disparities in cardiovascular care access and delivery in India: insights from the American College of Cardiology's Pinnacle India Quality Improvement Program (Piqip). J Am Coll Cardiol 67(13):1849. https://doi.org/10.1016/s0735-1097(16)31850-2

Kaufman JS (2008) Social epidemiology. In: Rothman KJ, Greenland S, Lash TL (eds) Modern epidemiology, 3rd edn. Lippincott Williams & Wilkins, Philadelphia, pp 532–548

Kishk NA (2002) Knowledge, attitudes and practices of women towards antenatal care: rural–urban comparison. J Egypt Public Health Assoc 77:479–498

Krieger N (2011) Epidemiology and the people's health. Oxford University Press, New York

Kronfol NM (2012a) Access and barriers to healthcare delivery in Arab countries: a review. East Mediterr Health J 18(12):1239–1246. http://www.emro.who.int/emhj-volume-18-2012/issue-12/09.html

Kronfol NM (2012b) Delivery of health services in Arab countries: a review. East Mediterr Health J 18(12):1229–1238

Kronfol NM (2012c) Health services to groups with special needs in the Arab world: a review. East Mediterr Health J 18(12):1247–1253

Last F, Fowler D, Freer-Smith PH (1985) Effects of air pollutants on agricultural crops. Burlington Press, Cambridge

Lavizzo-Mourey R (2015) In it together—building a culture of health. http://www.rwjf.org/en/library/annual-reports/presidents-message-2015.html

Lee L (2004) The current state of public health in China. Annu Rev Public Health 25(1):327–339. https://doi.org/10.1146/annurev.publhealth.25.101802.123116

Lewis O (1966) La vida; a Puerto Rican family in the culture of poverty—San Juan and New York. Secker & Warburg, London

Leyva B, Allen JD, Tom LS et al (2014) Religion, fatalism, and cancer control: a qualitative study among Hispanic Catholics. Am J Health Behav 38(6): 839–849. https://doi.org/10.5993/AJHB.38.66

Lin A, Harris D (2009) The colors of poverty: why racial and ethnic disparities persist (National Poverty Center, Poverty Brief # 16). http://npc.umich.edu/publications/policy_briefs/brief16/PolicyBrief16.pdf

Liu X, Sun H, Feike T et al (2016) Assessing the impact of air pollution on grain yield of winter wheat—a case study in the North China Plain. PLoS One 11:1–15. https://doi.org/10.1371/journal.pone.0162655

Marmot MG (2006) Status syndrome, a challenge to medicine. JAMA 295(11):1304–1307

Marmot MG, Bell R (2009) Action on health disparities in the US: Commission on Social Determinants of Health. JAMA 301(11):1169–1171

Marmot MG, Rose G, Shipley M et al (1978) Employment grade and coronary heart disease in British civil servants. J Epidemiol Community Health 32(4):244–249. https://doi.org/10.1136/jech.32.4.244

Marmot MG, Smith GD, Stansfeld S et al (1991) Health inequalities among British civil servants: the Whitehall II study. Lancet 337(8754):1387–1393. https://doi.org/10.1016/0140-6736(91)93068-K

McEwen B, Nasca C, Gray JD (2015) Stress effects on neuronal structure: hippocampus, amygdala and prefrontal cortex. Neuropsychopharmacology 41(1):3–23. https://doi.org/10.1038/npp.2015.171

Mendoza R (2011) Why do the poor pay more? Exploring the poverty penalty concept. J Int Dev 23(1):1–28

Mikkonen J, Raphael D (2010) Social determinants of health: the Canadian facts. York University School of Health Policy and Management, Toronto

Miranda ML, Messer LC, Kroger GL (2012) Associations between the quality of the residential environment and pregnancy outcomes among women in North Carolina. Environ Health Perspect 120(3):471–477

Mohan I, Gupta R, Misra A et al (2016) Disparities in prevalence of cardiometablic risk factors in rural, urban-poor and urban-middle class women in India. PLoS One 11(2):e0149437. https://doi.org/10.1371/journal.pone.0149437

Moy E, Barrett M, Ho K (2011) Potentially preventable hospitalizations—United States, 2004–2007. MMWR 60(Suppl):80–83

Murguia-Peniche T, Illescas-Zarate D, Chico-Barba G et al (2016) An ecological study of stillbirths in Mexico from 2000 to 2013. Bull World Health Organ 94:322–330A. https://doi.org/10.2471/BLT.15.154922

National Coalition on Black Civic Participation (2014) Black Women in the United States, 2014: progress and challenges 50 years after the war on poverty,

50 years after the civil rights act of 1964, 60 years after Brown v. Board of Education. ncbcp.org/news/releases/BWRReport.BlackWomeninU.S.2015.3.26.15FINAL.pdf

OECD (2014a) OECD health statistics 2014. How does the US compare? http://www.oecd.org/unitedstates/Briefing-Note-UNITED-STATES-2014.pdf

OECD (2014b) Education at a glance 2014: OECD indicators. https://doi.org/10.1787/eag-2014-en. Accessed 2 Apr 2017

Pacquiao DF (2016) Cultural competence in ethical decision-making. In: Andrews MM, Boyle JS (eds) Transcultural concepts in nursing care, 7th edn. Wolters Kluwer, Philadelphia, pp 447–464

Pan X, Li G, Gao T (2012) Dangerous breathing P.M 2.5: measuring the human health and economic impacts on China's largest cities, Beijing, China. China Environmental Science Press. Guardian News and Media Limited

Population Reference Bureau (2012) India's aging population. Today's research on aging. http://www.prb.org/pdf12/TodaysResearchAging25.pdf

Poss J, Jezewski MA (2002) The role and meaning of susto in Mexican Americans' explanatory model of type 2 diabetes. Med Anthropol Q 16(3):360–377

Powers M, Faden R (2008) Social justice: the moral foundations of public health and health policy. Oxford University Press, New York

Putnam RD (2000) Bowling alone: the collapse and revival of American community. Simon & Schuster, New York. ISBN: 0-7432-0304-6

Ramachandran A, Snehalatha C, Vijay V (2003) Explosion of type 2 diabetes in the Indian subcontinent. Int Diabet Monit 15:1–6

Rao N (2014) Women in India—longevity, health disparities and empowerment. https://globalhealthaging.org/2014/07/26/women-in-india-longevity-health-disparities-empowerment/

Raphael D (2004) Introduction to the social determinants of health. In: Raphael D (ed) Social determinants of health: Canadian perspectives. Scholars Press, Toronto, pp 2–19

Rawls J (1971) A theory of justice. Harvard University Press, Cambridge

Rohde RA, Muller RA (2015) Air pollution in China: mapping concentrations and sources. http://berkeleyearth.org/wp-content/uploads/2015/08/China-Air-Quality-Paper-July-2015.pdf

Romdhane HB, Grenier FR (2009) Social determinants of health in Tunisia: the case analysis of Ariana. Int J Equity Health 8:9. https://doi.org/10.1186/1475-9276-8-9. © World Health Organization

Sampson RJ, Raudenbush SW (1999) Systematic social observation of public spaces: a new look at disorder in urban neighborhoods. Am J Sociol 105(3):603

Seith D, Kalof C (2011) Who are America's poor children? Examining health disparities by race and ethnicity. National Center for Children in Poverty, Columbia University

Sengupta R, Jena N (2009) The current trade paradigm and women's health concerns in India: with special reference to the proposed EU-India Free Trade Agreement. SSRN Electron J. https://doi.org/10.2139/ssrn.1757785

Setse RW, Euler GL, Gonzalez-Feliciano AG et al (2011) Influenza vaccination coverage—United States, 2000–2010. MMWR 60(Suppl):38–41

Slaughter MJ, Swagel P (1997) Does globalization lower wages and export jobs? Econ Issues (11):1–13. IMF, Washington, DC

UN (1948) Universal Declaration of Human Rights. UN General Assembly, 10 Dec 1948

UNESCO (2015) Gender and EFA 2000-2015: achievements and challenges. Author, Paris

United Nations (2004) World urbanization prospects: the 2003 revision. UN publication sales no. E.04.XlII.6.ISBN 92-1-141396-0. UN, New York

US Census (2016) Income and poverty in the US:2015. https://www.census.gov/library/publications/2016/demo/p60-256.html

USDA (2017) Poverty demographics. https://www.ers.usda.gov/topics/rural-economy-population/rural-poverty-well-being/poverty-demographics/

USDHHS (2010) Healthy people 2020. Author, Washington, DC

USDHHS (2015) Key features of the ACA. http://www.hhs.gov/healthcare/facts-and-features/key-features-of-aca-by-year/index.html#

USDHHS, HRSA-MCHB (2013) Child Health USA, 2013. http://mchb.hrsa.gov/chusa13/perinatal-health-status-indicators/perinatal-health-status-indicators.html

USDHHS, Office of Minority Health (2001) National standards for culturally and linguistically appropriate services in health care: final report. http://www.omhrc.gov/clas/. Accessed 15 Apr 2004

USDHHS-OMH (2014) Diabetes and African Americans. http://minorityhealth.hhs.gov/omh/browse.aspx?lvl=4&lvlID=18

Washington DL, Bowles J, Saha S et al (2008) Transforming clinical practice to eliminate racial-ethnic disparities in healthcare. J Gen Intern Med 23(5):685–691

Whitehead M (1992) The concepts and principles of equity and health. Int J Health Serv 22:429–445

WHO (2015a) Health Impact Assessment (HIA). http://www.who.int/hia/evidence/doh/en/

WHO (2015b) Health in the post-2015 development agenda: need for a social determinants of health approach. http://www.who.int/social_determinants/advocacy/health-post-2015_sdh/e

WHO (2016) Measuring the adequacy of antenatal health care: a national cross-sectional study in Mexico. Bull WHO 94:452–461. https://doi.org/10.2471/BLT.15.168302

Wilkinson R, Pickett K (2010) The spirit level, why greater equality makes societies stronger. Penguin Books, New York

Williams DR, John DA, Oyserman D et al (2012) Research on discrimination and health: an exploratory study. Am J Public Health 102(5):973–978

Wilson W (1996) When work disappears: the world of the new urban poor. Alfred A. Knopf, Inc., New York

Part I

Guideline: Knowledge of Cultures

Knowledge of Cultures

2

Larry Purnell

Guideline: Nurses shall gain an understanding of the perspectives, traditions, values, practices, and family systems of culturally diverse families, communities, and populations they care for, as well as knowledge of the complex variables that affect the achievement of health and well-being.

Douglas et al. (2014: 110)

2.1 Introduction

As globalization and immigration increase, it has become more important for nurses, other healthcare providers, and organizations to become culturally competent in order to decrease healthcare disparities of vulnerable populations. Many definitions of culture and culture care exist. A definition for individuals and groups is the totality of socially transmitted behavior patterns, arts, beliefs, values, customs, lifeways, and all other products of human work and thought characteristics of a population that guides their worldview and decision-making. The patterns may be explicit or implicit and are shared by the majority, but not all, of the culture (Purnell 2013). Culture is primarily learned in the family followed by schools, churches, and other organizations where people gather. A popular definition of culturally competent care more specific to organizational cultural competence is "cultural competence is defined as a set of congruent behaviors, attitudes, and policies that come together in a system, agency, or among professionals and enables that

system, agency, or those professionals to work effectively in cross-cultural situations" (Cross et al. 1989, para 1).

Whereas this chapter does not address specific models and theories of culture care, nurses and other healthcare professionals are encouraged to seek models that fit their needs. A plethora of images of models for culturally competent care exist. Some are similar but others are more complex (Images of Cultural Models n.d.). The most popular theories and models include Campinha-Bacote's Model The Process of Cultural Competence in the Delivery of Healthcare Services (http://transculturalcare.net/the-process-of-cultural-competence-in-the-delivery-of-healthcare-services/), Jeffrey's Cultural Competence and Confidence (CCC) Model: Transcultural Self-Efficiency (Jeffreys 2010a, b), Leininger's Culture Care Diversity and Universality Theory (McFarland and Wehbe-Alamah 2015), the Papadopoulos Model for Developing Culturally Competent and Compassionate Care for Healthcare Professionals (Papadopoulos et al. 2016), the Purnell Model for Cultural Competence (Purnell 2014), and Shim's Dimensional Puzzle Model of Culturally Competent Care (Schim et al. 2005). Some of the theories and models are used for research, some are primarily used for education, and some are used for both education and research.

L. Purnell, Ph.D., R.N., FAAN
School of Nursing, University of Delaware, Newark, DE, USA

Florida International University, Miami, FL, USA

Excelsior College, Albany, NY, USA
e-mail: lpurnell@udel.edu

© Springer International Publishing AG, part of Springer Nature 2018
M. Douglas et al. (eds.), *Global Applications of Culturally Competent Health Care: Guidelines for Practice*, https://doi.org/10.1007/978-3-319-69332-3_2

2.2 The Complexity of Culture: Individual, Group, and Organizational Culture

Culture is both objective and subjective. Every culture creates a system of shared knowledge if it is to survive as a group and foster communication among its members. These shared patterns of information are both objective and subjective (obvious and hidden). Objective culture, also considered visible elements of culture, are things an outsider can see but may not understand "why things are the way they are." Objective culture includes things that people make such as art, music, and styles of clothing and dress; objective culture can be shared and appreciated by others. For example, art from an indigenous population may be quite different from Renaissance, Cubism, Expressionism, Surrealism, or Abstract art. However, one can appreciate all objective forms of culture, especially their differences.

Subjective culture, on the other hand, is largely unconscious and is a way of perceiving the social environment which includes behavioral norms, social roles, ideas, beliefs, and values (Triandis 2002), including those related to health and healthcare that can vary within and among groups. Furthermore, subjective culture has two lenses, *etic* and *emic*. *Etic* culture refers to general categories that can be found in all cultures that serve as common grounds for comparison. *Emic* refers to categories that might only make sense in a specific culture and makes a culture unique and meaningful to those who belong to it (Olive 2014). As with objective culture, one can appreciate and value the subjective cultural values of many diverse groups of people.

Moreover, culture as an anthropological and social construct has three levels. A primary level that represents the deepest level in which rules are known by all, observed by all, implicit, and taken for granted. A secondary level in which only members know the rules of behavior and can articulate them. The healthcare provider must make a conscious effort to uncover them. A tertiary level that is visible to outsiders, such as things that can be seen, worn, or otherwise observed, also known as the objective culture (Koffman 2006; Purnell 2013).

Culture and cultural competence are dynamic, characterized by constant change and require healthcare providers to engage in a lifelong learning process (Jeffreys 2010a, b). Cultural attributes and values that influence individual and group differences are critical in preventing overgeneralizing and stereotyping. Much of what applies to a patient's individual and group culture also applies to organizational culture. Awareness of culture progresses along four stages: unconscious incompetence, conscious incompetence, conscious competence, and unconscious competence (Nursing Best Practice Guidelines: Summary of Key Models Related to Cultural Competence n.d.; Purnell 2013).

In unconscious incompetence, the healthcare provider is not aware of cultural differences, and the healthcare provider might do something culturally wrong or even offensive and not realize it. For example, a male nurse may extend his hand in an attempt to shake hands with a traditional female Muslim or Orthodox Jewish patient. In traditional Islam and Orthodox Jewish religion, a male is forbidden to touch a female unless it is an emergency situation (Kulwicki and Ballout 2013; Selekman 2013).

In conscious incompetence, the nurse is aware that differences exist but not understand what they are and might mean. In this case, the nurse knows he/she is doing something wrong but not know exactly what is wrong. For example, a nurse greets a patient by his/her first name, a practice that is considered rude and culturally unacceptable among some, especially in collectivistic cultures. The patient might inform the nurse to use Mr., Mrs., or Miss before the name or give some nonverbal reaction that something is unacceptable. When this happens, the nurse needs to ask about the patient's reaction, apologize, and provide the preferred name of address in the patient's medical record.

In conscious competence, the nurse knows that differences exist, knows some of the differences, and attempts to know more of these differences and how the provider can use and apply them for culturally congruent care. The nurse knows he/she is doing something right but has to consciously focus on doing it the correct way.

For example, in a collectivistic culture where it is rude or unacceptable to give a "no" answer to a question, the only acceptable answer is to respond affirmatively to "save face," one's own sense of dignity or prestige in social contexts. The nurse learns to ask questions that cannot be answered with a "yes" or "no." When asking about medication adherence, instead of asking if the patient takes a medicine as prescribed, ask the patient at what time he/she took the medicine that day. Another way to ask is how many days did you miss taking your medicine this week.

Unconscious competence is where cultural appropriate behavior becomes automatic. The nurse knows he/she is doing something culturally congruent without having to think about it. However, this can be problematic and even stereotypic because individual differences can exist greatly among individuals in each culture.

A culturally competent healthcare organization shares most of the concepts related to individual and group cultures. Cultural competence in healthcare has been defined as "a set of congruent behaviors, attitudes, and policies that come together in a system, agency, or among professionals and enable that system, agency, or those professionals to work effectively in cross-cultural situations" (Health Resources and Services Administration 2002: 3). The tenets of organizational cultural competency are inclusive of all professional groups as well as clerical, technical, and unlicensed assistive personnel. The overall responsibility of providing culturally safe and culturally congruent care is the responsibility of the organizations' managers and administrators (Marrone 2013).

Organizational cultural competence is a process and is responsible for assuring that culture is incorporated at all levels to meet culturally unique needs, thereby increasing quality care. Enhanced quality care reduces health disparities and improves health outcomes for vulnerable and underserved populations.

Culturally competent healthcare organizations provide consumers with effective, understandable, and respectful care provided in ways that fit with their cultural values and beliefs and in the consumer's preferred language if at all possible. To achieve this goal, the organization must integrate cultural and linguistic competence-related measures into internal audits, performance improvement programs, patient satisfaction assessments and surveys, and outcomes-based evaluations. In addition, it requires collecting and updating information related to consumers' race and ethnicity and spoken, written, and sign languages. These data help maintain a current demographic, cultural, and epidemiological profile of the community to plan for and implement services that respond to its cultural and linguistic characteristics (Office of Minority Health 2001).

To provide effective patient education, a requisite is to review the language literacy level of consumers and use culturally respectful images in written and television or video patient education materials. In addition, a system must be in place that indicates whether language assistance is needed prior to or at the point of entry into the organization if at all possible. Organizations have values espoused by the leaders and most often are grounded in shared assumptions of how the organization should be run. While the espoused values are often prescribed at the highest level in an organization, each community may have its own norms, perspectives, and collective understandings. Their willingness to share and to seek knowledge will be influenced by these collective views. Furthermore, culturally competent human resources departments should promote patient-centered care by including patient satisfaction measures in employee performance appraisals.

To be effective, written satisfaction surveys should be translated into the languages that represent the catchment area for the organization; otherwise, the data collection process is incomplete. It may not be possible to translate satisfaction surveys into all the languages (some are only verbal) and dialects spoken by consumers, but at least some should be.

Andrews (1998) provides a six-step framework for ensuring organizational cultural competency.

1. Collect demographic and descriptive data of the prevalent cultural, ethnic, linguistic, and spiritual groups represented among patients, families, visitors, the community, and the staff in the service area.

2. Describe the effectiveness of current systems and processes in meeting diverse needs.
3. Assess the organization's strengths and limitations by examining the institution's ethos toward cultural diversity and the presence or absence of a corporate culture that promotes accord among its constituents.
4. Determine organizational need and readiness for change through dialogue with key stakeholders aimed at discovering foci of anticipated support and recognizing areas of potential resistance.
5. Implement strategic plans, policies, and procedures that include measurable benchmarks of success and an ongoing process to ensure that change is maintained.
6. Evaluate actual outcomes against established benchmarks utilizing performance improvement, quality, and customer satisfaction data.

Culturally competent healthcare organizations implement strategies to recruit, retain, and promote at all levels of the organization a diverse staff and leadership team that are representative of the demographics of the service area. The goal of recruiting and retaining a diverse workforce that matches the demographics of the service area is to reduce health disparities among vulnerable and underserved populations that often results from discordant consumer–provider relationships. Culture and language discordance can lead to decreased access to care, decreased quality of care, increased cost of care, decreased patient satisfaction, recidivism, discrimination, and poor health outcomes (American Association of Critical Care Nurses 2008; Europa 2010). To reduce discordance between consumers and providers, an organization needs to integrate diversity into the organization's mission statement, strategic plans, and goals. A diverse workforce program includes mentoring programs, community-based internships, and collaborations with academic partners such as universities, local schools, training programs, and faith-based organizations. To expand the recruitment base, organizations should recruit at minority health and recruitment fairs, advertise in multiple languages, and list job opportunities in minority publications such as local newspapers and community newsletters. It also requires that the availability of language assistance services include sign language, the translation of critical documents such as consents and patient education materials, pain scales, and communication boards/aids for patients who are not able to speak or understand the dominant language.

2.3 Essential Knowledge to Provide Evidence-Based, Culturally Competent Nursing Care

Nurses, as well as other healthcare providers, need essential basics to practice culturally competent and congruent care. All healthcare providers must understand that culture has a strong effect on attitudes, values, traditions, and behavior, and they vary within the culture according to age, generation, nationality, race and ethnicity, color, gender, religion, educational status, socioeconomic status, occupation, military status, political beliefs, urban versus rural residence, enclave identity, marital status, parental status, physical characteristics, sexual orientation, gender issues, and reason for migration (sojourner, immigrant, or undocumented) (Purnell 2005, 2013; Purnell and Fenkl 2018).

Learning health-seeking behaviors of culturally diverse individuals, families, communities, and populations is essential for providing culturally competent and culturally congruent care. These skills can be learned through formal educational programs, in-services on specific cultural and ethnic groups, and immersion experiences in diverse cultures in the home environment as well as immersion experiences in the patient's home country. In addition, some travel blogs, although they may not be peer reviewed or research based, provide basic etiquette, and nonverbal information on gesturing in a specific culture can have value.

Culture and language are closely related; through language, culture is passed onto each generation. Although language is a communication medium that allows individuals to pass ideas between them, sharing a language does not necessarily mean sharing a culture; nor does a culture necessarily share a language. See Chap. 5 for a more extensive information on communication.

Health policy can affect culturally diverse groups, particularly those who are economically disadvantaged, vulnerable, and/or underserved. Nurses can help ensure social justice by identifying personal and familial social support networks, by working with professional community human resources, and by engaging in political advocacy (see Chap. 8) (International Council of Nurses 2011; National Association of Social Workers 2007).

Professional nurses need specific knowledge about the major groups of culturally diverse individuals, families, and communities they serve, including but not limited to specific cultural practices regarding health and determining beliefs about health and illness, biological and genetic variations, cross-cultural worldviews, and acculturation and life experiences such as refugee and immigration status as well as a history of oppression, violence, and trauma suffered (Andrews and Boyle 2016; Douglas et al. 2014; United Nations 2015). Culturally competent assessment skills (see Chap. 19) are essential to facilitate communication, to demonstrate respect for cultural diversity, and to ask culturally sensitive questions about beliefs and practices that need to be considered in the delivery of health and nursing care. The more knowledge a healthcare provider has about a specific culture, the more accurate and complete the cultural assessment will be. For example, if the nurse is not aware that many patients use traditional healers, the nurse might not ask specific and appropriate questions about the individual's use of these traditional practitioners and their therapies. Because nurses cannot know the attributes of all cultures, it is essential to use a cultural assessment model or framework (see Chap. 19). Thus, nurses should seek specialized knowledge from the body of literature in transcultural nursing practice that focuses on specific and universal attitudes, knowledge, and skills used to assess, plan, implement, and evaluate culturally competent nursing care (McFarland and Wehbe-Alamah 2015; Papadopoulos 2006).

In addition, nurses need knowledge of the types of institutional, class, economic, cultural, and language barriers that may prevent individuals and families from accessing healthcare. Knowledge can also be gained from associated disciplines such as anthropology, sociology, and communication arts.

2.4 Essential Knowledge of Cultural and Anthropological Concepts

Culture is based in anthropology; therefore, a working knowledge of the following terms is essential. These terms and their definitions related to cultural competence follow: enculturation, ethnocentrism, acculturation, assimilation, cultural awareness, culture sensitivity, cultural competence, cultural congruence, generalization versus stereotype, cultural imperialism, cultural imposition, cultural relativism, ethnic group, and subculture. A brief description of each of these terms is defined providing a starting point for a broad understanding of culture so the healthcare provider can be aware of them in practice.

An ethnohistory (the history of peoples and cultures) and the social context of the cultural/ethnic group under care are essential. One might have a good knowledge base of the group but must still take extreme caution and not stereotype the individual. At a minimum, nursing curricula need to include the ethnic and cultural populations where students take their clinical practice. Moreover, because we live in a global society, upon graduation, students might practice in settings where different populations are present. Thus, the curricula should also include case studies that are not in the program's catchment area.

The literature reports many definitions of the terms cultural awareness, cultural sensitivity, and cultural competence. Sometimes, these definitions are used interchangeably, but each has a distinct meaning. Cultural awareness has to do with an appreciation of the external signs of diversity, such as the arts, music, dress, foods, and physical characteristics. There are four levels of cultural awareness that reflect how people grow to perceive cultural differences (Quappe and Cantatore 2007).

In the first level of cultural awareness, known as the parochial stage, people are aware of their way of doing things, and their way is the only way. I know their way, but my way is better. Thus, they ignore the impact of cultural differences.

In the second level of cultural awareness, known as the ethnocentric state, people are aware of other ways of doing things but still consider their way as the best one. Thus, cultural differences are perceived as a source of problems and ignore them or reduce their significance.

The third level of cultural awareness, known as the synergistic stage, becomes my way and their way. People are aware of their own ways of doing things and others' ways of doing things and chose the best way according to the situation. This stage can lead to benefits, and people are willing to use cultural diversity to create new solutions and alternatives.

The fourth and final stage of cultural awareness, our way, is also known as participatory third stage. This stage brings people from different cultural background together for creating a culture of shared meanings. People dialogue repeatedly with others, creating new meanings and new rules to meet the needs of a particular situation (Quappe and Cantatore 2007).

Cultural sensitivity has to do with personal attitudes and not saying things that might be offensive to someone from a cultural or ethnic background different from the healthcare providers. Cultural sensitivity is being aware that cultural differences and similarities between people exist without assigning them a value—positive or negative, better or worse, and right or wrong. It does not mean that the provider can apply this knowledge and deliver care congruent with the patient's cultural beliefs and practices (Campinha-Bacote 2002; Giger et al. 2007; Purnell 2016).

Ethnocentrism—the universal tendency of human beings to think that their ways of thinking, acting, and believing are the only right, proper, and natural ways (which most people practice to some degree)—can be a major barrier to pro-

viding culturally competent care. Ethnocentrism perpetuates an attitude (sometimes unconsciously) in which beliefs that differ greatly from one's own are strange, bizarre, or unenlightened and, therefore, wrong. The extent to which one's cultural values are internalized influences the tendency toward ethnocentrism (Zikargae 2013). In the healthcare arena, ethnocentrism can prevent effective therapeutic communication when the healthcare provider and patient are of different cultural or ethnic backgrounds, and each perceives their own culture to be superior (Douglas et al. 2014; Singelis 1998). While it may be natural to believe otherwise, all humans are ethnocentric, at least to some degree. This is not necessarily always a bad thing because a certain amount of love for one's own culture is necessary to hold societies together. However, anything that is positive at a certain level can become negative and dysfunctional when taken too far (McKeiver et al. 2013). However, culturally competent healthcare providers can train themselves not to judge one culture by the standards of another.

Although generalizing and stereotyping are similar, functionally, they are very different. Generalizing, basically a research principle is a starting point, whereas stereotyping is an endpoint. A generalization, reducing numerous characteristics of an individual or group of people to a general form that renders them indistinguishable, is almost certain to be an oversimplification. However, generalizations can lead to stereotyping, an oversimplified conception, opinion, or belief about some aspect of an individual or group. The healthcare provider must specifically ask questions to determine values and beliefs and avoid stereotypical views of patients (see the Sect. 2.5 in this chapter).

Within all cultures are subcultures and ethnic groups whose values and experiences differ from those of the dominant culture with which they identify. In sociology, anthropology, and cultural studies, a subculture is defined as a group of people with a culture that differentiates them from the larger culture of which they are a part. Subcultures may be distinct or hidden such as gay, lesbian, bisexual, and transgendered populations in some countries. The subculture can include members from the European American, Thai, Chinese, Hispanic, etc. cultures. Alcoholic Anonymous is another example of a subculture. The membership in Alcoholics Anonymous may include African/Americans and Blacks from different countries, Asians, Arabs, etc. creating a subculture. If the subculture is characterized by a systematic opposition to the dominant culture, then it may be described as a counterculture. Examples of subcultures are Goths, punks, and stoners, although popular lay literature might call these groups cultures instead of subcultures. A counterculture would include cults (What is the difference between culture and subculture? 2017).

Acculturation occurs when a person gives up some, but not all of the traits of his or her culture of origin as a result of contact with another culture. Acculturation is not an absolute, and it has varying degrees. Traditional people hold onto the majority of cultural traits from their culture of origin that is frequently seen when people live in ethnic enclaves and can get most of their needs met without mixing with the outside world. Bicultural acculturation occurs when an individual is able to function equally in the dominant culture and in one's own culture. People who are comfortable working in the dominant culture and return to their ethnic enclave without taking on most of the dominant culture's traits are usually bicultural. Marginalized individuals are not comfortable in their new culture or their culture of origin, sometimes because the new culture does not accept them.

Assimilation is the gradual adoption and incorporation of characteristics of the prevailing culture (Portes 2007; Rudmin 2003). Assimilation is a process in degrees where people gradually adapt to the ways of the majority culture and giving more value to the cultural aspects of the majority community in which they live. Full assimilation occurs when it becomes hard to tell that the person belongs to or is from a minority culture.

Enculturation is a natural conscious and unconscious conditioning process of learning accepted cultural norms, values, and roles in society and achieving competence in one's culture through socialization. Enculturation is facilitated by growing up in a particular culture, and it can be through formal education, apprenticeships, mentorships, and role modeling (Clarke and Hofsess 1998; Rudmin 2003). Enculturation is the process of teaching an individual the norms and values of a culture through unconscious repetition. The totality of actions within a culture establishes a context that sets the conditions for what is possible within the society. Learning in this context becomes a lifelong process developed through rhetoric in the form of speech, texts, images, gestures, and practices that reaffirm the technological, economic, political, social, ideological, and philosophical bases of the culture. This is a critical concept for anyone working in the areas of rhetoric, culture, and education. The process of enculturation sets both possibilities and limits, so healthcare providers cannot automatically assume the contexts they create are unproblematically positive (Rudmin 2003).

As globalization and immigration increase, providers must also address very crucial issues such as cultural imperialism, cultural relativism, and cultural imposition. Cultural imperialism is the practice of extending the policies and practices of one group (usually the dominant one) to disenfranchised, minority, and vulnerable groups. An example is the US government's forced migration of Native American tribes to reservations with individual allotments of lands (instead of group ownership), as well as forced attendance of their children at boarding schools attended by predominantly White people. Proponents of cultural imperialism appeal to universal human rights, values, and standards (Purnell 2011).

Cultural relativism is the belief that the behaviors and practices of people should be judged only from the context of their cultural system. Proponents of cultural relativism argue that issues such as abortion, euthanasia, female circumcision, and physical punishment in child rearing should be accepted as cultural values without judgment from the outside world. Opponents argue that cultural relativism may undermine condemnation of human rights violations, and family violence cannot be justified or excused on a cultural basis (Ineneche 2010).

Cultural imposition is the intrusive application of the majority group's cultural view upon individuals and families (Forte 2016; United Nations 2015). Every person, regardless of native culture or local community possesses universal rights simply as humans, regardless of differences among cultures. Anthropology assertions of universal human rights and imperialism are intimately connected. A declaration about human rights can come close to advocacy of another country's ideological imperialism (Forte 2016). Examples of cultural imperialism in health are prescribing special diets without regard to patients' cultures and limiting visitors to immediate family.

2.5 Variant Characteristics of Culture

Whereas there is value in learning the health beliefs, practices, and values of the myriad cultures such as American, Amish, Arab, British, Chinese, Filipino, Gypsy, German, Guatemalan, Haitian, Irish, Japanese, Peruvian, Turkish, etc., great diversity exists within each of these broad cultural groups. Their health beliefs, practices, and values should be seen as generalizations to be validated rather than stereotyping each individual. The major influences that shape people's worldviews and the degree to which they identify with their cultural group of origin are called the "variant characteristics of culture." The variant characteristics include but are not limited to age, generation, nationality, race and ethnicity, color, gender, religion, educational status, socioeconomic status, occupation, military status, political beliefs, urban versus rural residence, enclave identity, marital status, parental status, physical characteristics, sexual orientation, gender issues, and reason for migration such as sojourner, immigrant, asylee, or undocumented (Purnell 2005, 2013; Purnell and Fenkl 2018). Some variant characteristics cannot be changed but others can.

Nationality cannot be changed; however, throughout history, immigrants have changed their names to disguise their ethnic origins to better fit into society or to decrease prejudice or discrimination. For example, many Jews changed the spelling of their last names during and after World War II to avoid discrimination. Race cannot be changed, but people can and do make changes in their appearance to better fit into society, including with cosmetic surgery. Whereas many researchers argue that there's no scientific basis for race, the term is still used for data collection and used in different ways, including exploring the rates of disease and infections in vulnerable populations. Skin color cannot usually be changed on a permanent basis.

Age cannot be changed, but many people go to extensive lengths to make themselves look younger. One's worldview changes with age. In some cultures, older people are looked upon with reverence and increased respect. Age differences, beliefs, and values with the accompanying worldview are frequently called the generation gap. More organizations are including the term "diversity and inclusivity" in mission statements to include different age groups.

Religious affiliation has an impact on people's beliefs and practices, including health beliefs and practices according to how devout they are. Moreover, people can and do change their religious affiliations or self-identify as atheists. However, if someone changes his or her religious affiliation— for example, from Judaism to Pentecostal or Baptist to Islam—a significant stigma may occur within their family or community. Worldwide, people have migrated to accommodate their religion that was discriminated upon in their home country. The Amish immigrated to the United States from Europe for religious freedom. Many Jews immigrated to the United States, Argentina, and other countries because of discrimination in their home country. Religion can also advise or prescribe dietary practices such as Seventh-day Adventists who have long prescribed a vegetarian diet and abstinence from alcohol and, for many, even coffee.

Educational status can also have a major impact on an individual's cultural beliefs and practices. As education increases, people's worldview changes and increases their knowledge base for decision-making. However, formal education does not necessarily increase health literacy but does provide the ability to think critically. For example, someone with an advance degree in history might not have good health literacy.

Socioeconomic status can change either up or down and can be a major determinant for access to and use of healthcare. Low socioeconomic status may dictate if or where a person can get healthcare as well as the type of procedures they can afford if not covered by health insurance.

One's occupation can change. A common omission on intake assessments is to ask about a consumer's occupation but not delve into past occupations. In addition, if the patient said he/she was retired, no follow-up is done. For example, a patient may currently be a teacher but was previously employed in a high-risk job such as in a coal mine, on a farm, or in a laboratory collecting or handling specimens from known or suspected pandemic patients (US Department of Labor: Occupational Safety and Health Administration 2009). In addition, someone may have worked near a superfund site or swamps exposing them to additional health risks.

People who have had military experience may be more accustomed to hierarchical decision-making and rules of authority. As military people travel with their government, they can be exposed to chemical warfare resulting in health conditions such as agent orange that do not surface for years later and are exposed to all the war traumas resulting in post-traumatic stress syndrome that are not assessed on intake interviews after their military leave is over.

Political beliefs of consumers and health professionals can also affect the delivery of healthcare. One of the major reasons for worldwide migration is ideological and political beliefs. However, they can change over time. Issues like marijuana, medical or recreational, and birth control and abortion can have an effect on a patient's health as well as how health providers choose to proceed with advising patients and their treatment options.

Urban versus rural residence can affect patients' health risks and access to healthcare. In urban environments, people are more likely be exposed to pathogens and infectious diseases due to overcrowding, air pollution from vehicle and industrial emissions, and pollution from waste and sewage contaminating water sources, violence, and traffic hazards to name a few. Rural residents are more likely to be exposed to chemical runoff into drinking water due to land or water pollution from waste dumping, ambient air pollution of chemicals used in farming, and the use of fossil fuels.

Enclave identity can be a deterrent to health and healthcare access. People who primarily live and work in an ethnic enclave where they can get their needs met without mixing with the outside world may be more traditional than people in their home country and rely almost entirely on complementary and alternative therapies.

Marital status: Married people and people with partners frequently have a different worldview than those without partners. Their worldview can change.

Parental status: Often, when people become parents—having children, adopting, or taking responsibility for raising a child—their worldview changes and they usually become more futuristic.

Sexual orientation: Sexual orientation is usually, but not always, stable over time. Some people are bisexual, while others may undergo transgendered surgery.

Gender issues: Men and women may have different concerns in regard to type of work and work hours, pay scales, health inequalities, and decision-making expectations. It is best to ask the patient who makes which decisions for healthcare and personal care and responsibilities at home.

Physical characteristics: One's physical characteristics may have an effect on how people see themselves and how others see them and include such characteristics as dress, height, weight, hair color and style, facial hair, skin color, and tattoos.

Immigration status (sojourner, immigrant, asylee, or undocumented status): Immigration status and length of time away from the country of origin also affect one's worldview. People who voluntarily immigrate generally acculturate and assimilate more easily. Sojourners who immigrate with the intention of remaining in their new homeland for only a short time on work assignments or refugees who think they may return to their home country may not have the need or desire to acculturate or assimilate. In addition, undocumented individuals (illegal immigrants) may have a different worldview from those who have arrived legally. Many in this group remained hidden in society so they will not be discovered and returned to their home country. Being undocumented limits a person's ability to get employment and health insurance as well as social engagements.

Length of time away from the country of origin: Usually but not always, the longer people are away from their culture of origin, the less traditional they become as they acculturate and assimilate into their new culture.

2.6 Recommendations

Recommendations for clinical practice, administration, education, and research follow.

2.6.1 Recommendations for Clinical Practice

All clinical staff must address culture on intake assessments and add to the assessment on a continual basis (see Chap. 6). Pertinent cultural characteristics should be included on the patient's plan of care. Clinical staff must become knowledgeable about the cultural attributes of diverse patients that include the variant characteristics of culture. Professional staff can use search engines and libraries to help identify culturally congruent practices of the populations served. A special attempt must be made to remember that the practices identified are generalizations to avoid stereotyping. As staff provides care to specific ethnic and cultural individuals, encourage them to keep a journal log of practices and share them with all staff.

2.6.2 Recommendations for Administration

Organizational cultural competence must be included in the overall mission and philosophy and extended into every department and unit. Administration must facilitate staff participation in classes on culturally competent care and knowledge of cultural groups served. A budget must be provided to help organize cultural awareness activities such as community fairs and heritage days with culturally diverse speakers, media, ethnic foods, and spirituality. The budget must also be sufficient to provide accessible resources for staff to learn about specific cultures and common language terms used by populations served. A cultural calendar can be developed that includes diverse patients' religious holidays, Emancipation days, Independence days, and other important events celebrated such as *quinceanera*, the celebration of a young woman's 15th birthday marking her passage from girlhood to womanhood. This social event emphasizes the importance of family and society in the life of a young woman.

2.6.3 Recommendations for Education

The education department should provide in-service classes on the basic terminology related to culture and anthropology as described previously in this chapter. During informal in-services and staff meetings, staff at all levels could be encouraged to give specific examples of patients' cultural practices as well as their own cultural practices. A "Train the Trainer" program could be instituted for staff to provide cultural-related information on a 24-hour basis. An internal web site could be developed where staff can access cultural general and culturally specific information. Staff should also be encouraged to attend formal courses and conferences related to culture.

2.6.4 Recommendations for Research

As staff identifies gaps in the evidence-based literature on culturally diverse patients in their practice, they can make recommendations to researchers in the facility. If research assistance is needed, educators in the organization can partner with local colleges, universities, and culturally based communities to help them conduct research (see Chap. 39). Staff should be encouraged to be active participants with researchers conducting the research.

Conclusion

Minority communities and those at the lower socioeconomic rungs still remain disproportionately burdened by chronic disease and are much more likely to succumb to certain diseases and illnesses. Caring for culturally diverse patients and families has become more commonplace throughout the world as global movement occurs because of economic reasons, politics, and warfare. Health disparities adversely affect groups of people who have systematically experienced social and/or economic obstacles to health based on their race or ethnicity, religion, socioeconomic status, gender, age, physical disability, sexual orientation, geographic location, and/or other characteristics historically linked to discrimination or exclusion. Asylees and refugees are included in health disparities and have increased the need for culturally congruent care (Office of Minority Health 2017).

To decrease health and healthcare disparities, providers must have a working knowledge of cultural values, beliefs, and practices. If healthcare providers and the healthcare delivery system do not become culturally competent and congruent, patient and family care are compromised, resulting in poorer health outcomes, an increase in cost, and lower satisfaction with care.

Culturally competent providers value diversity and respect individual differences regardless of one's race, religious beliefs, or cultural background. Respect for cultural differences is essential to the development of dynamic interpersonal relationships that promote a positive influence on each person's interpretation of and responses to healthcare in a multicultural environment.

References

American Association of Critical Care Nurses (2008) Safeguarding the patient and the profession: the value of critical care nurse certification. Am J Crit Care 12:154–164

Andrews MM (1998) A model for cultural change: nurse leaders must realize the importance of transculturally based administrative practices. Nurs Manag 29(10):62–66

Andrews MM, Boyle JS (eds) (2016) Transcultural concepts and nursing care, 7th edn. Wolters Kluwer, Philadelphia

Campinha Bacote's Model the Process of Cultural Competence in the Delivery of Healthcare Services. http://transculturalcare.net/the-process-of-cultural-competence-in-the-delivery-of-healthcare-services/. Accessed 5 Nov 2017

Campinha-Bacote J (2002) The process of cultural competence in the delivery of healthcare services: a model of care. J Transcult Nurs 13(3):181–184

Clarke L, Hofsess L (1998) Acculturation. In: Loue S (ed) Handbook of immigrant health. Plenum Press, New York

Cross T, Bazron B, Dennis K, Isaacs M (1989) https://population-based-intervention.wikispaces.com/Cultural+Competence-Collaboration. Accessed 24 Aug 2017

Douglas M, Rosenketter M, Pacquiao D, Clark Callister L, Hattar-Pollara M, Lauderdale J, Milsted J, Nardi D, Purnell L (2014) Guidelines for implementing culturally competent nursing care. J Transcult Nurs 25(2):109–221

Europa (2010) Commission takes steps to promote patient safety in Europe [Press release]. http://europa.eu/rapid/pressReleasesAction.do?reference=IP/08/1973&format=HTML&aged=0&language=EN&guiLanguage=en. Accessed 23 Aug 2017

Forte C (2016) Canadian anthropology or cultural imperialism? https://openanthropology.files.wordpress.com/2016/01/forte_canadian_anthropology2.pdf. Accessed 22 Aug 2017

Giger J, Davidhizar R, Purnell L, Harden J, Phillips J, Strickland O (2007) American Academy of Nursing Expert Panel Report: developing cultural competence to eliminate health disparities in ethnic minorities and other vulnerable populations. J Transcult Nurs 18(2):95–102

Health Resources and Services Administration (2002) Indicators of cultural competence in health care delivery organizations: an organizational cultural competence assessment profile. U.S. Department of Health and Human Resources. http://www.hrsa.gov/CulturalCompetence/healthdlvr.pdf. Accessed 24 Aug 2017

Images of Cultural Models (n.d.) https://www.bing.com/images/search?q=images%20purnell%20and%20cultural%20models&qs=n&form=QBIR&sp=-1&pq=images%20purnell%20and%20cultural%20models&sc=0-34&sk=&cvid=780636C5D-A5743AEA105773D206A17CE. Accessed 24 Aug 2017

Ineneche E (2010) Cultural diversity and cultural competency: new issues for elderly care and services. http://www.theseus.fi/bitstream/handle/10024/7063/Iheneche_Ernest.pdf?sequence=134&sk=&cvid=780636C5DA5743AEA105773D206A17CE. Accessed 22 Aug 2017

International Council of Nurses (2011) Position statements. Nurses and human rights. http://www.icn.ch/images/stories/documents/publications/position_statements/E10_Nurses_Human_Rights.pdf. Accessed 29 July 2017

Jeffreys MR (ed) (2010a) Teaching cultural competence in nursing and health care. Springer, New York

Jeffreys MR (2010b) A model to guide cultural competence (CCC): transcultural self-efficiency. In: Jeffreys MA (ed) Teaching cultural competence in nursing and health care. Springer Publishing Company, New York

Koffman J (2006) Transcultural and ethical issues at the end of life. In: Cooper J (ed) Stepping into palliative care. Radcliffe Publishing Ltd, Abington

Kulwicki A, Ballout S (2013) People of Arab heritage. In: Purnell L (ed) Transcultural health care: a culturally competent approach. F. A. Davis, Philadelphia

Marrone S (2013) Organizational cultural competence. In: Purnell L (ed) Transcultural health care: a culturally competent approach. F. A. Davis, Philadelphia

McFarland MR, Wehbe-Alamah HB (eds) (2015) Culture care diversity and universality, 3rd edn. Jones & Bartlett Learning, Burlington

McKeiver K, Dreasher L, Halden Y (2013) Developing intercultural communication skills for academic advising. NACADA Webinar recording. http://www. nacada.ksu.edu/Resources/Product-Details/ID/REC053CD.aspx. Accessed 26 Aug 2017

National Association of Social Workers (2007) Indicators for the achievement of the NASW standards for cultural competence in the social work profession. http://www.naswpress.org/publications/standards/indicators.html. Accessed 29 July 2017

Nursing Best Practice Guidelines: Summary of Key Models Related to Cultural Competence (n.d.) http://pda.rnao.ca/content/summary-key-models-related-cultural-competence. Accessed 29 July 2017

Office of Minority Health (2001) National standards for culturally and linguistically appropriate services. https://minorityhealth.hhs.gov/omh/browse. aspx?lvl=2&lvlid=53OMH. Accessed 24 Aug 2017

Office of Minority Health (2017) Working to raise awareness and reduce health disparities. https://www.minorityhealth.hhs.gov/Blog/BlogPost.aspx?BlogID=194. Accessed 2 Sept 2017

Olive JL (2014) Reflecting on the tensions between emic and etic perspectives in life history research: lessons learned. Forum Qual Soc Res 15(2). http://www.qualitative-research.net/index.php/fqs/article/view/2072/3656. Accessed 22 Aug 2017

Papadopoulos I (ed) (2006) Transcultural health and social care: development of culturally competent practitioners. Churchill Livingstone, London

Papadopoulos I, Shea S, Taylor G, Pezzella A, Foley L (2016) Developing tools to promote culturally competent compassion, courage, and intercultural communication in healthcare. J Compassion Health Care 3(2). https://doi.org/10.1186/s40639-016-0019-6

Portes A (2007) Migration development and segmented assimilation: a conceptual review of evidence. Am Acad Pol Soc Sci 610:73–97

Purnell L (2005) The Purnell model for cultural competence. J Multicult Nurs Health 11(2). http://files.midwestclinicians.org/sharedchcpolicies/Policies_Forms/Cultural%20Competency/PURNELL'S%20MODEL.pdf. Accessed 22 Aug 2017

Purnell L (2011) Cultural competence in a changing healthcare environment. In: Chaska NL (ed) The nursing profession: tomorrow and beyond. Sage Publications, Thousand Oakes

Purnell L (ed) (2013) Transcultural health care: a culturally competent approach, 4th edn. F. A. Davis, Philadelphia

Purnell L (2014) Guide to culturally competent health care.3rd edn. F.A. Davis, Philadelphia

Purnell L (2016) Invited scholarly inquiry article: are we really measuring cultural competence? Nurs Sci Q 29(2):124–127

Purnell L, Fenkl E (2018) Guide to culturally competent health care. F.A. Davis Co., Philadelphia

Quappe S, Cantatore G (2007) http://www.culturosity.com/articles/whatisculturalawareness.htm. Accessed 22 Aug 2017

Rudmin FW (2003) Critical history of the acculturation psychology of assimilation, separation, integration, and marginalization. Rev Gen Psychol 7(1):3–37

Schim SM, Doorenbos AZ, Borse NM (2005) Cultural competence among Ontario and Michigan healthcare providers. J Nurs Scholarsh 37(4):354–360

Selekman J (2013) People of Jewish heritage. In: Purnell L (ed) Transcultural health care: a culturally competent approach. F. A. Davis, Philadelphia

Singelis TM (ed) (1998) Teaching about culture, ethnicity, and diversity. Sage Publications, Thousand Oakes

Triandis HC (2002) Subjective culture. Online Read Psychol Cult 2(2). https://doi.org/10.9707/2307-0919.1021. Accessed 22 Aug 2017

U.S. Department of Labor: Occupational Safety and Health Administration (2009) https://www.osha.gov/Publications/exposure-risk-classification-factsheet.html. Accessed 27 Aug 2017

United Nations (2015) Universal declaration of human rights. http://www.un.org/en/udhrbook/pdf/udhr_booklet_en_web.pdf. Accessed 29 July 2017

What is the difference between culture and subculture? (2017) https://www.reference.com/world-view/difference-between-culture-subculture-66c90a38bfcd070. Accessed 29 July 2017

Zikargae MH (2013) The impacts of ethnocentrism and stereotype on inter-cultural relations of Ethiopian higher education students. Online J Commun Media Technol 3(4). http://www.ojcmt.net/articles/34/348.pdf/. Accessed 22 Aug 2017

Case Study: Building Trust Among American Indian/Alaska Native Communities—Respect and Focus on Strengths

Janet R. Katz and Darlene P. Hughes

Maria, a community health registered nurse, was living in rural Northwestern USA. She was seeking a position in an Indian Health Services (IHS) clinic. Maria knew that Native Americans suffered some of the worst health disparities in the USA, as did most indigenous peoples around the world (Katz et al. 2016), and she wanted to help. Maria had met several Native American nurses when she was in school but had never talked to them about their communities. She would later see this as a great missed opportunity.

In her new job, Maria noticed a high rate of diabetes, hypertension, heart disease, depression, and alcohol misuse similar to other clinics in which she had worked. But, one family represented a turning point for her. She realized she did not know much about the people, culture, setting, and community that the clinic served. The family included a grandmother (Sadie), Sadie's daughter (Violet), Sadie's grandchildren (Kyla, age 5 years; Charles, age 6 years; Martha, age 8 years; and John, age 15 years), and the children's father (Raymond). After multiple visits,

Maria learned the grandmother and both parents had diabetes, obesity, hypertension, and expressed signs of depression. Maria would often see the three younger children for common cold viruses, minor injuries, and common health issues that is nothing out of the ordinary for growing children. The children were always cheerful when they came to the clinic; however, Maria did notice their clothes were often threadbare. The older son, John, seldom came to the clinic, but when he did, he said he was okay. Maria was concerned; she knew alcohol and drug misuse was prevalent in this area. Raymond worked seasonally as a smoke jumper and a trucker the remainder of the year. Due to his schedule, he rarely came to appointments. When he did, Maria noticed he stood quietly in the background.

On one visit, Sadie came to the clinic alone. She confided that she was very tired and was feeling overwhelmed. Her daughter was traveling searching for work and was leaving the grandchildren with her more often, sometimes for multiple days at a time. She said she might have to take the children into her home permanently if her daughter could not find work locally. Sadie also confided that Kyla was not Violet's biological child but her cousin's. Sadie knew her daughter was trying hard to be a good parent to all of the children. Raymond was away every 2 weeks and so was unable to help much. Sadie stated she no longer had the energy to care for young

J. R. Katz, R.N., Ph.D., FAAN (✉)
D. P. Hughes, M.S.N., R.N.
College of Nursing, Washington State University, Spokane, WA, USA
e-mail: jkatz@wsu.edu; darlene.hughes@wsu.edu

© Springer International Publishing AG, part of Springer Nature 2018
M. Douglas et al. (eds.), *Global Applications of Culturally Competent Health Care: Guidelines for Practice*, https://doi.org/10.1007/978-3-319-69332-3_3

children. She also voiced concern about John. She stated that he was home less often and appeared to have been drinking. She told Maria she had struggled with alcohol misuse several years ago.

Over the next month, Maria saw the grandmother several times for uncontrolled hypertension and medication changes. This made her more fatigued. Maria was concerned that Sadie was at increased risks for stroke or heart attack. Maria decided she really needed to talk to Violet. At first, Violet was unable to come in. When Violet was able to make it to the clinic, Maria noted she appeared tired and frustrated. She seemed depressed and overwhelmed. She was unable to find work, Raymond was often away, Sadie was not well, John was partying with his friends more, and she didn't have money to buy the children new school clothes. There had been several suicides in the community this last winter, and Violet was very worried about John. Maria asked her if she wanted to speak to a mental health provider. Violet stated, "Oh, I don't need that; they can't help me anyway; they don't understand what we go through, how hard it is; and they talk all the time, but talk doesn't find us jobs." Maria did not want to breach Sadie's confidentiality, so she tried to ask Violet about care of the children. Violet said, "I am worried about the kids, I know mom is having a hard time." "I wish I knew what to do."

3.1   Cultural Issues

There are 562 federally recognized tribes in the USA (Bureau of Indian Affairs 2015). American Indian or Alaskan Native identity does not imply a homogeneous but instead is represented by unique cultures from multiple regions and tribes (Champagne 2014). However, there are some general cultural principles tied to a common history of colonization, boarding schools, loss of culture, trauma, exploitation by researchers and academics, broken treaties, poverty, and under funded health care (Evans-Campbell 2008). It is important to understand that the exploitation, broken agreements, and negative stereotypes imposed on American Indian/Alaska Native (AI/AN) people have led to much mistrust in institutions and non-native people. A community nurse, like Maria, needs to learn and understand cultural specifics to adequately care for the people in her clinic service area. Although native people experience many health, economic, and social disparities, tribal family and community structure often provide advantages for their members' community ties, family bonds that span centuries, and a persistence for survival translate to deep resiliency and strength (Kicza and Horn 2016). Building trust and relationships with a tribal community and its members is essential. Understanding the impact of historical and sociopolitical harms on present-day life includes a solid understanding of how broken cultural traditions impacts present-day childcare.

Communication is predicated on trust and follows sociocultural norms. When erroneous generalizations are made by the nurse or other health-care providers, trusting communication can break down. For tribal communities in the northwestern area of the USA, a handshake may be most often used when greeting people. Remember that many stereotypes or generalizations, such as handshaking, may or may not be true for any one individual; taking cues from the person being greeted is important (Mihesuah 2013).

Another factor to be cognizant of is the concept of family and the extensive familial relationships within communities. It is not uncommon to be told a person is a cousin, sister, or auntie, when there is no biological connection. This does not diminish the familial bond. Over many hundreds of years, extensive family networks have developed. You may find people with the same last name who are distant cousins. Although there are close family ties throughout a community, privacy and confidentiality are imperative to build trust (Evans-Campbell 2008; Lonczak et al. 2013). Greetings and introductions often begin with establishing what family a person belongs to rather than in European/American society where the first question is "What do you do?" the questions may be "Who are your parents, grandparents, great-grandparents." And "Where you are from?" These are important questions for establishing connections. People often identify themselves with their name, tribal affiliation, and family connections.

Elders are given added respect by all members of the community (Braun et al. 2014). If Elders are present, younger people may defer to them rather than talk for themselves. At family and community events, elders are always served first. It is not uncommon for a community to regard a community health nurse over 50 years of age as an elder. Patients may want to talk to family or even tribal elders before making health-care decisions.

The use of medicinal plants remains a common practice by many tribal people (Wendt and Gone 2016). To determine if a patient is using traditional plant medicine, questions must be asked in respectful ways to understand non-Western treatments. Spirituality and religion also vary greatly among tribes and individuals. A community's religion is likely influenced by colonization. The religious order that is dominant in the community may have been determined by first contact or by the practices of original religious leaders. In many Alaska Native villages, the Russian Christian Orthodox Church remains a strong influence due to the humanitarian actions the original priest showed the Alaska Native peoples (Oleska 2010). There are also people and bands (groups that now make up larger tribes) who practice traditional spiritual ways.

3.2 Social Structural Issues

Tribal sovereignty was present among all North American tribes long before European contact. It is estimated in 1492 there were about 75 million indigenous people in North and South America, representing 15% of the world's population (Thornton 1997). Yet, with colonization came a policy of conquest and control that lasted to the early 1800s, severely reducing the population. It is estimated today AI/AN make up 2% of the US population or about 5.4 million people (U.S. Census 2015). Beginning in the early 1800s, treaty making was predominantly US policy. Treaties were based

on taking over vast tracts of land in exchange for services such as food and health care (Barbero 2005). Health-care funding was first appropriated in 1832, specifically for small pox epidemics (Shelton 2004). Treaties promised these services "in perpetuity" (Shelton 2004).

Boarding schools were enforced to ensure assimilation. Many children were taken from their homes and sent to distant boarding schools where they were forbidden to practice traditional ways (clothing, prayer, language, food, or medicine) and were severely punished when they did so (Bigfoot and Schmidt 2010; Charbonneau-Dahlen et al. 2016). Boarding schools have left a legacy of emotional, sexual, and physical abuse which are regarded today as factors in high suicide rates, depression, substance misuse, and domestic violence (Heart 2003; Thomas and Austin 2012). Assimilation may have been well-intentioned by some, but it leads to a rupture in culture, disconnection in knowledge of traditions, and a profound sadness that is being felt today. Many cite boarding schools and general assimilation policies as directly related to today's social determinants of health disparities.

Assimilation policies were followed by laws that allowed non-native people to buy land on reservations leading to what is called checker boarding (Deyo et al. 2014). Many communities are working on buying back that land to make their reservations whole again. The Indian Health Service was officially formed in the early 1900s; it had formally been under the War Office (Barbero 2005). In 1975 the Indian Self-Determination and Education Assistance Act and the Indian Health Care Improvement Act were enacted to protect native people's rights to education and health care, essentially to fulfill treaty promises made years earlier (Barbero: Indian Health Services 2007).

3.3 Culturally Competent Strategies Recommended

Health disparities and historical atrocities greatly impact individual and community health outcomes. AI/AN people have made tremendous strides in healing. They continue to realize more tribal sovereignty through controlling their own health services, acting as their own gatekeepers, and educating their children to become community leaders.

3.3.1   Individual-/Family-Level Interventions

- Familiarize yourself with health disparity issues relevant to tribal communities.
- Learn about historical and intergenerational trauma without making assumptions about individuals or their families. Just be aware.
- Upon meeting your client for the first time, be patient, *don't appear rushed.* Offer your hand to shake, don't force it. If appropriate for culture, make eye contact, nod, and welcome them to your office. Ask general questions about how they are doing.
- Assess family structure through introduction beginning with yourself. Acknowledge elders with respect asking them if they would like to sit or need anything. When asking questions in a group, be sure to ask elders first.
- Obtain a detailed assessment of any unique cultural needs, i.e., religious and language preferences; normal health-care provider; childcare options, if applicable; environment (home and community); and occupation (training, education, and work opportunities). Allow client/s the opportunity to decline giving information.
- Respect patient's privacy and potential reluctance to share information with a non-native health-care provider.
- Ask most pressing questions relevant to specific visit. Don't try or expect to get all background information at first visit. *Be patient. Know you will need to build trust.*
- Provide a thorough explanation of confidentiality.
- When appropriate, provide information about transportation to a more comprehensive health-care facility for testing if elder (Sadie) needed.

- When appropriate, gently discuss concerns about teenage son, recent community losses to suicide, and inquire if parents would like you or another provider to talk to son such as a teacher or a counselor.
- Provide education and resources on job opportunities, parenting classes, alcohol or drug misuse programs, adolescent support programs, childcare services, and CNA services (for elder if needed).

3.3.2   Organizational-Level Interventions

- Be familiar with current politics that may be impacting the tribe.
- Establish a cultural competency program. Do not assume your facility has cultural understanding for the client base, even if it is an IHS clinic.
- Advocate for hiring a community member to consult on unique tribal culture and traditions.
- If some elders still speak the native language, enlist them to help translate some health information.
- Propose to host an elder men or women's group meeting monthly.
- Develop a committee to design and produce education materials inclusive of traditional foods, practices, dress, and activities.

3.3.3   Community Societal-Level Interventions

- Determine the strengths of community to include cultural practices and traditions, family support and caring, and events to attend.
- Collaborate with elder men or other men's groups to learn about fathering and steps to assisting fathers in becoming more involved in parenting.
- Don't be afraid to ask questions about the local culture and how the tribal members would like your help. Be humble and respectful.

Conclusion

Working with a Native American tribe as a non-native nurse requires learning a great deal of new information about Native American culture. Most importantly, be aware of the comfort level of each individual in the family to speak with you. Don't push, be patient. Develop a trusting relationship. Be comfortable with admitting you do not know everything about their culture. Use and accept humor.

References

Barbero CL (2005) The federal trust responsibility: justification for Indian-specific heath policy. https://uihi.us/Shared%20Documents/Health%20Policy/Federal%20Trust.doc. Accessed 30 June 2017

Bigfoot DS, Schmidt SR (2010) Honoring children, mending the circle: cultural adaptation of trauma-focused cognitive-behavioral therapy for American Indian and Alaska Native children. J Clin Psychol 66(8):847–856

Braun KL, Browne CV, Ka'opua LS, Kim BJ, Mokuau N (2014) Research on indigenous elders: from positivistic to decolonizing methodologies. The Gerontologist 54(1):117–126

Bureau of Indian Affairs (2015) Indian entities recognized and eligible to receive services from the United States Bureau of Indian Affairs. Federal basis for health services. Federal Register: Bureau of Indian Affairs. https://www.ihs.gov/aboutihs/eligibility/. Accesses 11 April 2017

Champagne D (2014) The term 'American Indian', plus ethnicity, sovereignty, and identity. Indian Country Today. June 2014. https://indiancountrymedianetwork.com/history/events/the-term-american-indian-plus-ethnicity-sovereignty-and-identity/#. Accessed 3 July 2017

Charbonneau-Dahlen BK, Lowe J, Morris SL (2016) Giving voice to historical trauma through storytelling: the impact of boarding school experience on American Indians. J Aggress Maltreat Trauma 25(6):598–617

Deyo N, Bohdan M, Burke R, Kelley A, van der Werff B, Blackmer ED et al (2014) Trails on tribal lands in the United States. Landsc Urban Plan 125:130–139

Evans-Campbell T (2008) Historical trauma in American Indian/Native Alaska communities: a multilevel framework for exploring impacts on individuals, families, and communities. J Interpers Violence 23(3):316–338

Heart MYHB (2003) The historical trauma response among natives and its relationship with substance abuse: a Lakota illustration. J Psychoactive Drugs 35(1):7–13

Indian Health Services (2007) Federal basis for health services. Indian Health Service. https://www.ihs.gov/newsroom/factsheets/basisforhealthservices/. Accessed 30 June 2017

Katz JR, Barbosa-Leiker C, Benavides-Vaello S (2016) Measuring the success of a pipeline program to increase nursing workforce diversity. J Prof Nurs 32(1):6–14. https://doi.org/10.1016/j.profnurs.2015.05.003

Kicza JE, Horn R (2016) Resilient cultures: America's native peoples confront European colonialization 1500–1800. Routledge

Lonczak HS, Thomas LR, Donovan D, Austin L, Sigo RL, Lawrence N, Tribe S (2013) Navigating the tide together: early collaboration between tribal and academic partners in a CBPR study. Pimatisiwin 11(3):395

Mihesuah DA (2013) American Indians: stereotypes & realities. SCB Distributors

Oleska MJ (2010) Alaskan missionary spirituality. https://www.amazon.com/Alaskan-Missionary-Spirituality-Michael-2010-02-01/dp/B01K3OUGVU

Shelton LB (2004) Legal and historical roots of health care for American Indians and Alaska Natives in the United States. Henry J Kaiser Family Foundation. Pub. #7021

Thomas L, Austin L (2012) Recognized American Indian Organizations (RAIOs) Health Priorities Summit. Summary Report, Cradleboard to Career. http://uwashington.uberflip.com/i/106618-from-cradleboard-to-career-summary-report/3. Accessed 30 June 2017

Thornton R (1997) Population: precontact to the present. In: Hoxie, Encyclopedia of North American Indians, 501

U.S. Census (2015) FFF: American Indian and Alaska Native Heritage Month: November 2015. https://www.census.gov/newsroom/facts-for-features/2015/cb15-ff22.html/. Accessed 30 June 2017

Wendt DC, Gone JP (2016) Integrating professional and indigenous therapies: an urban American Indian narrative clinical case study. Couns Psychol 44(5):695–729

Case Study: An 85-Year-Old Immigrant from the Former Soviet Union

4

Lynn Clark Callister

Katerina Fyodorova, an 85-year-old Russia immigrant, came to the United States in 1998 with the wave of immigrants coming from the former Soviet Union (FSU) with the collapse of the Soviet regime. Katerina is commonly referred to as a *babushka* or grandmother. She is widowed, her parents are deceased, and she has no living siblings and has no children.

Despite living in the United States for nearly 30 years, her primary language is still Russian. She speaks Russian in her home and associates mostly with other immigrants from the FSU. She lives alone in a high-rise, low-income housing in a poor-quality neighborhood in a large metropolitan area on the east coast of the United States. This area and surrounding environs have the largest people from the FSU, although Alaska and cities on the East and West coast also have large populations of such immigrants. Katerina enjoys accessing New York's daily *Novoye Russkoye Slovo* newspaper and the cable television channels and radio stations available in Russian in the New York area.

Katerina is subsisting on a very limited income. At times she feels depressed and lonely and doesn't know where to turn to. She sometimes feels a sense of hopelessness about her situation. She does not feel comfortable confiding in

physicians because of the stigma associated with major depressive disorders in the USSR.

Speaking in a circular fashion, Katerina may describe her bittersweet memories of life under communism in her homeland and her current feelings of social needlessness, loneliness, and isolation. The unmet need for diagnosis and treatment of depression among immigrants from the former USSR now living in the United States has been reported in the literature (Landa et al. 2015). In study participants seen in a primary care clinic, 26.5% had a probable major depressive disorder. It is noted that such depression does not diminish in those who have lived in the United States for decades and is often underdiagnosed and untreated (Landa et al. 2015: 283).

4.1 Cultural Issues

Like many of her aging peers, Katerina's healthcare can be characterized by a pattern of *begat' po racham* or "running between doctors." This includes a variety of both biomedical and traditional therapies. This pattern of healthcare has led to weaker patient-provider communication and lower levels of satisfaction with healthcare. She does not appear to have any serious medical problems, but has little to do, having much time on her hands, and is living in social isolation, in addition to not having a basic understanding of the normal aging processes. Such a non-systematic

L. C. Callister, R.N., Ph.D., FAAN
School of Nursing, Brigham Young University,
Provo, UT, USA
e-mail: callister-lynn@comcast.net

© Springer International Publishing AG, part of Springer Nature 2018
M. Douglas et al. (eds.), *Global Applications of Culturally Competent Health Care: Guidelines for Practice*, https://doi.org/10.1007/978-3-319-69332-3_4

pattern of seeking healthcare among FSU immigrants to the United States has been described in the literature (Chudakova 2016).

In a recent visit at the clinic, she offered the clinic nurse an informal payment in the hopes of getting a "higher" level of care and bypassing the lines at the clinic as well as required paperwork, not understanding that such practices are not appropriate or expected in healthcare facilities in the United States (Gordeev et al. 2014). Such practice is an important health policy issue for those caring for immigrants from the FSU.

When Katerina sees a healthcare provider, she is likely to report only fair or poor health than her American counterparts which is also reported in the literature (Hofmann 2012). In Slavic cultures, "speaking positively about one's own well-being is thought to bring misfortune" (Hofmann 2012: 319; Paxson 2005). However, her complaints are very vague and general.

When Katerina has a conversation with an American healthcare provider, she is often uncomfortable. She would prefer that providers should communicate with her in a paternalistic manner because this is what she was used to in the FSU (Younger 2016). This has also been reported in the literature in a study of immigrants from the FSU living in Germany (Bachmann et al. 2014).

When possible, Katerina prefers to use complementary therapies because they are less expensive, come from nature and thus come from God, and are available without prescription. She also perceives them as having fewer complications than biomedical therapies which are "too strong, chemical, and not natural" (Van Son and Stasyuk 2014: 546). Dietary proscriptions include onions, garlic, lemons, and beets. Herbs most commonly used include valerian, kava, Siberian ginseng, St. John's Wort, pheasant's eye, and yarrow (Tagintseva 2005). She makes decisions about these therapies by conferring with neighbors and friends who are also from the former FSU (Van Son and Stasyuk 2014). This kind of inappropriate self-care (samolechenie) is problematic as Katerina seeks to "become her own doctor," characterized by dismissing potential health concerns by saying fatalistically, "it is as it is" (kakoye est).

4.2 Social Structural Issues

There are 15 Soviet republics, which include the Slavic states (Russian Federation, Ukraine, and Belarus; the Baltic States (Estonia, Latvia, and Lithuania); the Caucasus states (Armenia, Azerbaijan and George; the Central Asian republics (Kazakhstan, Uzbekistan, Turkmenistan, Kyrgyzstan, and Tajikistan) as well as Moldova. Many of these states have large populations of ethnic Russians. Katerina came from an ethnically and culturally diverse background, with a population of more than 150 minority nationalities and 100 different languages besides Russian living in Russia (Younger 2016).

Since 1991, many immigrants from the newly independent states of the FSU have come to the United States, including those from the Russian Federation. The 2015 estimate of the US population born in the former USSR is 1,066,944 (American FactFinder 2017a). New York State and surrounding areas have the largest percentage of people from the FSU, although Alaska and cities on the East and West Coasts of the United States also have large populations of such immigrants (American FactFinder 2017b).

Like many immigrants from the FSU, Katerina is an ethnic Jew who came because of an American program granting asylum to Soviet Jews because of anti-Semitism in the USSR (Landa et al. 2015). Katerina is secularized and religiously non-observant. The majority of former Soviet Jewish immigrants were over 55 years of age when they came to the United States, which is much older than other immigrant populations. Like many Jewish immigrants from the FSU, Katerina has close relatives living in Israel because of the divided destinations of Jews leaving the FSU after the fall of the Soviet Union.

4.3 Culturally Competent Strategies Recommended

The following are recommendations to enable the development culturally congruent and effective strategies to improve the quality of life in immigrants from the FSU living in the United States such as Katerina.

on her strengths and resiliency as a survivor of challenging life circumstances.

4.3.1 Individual/Family Level Interventions

- In the primary care clinic, a physical and psychosocial-cultural assessment should be conducted with Katerina using a certified interpreter. This should include learning about language preference, how healthcare decisions are made, preferred communication style with healthcare providers, perceptions of the promotion of health and causes of illness, knowledge about community resources, and culturally preferred treatments for illness (Bachmann et al. 2014; Douglas et al. 2014). The more knowledge professional nurses have about specific cultural groups, the more accurate and complete the cultural assessment will be (Douglas et al. 2014).
- Consult with social services to assist Katerina in accessing resources such as English classes, health education (including media presentations that have been translated into Russian), smoking cessation initiatives, and community services for seniors including meals and exercise programs.
- Provide connection with any community organizations and other community resources for immigrants from the FSU.
- Help Katerina understand the difference between normal aging and symptoms that may indicate underlying health conditions.
- Help Katerina understand the potential health risks associated with combining biomedical and complementary therapies.
- Help her to understand how to communicate effectively with healthcare providers.
- Assess Katerina for a major depressive disorder using tools translated into Russian.
- The Patient Health Questionnaire-I (PHQ) is a screening tool for depression which is available in Russia (Kroenke et al. 2001) (www phqscreeners.com).
- Help Katerina access resources to overcome feelings of despair and hopelessness, focusing

4.3.2 Organizational Level Interventions

- Provide a certified interpreter during healthcare encounters.
- Provide staff with current literature on immigrants from the FSU living in the United States and meet to discuss the implications of that literature on their clinical practice.
- Provide cultural competency education for providers serving populations of immigrants from the FSU such as the interprofessional education Russian cultural competence course at Washington State University described in the literature (Topping 2015).
- Access, or develop, produce, and disseminate patient education material translated into English.
- Collaborate with Russian focused media outlets to provide health messages on the radio and television stations and in print media.

4.3.3 Community Level Interventions

- Collect quantitative and qualitative data in mixed methods studies on the challenges and needs of immigrants from the FSU to increase understanding and facilitate the development of appropriate interventions. This may be done in collaboration with resources such as the Davis Center for Russian and Eurasian Studies at Harvard or utilize local universities. This could include an oral history project with older immigrants such as Katerina which would increase our outstanding of the lives of immigrants from the FSU. These immigrants have stories to share that are richly descriptive and potentially helpful in facilitating quality healthcare delivery to them.
- Collaborate with low-income housing facilities to work toward improving the environment

in a way that helps Katerina and other FSU immigrants feel safe and connected.

Conclusion

Cultural issues specific to caring for immigrants from the FSU may include poor patient-provider relationships because of linguistic issues and differences in communication styles, help-seeking patterns of accessing multiple providers, the use of complementary rather than biomedical therapies, the potential use of informal payment, a lack of knowing the difference between natural aging processes and potential illness, and the significant potential for major depressive disorders. Strategies for culturally competent healthcare delivery at the individual, organizational, and societal levels should be designed and implemented to address Katerina and other immigrant's vulnerability due to the social determinants of health related to the health and well-being of immigrants from the FSU (Douglas et al. 2014).

References

American FactFinder (2017a) Place of birth for the foreign-born population in the United States. http://factfinder.census.gov/faces/tableservices/jsf/pages/productview.xhtml?pid=ACS_1 5_1YR_B05006. Accessed 16 July 2017

American FactFinder (2017b) Top 101 cites with the most residents born in Russia (populations 500+). http://factfinder.census.gov. Accessed 16 July 2017

Bachmann V, Volkner M, Bosnerr S, Doner-Banzhoff N (2014) The experiences of Russian-speaking migrants in primary care consultations. Dtsch Arztebl Int 111(5):51–52

Chudakova T (2016) Caring for strangers: aging, traditional medicine, and collective self-care in post-socialist Russia. Med Anthropol Q 31(1): 78–96

Douglas MK, Rosenkoetter M, Pacquiao DF, Callister LC, Hattar-Pollara M, Lauderdale J, Milsted J, Nardi D, Purnell L (2014) Guidelines for implementing culturally competent nursing care. J Transcult Nurs 25(2):109–121

Gordeev VS, Pavloa M, Groot W (2014) Informal payments for health care services in Russia: old issue in new realities. Health Econ Policy Law 9:25–48

Hofmann ET (2012) The burden of culture? Health outcomes among immigrants from the Former Soviet Union in the United States. J Immigr Minor Health 14:315–322

Kroenke K, Spitzer RL, Williams JBW (2001) The PHQ-i: validity of a brief depression severity measure. J Gen Intern Med 16:606–613

Landa A, Skristskaya N, Nicasio A, Humensky J, Lewis-Fernandez R (2015) Unmet need for treatment of depression among immigrants from the former USSR in the US: a primary care study. Int J Psychiatry Med 50(3):271–289

Paxson M (2005) Solovyovo: the story of memory in a Russian village. Woodrow Wilson Center Press, Washington, DC

Tagintseva TY (2005) The use of herbal medicine by U.S. immigrants from the Former Soviet Union [Master's Thesis]. https://research.wsulibs.wsu.edu/xmlui/bitstream/handle/2376/381/t_tagintseva_072205.pds?sequence=1. Accessed 30 July 2017

Topping D (2015) An inter-professional education Russian cultural competence course: implementation and follow-up perspectives. J Interprof Care 29(5): 501–503

Van Son CR, Stasyuk O (2014) Older immigrants from the former Soviet Union and their use of complementary and alternative medicine. Geriatr Nurs 35:S45–S48

Younger DS (2016) Health care in the Russian Federation. Neurol Clin 34:1085–1102

Case Study: Caring for Urban, American Indian, Gay, or Lesbian Youth at Risk for Suicide

5

Jana Lauderdale

Larry, a newly graduated baccalaureate-prepared nurse, has just moved to the Midwest from the upper northern United States (US). Being part Lakota Indian, he is interested in working with tribes different from his own and knows Oklahoma has the largest American Indian (AI) population of any state in the United States. His career plan is to get as much experience as possible working for tribal clinics, learning about, and caring for AI suicide victims in urban settings. He is aware of several suicides on his reservation as he was growing up, but no one talked much about them, so neither did he. Larry then plans to go to graduate school to become a psych-mental health nurse practitioner (PMHNP) and return to the Dakotas to work with his people to help reduce psych-mental health disparities. For this reason, he has just accepted a new position with the Indian Health Service (IHS) at the Oklahoma City Tribal Clinic in Oklahoma City, Oklahoma. This will be a new experience for Larry, not living on a reservation and working in an urban setting.

As a new graduate nurse in a new work environment, Larry has had a lot to learn in a short amount of time. As an AI growing up on a reservation, he was prepared for high rates of diabetes, cancer, cardiovascular disease, and strokes; however, as he had requested to work in the small mental health clinic, he quickly realized he had a poor understanding of the mental health issues facing urban Indians. Larry's first family to work with on his own had traveled 30 miles to the tribal clinic. They were there because they had lost their eldest son to alcohol and suicide at 19 years of age, and they were afraid their youngest son, 15-year-old Andy, was going to follow the same path.

Larry first interviewed Andy's parents while he waited in the reception area. His mother reported he had no appetite, was doing poorly in school, and had periods of negative, sad talk when he talked at all. He spent most of his time in his room on the computer. His dad said he noticed he has only one person he likes to talk with, an older adult called Henry, who lives several miles from their house. There are also two younger sisters in the family that his mother says, "Are taking up more and more of my time after school with their activities and with his father at work until 7pm and I am worried about leaving Andy at home in the afternoon for up to 3 hours at a time." Larry then excused the parents and spoke with Andy. Once they became comfortable with one another, Andy began to open up about his lack of friends, his disinterest in school, and how he missed talking to his grandfather who died 2 years ago. When asked what he missed most about his grandfather he said, "You know just someone to talk to that understands. My friend Henry is good to talk to also, but my parents won't let me go to his house. I have to sneak over to see him. But he under-

J. Lauderdale, Ph.D., R.N., FAAN
School of Nursing, Vanderbilt University, Nashville, TN, USA
e-mail: jana.lauderdale@vanderbilt.edu

stands me and can talk to me like my grandfather did." He sighed and said, "I am really tired of worrying about everything and being afraid. Sometimes I think, wouldn't it be nice if I could just go to sleep and not wake up."

When asked of what he was afraid, Andy looked at the floor and said, "That I am different." More probing resulted in Andy quietly saying, "I don't want to go on dates with girls; you know I am a 'Two-Spirit,' but I haven't told anyone because I am afraid of what will happen." Larry knows that for American Indians, Two-Spirit is the contemporary word used that means gay (Lang 1998). Larry encouraged him to talk to his parents, but he said, "No I can't do it; they are not strong enough." Larry could see Andy's case was going to require intensive outpatient therapy, so he quickly got to his computer to look up mental health providers in the family's community, but there was only one who was IHS affiliated. However, Andy said he did not want to go there because his brother had been a patient there and said, "And look how it turned out for him. No, I won't go there."

Larry then spoke with Andy's parents, confirming their fears that Andy had recently thought about suicide and his concern regarding Andy's resistance to go to the only IHS mental health facility in their area. Andy's father had panic in his eyes and whispered, "If dad were alive, he would be able to help. You know, he always knew how to explain things in a way the kids understood." Larry has many concerns on how to handle his new young patient's situation and has not yet been able to do anything beyond talking with him briefly confirming that indeed, Andy was experiencing suicide ideations. He felt rushed as he tried to find a clinic that was good for both him and his family.

5.1 Cultural Issues

American Indian Youth suicide has become a national health concern. The Centers for Disease Control and Prevention (2014) reports that AI youth suicide rates are the highest in the country, 62% above the national average for youth ages 10–25 years and is complicated by the fact that more AI youth are now living in urban areas, far from reservation or tribal communities (Burrage et al. 2016). Almost 70% of AIs live in urban areas; however, the US Census Bureau (2010) indicates there is still conflicting information regarding urban youth suicide rates. This is evident when comparing reports between reservation suicide rates, documented via the IHS system, and urban suicide rates reported by hospitals, many times using inaccurate identification of race or ethnicity on death certificates, which only further confounds the information (Middlebrook et al. 2001).

Common suicide predictors have been reported for both white and AI youth, including drug and alcohol misuse, family history of suicide or attempts, physical or sexual abuse, emotional issues, and weapon carrying (Ayyash-Abdo 2002; King and Merchant 2008; Mackin et al. 2012). However, many AIs believe suicide is a community problem related to loss of cultural beliefs and early colonial oppression rather than an individual problem (Wexler and Gone 2012), indicating suicide factors for this population may have deeper roots in the social, community, and societal realms than from the reported predictive factors. AI youth factors believed to promote suicide behavior include gender (Manzo et al. 2015), living in urban versus reservation areas (Freedenthal and Stiffman 2004), and the strength of the tribal culture (Novins et al. 1999). Losing one's culture can decrease cultural identity which eventually can impact health.

Historically, alternative gender roles and sexualities have been accepted by many tribes. However, today's AI people who are lesbian, gay, bisexual, and transgender (LGBT) or identify as Two-Spirit often still see their communities as non-accepting, encouraging isolation, discrimination, fear, and invisibility which may increase suicide risk factors. The term "Two-Spirits" was accepted in the 1990s at a Chicago conference as an acceptable term to describe LGBT AI individuals. Lang (1998) noted in his interviews with "Two-Spirit" AIs that culturally it is believed that the term means a male in a feminine role and a female in a masculine role. It is considered to be an all-encompassing term for the LGBT AI population (Medicine et al. 1997).

Newer program development in the area of suicide prevention focuses on a holistic approach, combining Western medicine with traditional Indian medicine to encourage individuals and families to improve their mental, physical, spiritual, and emotional well-being. Thus, establishing trust and respect is critical when working with LGBT and Two Spirit AI youth populations (Burrage et al. 2016).

5.2   Social Structure

With the majority of American Indians living in urban settings, healthcare providers must become sensitive to how people respond when living outside the comfort of their own culture. Support must be provided for cultural values and beliefs, respect for differences, and culturally congruent strategies when working with LGBT "Two Spirit" AI youth who are at risk for suicide.

Eighty-nine percent LGBT teens report verbal harassment; 55% report physical harassment. LGBT high school students are two times less likely to finish high school or pursue a college education. LGBT youth rejected by parents are more likely to attempt suicide, report depression, use illegal drugs, and have unprotected sex. Twenty to forty percent of homeless youth are LGBT.

5.3   Culturally Competent Strategies Recommended

5.3.1   Individual/Family Level Interventions

- Know the populations you serve. There are 566+ federally recognized tribes. Be aware of your population's commonalities and their individual nuances.
- Be aware of the most important factors leading to LGBT AI youth suicide attempts that include loneliness, isolation, and hopelessness which lead to lack of social support, social withdrawal, and victimization, causing social isolation, cognitive isolation, emotional isolation, and concealment of identity.

- Understand the LGBT or Two Spirit health concerns for pediatric or adolescents include mental health, unprotected health, drug and alcohol misuse, protective factors, illegal hormone injections (transgender), and self-isolation with loneliness and hopelessness that are the most important factors in suicide attempts in LGBT youth.
- Ensure protective factors that include family support.
- Understand AI perspectives of health and illness.
- Encourage informal support and use the teaching of the Seven Grandfathers as appropriate, as a way to exemplify living one's life according to the values of wisdom, love, respect, bravery, honesty, humility, and truth.
- Ensure your interventions are tailored for the youth and their family, with their tribal community in mind.
- Always take the history in person—not just via the intake form.
- Do not assume the adult who brings him/her to the clinic is the biological father. AIs have extended families, aunts, uncles, and grandparents that may be the caregiver.
- Do not make assumptions about sexual activity or practices. Specifically ask the following: Who are you dating? What are the genders of your sexual partners? What do you do with them? When you use condoms for anal or vaginal sex, how often do you use them?
- Screen for depression, alcohol, smoking, and drug use.
- Discuss protective factors and specifically ask the following: To whom do you turn when you feel sad or need someone to talk to? What is school like for you? How did your family react to your coming out?

5.3.2   Organizational Level Interventions

- Consider intervention approach that focus on getting support to people rather than people to services.
- Realize access to traditional healers may be as important as access to Western medicine.

- Recognize the importance of traditional AI culture to promote the well-being of youth.
- Realize the importance for informal support family, mentors, friends, youth leaders in the community, strong value of "Natives Helping Natives" vs. formal support (professional services).
- Make sure your referrals take into account travel time and that referrals are made to providers knowledgeable in the ways of AI populations.

5.3.3 Societal Level Interventions

- Identify community mentors for youth and provide suicide training.
- Mutual support is important and preferred to help AI youth struggling with suicide and is seen as part of AI identity and culture.
- Understand that peer support benefits emotional youth well-being.
- Involve as many community members as possible to help with education on youth suicide in AI communities. This will reduce the stigma of suicide and build a supportive community.
- Don't be surprised if the community, family, or youth does not want to talk about suicide openly as there is a b.elief that doing so invites negativity and may bring on harmful states.

5.4 Resources for LGBT Youth

- Gay and Lesbian Medical Association (GLMA) for finding a provider. Available at http://glma.org/
- Parents and Friends of Lesbians and Gays (PFLAG) for support for friends and family. Available at https://www.pflag.org/
- Gay, Lesbian, and Straight Education Network (GLSEN) for support in schools. Available at https://www.glsen.org/
- Children of Lesbian and Gays Everywhere (COLAGE) for children in LGBT families. Available at https://www.colage.org/
- Lambda Legal for legal support. Available at https://www.lambdalegal.org/

- American Civil Liberties Union (ACLU) for legal support. Available at https://www.aclu.org/
- The Trevor Project for LGBT-focused suicide hotline. Available at http://www.thetrevorproject.org/
- APA Lesbian, Gay, Bisexual and Transgender Concerns Office: www.apa.org/pi/lgbt/
- Association of Gay and Lesbian Psychiatrists: www.aglp.org/
- Fenway Institute: http://thefenwayinstitute.org/
- Gay and Lesbian Medical Association: www.glma.org
- The National Alliance on Mental Illness LGBT Resources & Fact Sheets: https://www.nami.org/Find-Support/LGBTQ

Conclusion

New AI graduates working for the first time in a suicide situation can become overwhelmed. The important point is to always gain trust, give respect, maintain a calm demeanor, and be a reassuring presence when working with Two Spirit, AI adolescents. Suicide or even thoughts of suicide can make families feel panicked and helpless. Always be culturally congruent in your approach and with interventions used. Understand that if prevention is viewed only as increasing access to clinical services and educating community members about suicide, little room is left for culturally congruent strategies (Burrage et al. 2016).

References

Ayyash-Abdo H (2002) Adolescent suicide: an ecological approach. Psychol Sch 39:459–475

Burrage R, Gone J, Momper S (2016) Urban American Indian community perspectives on resources and challenges for youth suicide prevention. Am J Community Psychol 58:136–149

Centers for Disease Control and Prevention (2014) Web-based injury statistics query and reporting system [Data File]. https://search.cdc.gov/search?query=Web-based+injury+statistics+query+and+reporting+system+&utf8=%E2%9C%93&affiliate=cdc-main. Accessed 20 Sept 2017

Freedenthal D, Stiffman AR (2004) Suicidal behavior in urban American Indian adolescents: a comparison with reservation youth in a Southwestern state. Suicide Life Threat Behav 34(2):160–171

King CA, Merchant CR (2008) Social and interpersonal factors relating to adolescent suicidality: a review of the literature. Arch Suicide Res 12:181–196

Lang S (1998) Men as women, women as men: changing gender in 'Native American culture'. University of Texas Press, Austin

Mackin J, Perkins T, Furrer CJ (2012) The power of protection: a population-based comparison of native and non-native youth suicide attempters. Am Indian Alsk Native Ment Health Res 19:20–54

Manzo K, Tiesman H, Stewart J, Hobbs GR, Knox S (2015) A comparison of risk factors associated with suicide ideation/attempts in American Indian and White youth in Montana. Arch Suicide Res 19:89–102

Medicine B, Jacobs SE, Thomas W, Lang S (eds) (1997) Changing Native American sex roles in an urban context. In: Two-Spirit people. Native American gender identity, sexuality, and spirituality. University of Illinois Press, Champaign-Urbana, pp 145–255

Middlebrook DL, LeMaster PL, Beals J, Novins DK, Manson SM (2001) Suicide prevention in American Indian and Alaska Native communities: a critical review of programs. Suicide Life Threat Behav 31(Suppl I):132–149

Novins DK, Beals J, Roberts RE, Manson S (1999) Factors associated with suicide ideation among American Indian adolescents: does culture matter? Suicide Life Threat Behav 29:332–346

Wexler LE, Gone JP (2012) Culturally responsive suicide prevention in indigenous communities: unexamined assumptions and new possibilities. Am J Public Health 102:800–806

Part II

Guideline: Education and Training

Education and Training in Culturally Competent Care

Larry Purnell

Guideline: *Nurses shall be educationally prepared to provide culturally congruent health care. Knowledge and skills necessary for assuring that nursing care is culturally congruent shall be included in global health care agendas that mandate formal education and clinical training, as well as required ongoing continuing education for all practicing nurses.*

Douglas et al. (2014: 110)

6.1 Introduction

In addition, to culture being incorporated into formal nursing programs, continuing education of nurses in culturally competent and congruent care is increasingly becoming a requirement for accreditation of healthcare organizations by agencies such as the Joint Commission (The Joint Commission 2010; The Joint Commission International 2011). Education for culturally competent care encompasses knowledge of the cultural values, beliefs, lifeways, and worldview of population groups as well as individuals (Papadopoulos 2006). Although Great Britain has encouraged culturally competent education in nursing and other healthcare professions, no official mandate has materialized (George et al. 2015). Whereas Australia and New Zealand has initiatives on cultural competence in education, a mandate for including cultural competence in nursing education could not be found. The same is true for other countries around the world.

L. Purnell, Ph.D., R.N., FAAN
School of Nursing, University of Delaware, Newark, DE, USA

Florida International University, Miami, FL, USA

Excelsior College, Albany, NY, USA
e-mail: lpurnell@udel.edu

6.2 Individualistic and Collectivistic Attributes as a Framework

A good starting point for staff at all levels is to gain an understanding of general principles of broad cultural groups and an understanding of individualistic and collectivistic cultures. All cultures that vary along a continuum of individualism and collectivism, subsets of broad worldviews, are somewhat context dependent.

Individualism versus collectivism scale									
Individualism									Collectivism
1		2	3	4	5	6	7	8	9	10

A degree of individualism and collectivism exists in every culture. Moreover, individualism and collectivism fall along a continuum, and some people from an individualistic culture will, to some degree, align themselves toward the collectivistic end of the scale. Some people from a collectivist culture will, to some degree, hold values along the individualistic end of the scale (see Table 6.1). The degree of acculturation and assimilation and the variant characteristics of culture (see Chap. 2) determine the degree of adherence to traditional individualistic and collectivist cultural values, beliefs, and practices (Hofstede and Hofstede 2005; Purnell 2013). They include orientation to self or group; decision-making; knowledge transmission;

Table 6.1 General collectivistic versus individualistic values

Collectivistic cultures	Individualistic cultures
Communication	
• Implicit indirect communication is most common. People are more likely to tell the professional what they think the professional wants to hear • More formal greeting is required by using the surname with a title. This can be a first step in gaining trust. The professional should always ask by what name the person wants to be called • Present temporality is most common, although balance is sought. The person usually wants to know how the illness/condition will affect them on a short-term basis. Address the individual's and family's concern before moving on • Punctuality is not valued except when absolutely necessary such as making transportation connections. If punctuality is required, explain the importance and the repercussions for tardiness such as a not being seen or a charge is made for being late • Truth telling may not be valued in order to "save face" • "Yes" may mean I hear you or I understand, not necessarily agreement. Do not ask questions that can easily be answered with "yes" or "no." The answer is invariably "yes." Instead of asking if the individual takes the medicine as prescribed, ask "what time do you take the medicine?" "How many times have you missed taking your medicine this week/month?" • Direct eye contact may be avoided with people in hierarchical positions as a means of respect, especially among older more traditional people but is maintained with friends and intimates. Do not assume that lack of eye contact means that the person is being evasive or not telling the truth • Sharing intimate life details of self or family is discouraged because it may cause a stigma for the person and the family. Ask intimate questions after a modicum of trust has been developed • Spatial distancing with non-intimates may be closer than 18 inches. Do not take offense if the person stands closer to you than what you have been accustomed to • Touch is readily and usually accepted between same-sex individuals but not necessarily between people of the opposite sex. Always ask permission and explain the necessity of touch • A diagnosis of depression is usually not acceptable. Do not use this diagnosis until a modicum of trust has been established	• Explicit, direct, straightforward communication is the norm • More informal greeting frequently use the given name early in an encounter. Professionals should introduce themselves by the name they preferred to be addressed. Ask the individual by what name they want to be addressed • Futuristic temporality is the norm. The person usually wants to know how the disease/condition will affect them on a long-term basis • Punctuality is valued. People are usually on time or early for formal appointments • Truth telling is expected at all times. Individuals will usually answer the professional truthfully or evade the question completely if they do not want to answer it • Questions requiring "yes" or "no" are usually answered truthfully • Direct eye contact is expected and is a sign of truth, respect, and trust • Sharing intimate life details is encouraged, even with non-intimates, and does not carry a stigma for people or their family • Spatial distancing with non-intimates is 18–24 inches. Sexual harassment laws encourage a low touch culture. Explain the necessity and ask permission before touching • A diagnosis of depression does not carry a stigma and can be shared with individuals and their families (if necessary) without a stigma

Table 6.1   (continued)

Collectivistic cultures	Individualistic cultures
Family roles and organization	
• Decision-making is a responsibility of the male or the most respected family member. The male is usually the spokesperson for the family, even though he may not be the decision-maker • Individual autonomy is not usually the norm • Older people's opinions are sought but not necessarily followed • Young adults and children are not expected to have a high degree of dependence until they leave their parent's home • Children are not usually encouraged to express themselves; they are expected to be seen, not heard • A stigma may result when a family member is placed in long-term care. Home care with the extended family is the norm • Alternative lifestyles are not readily accepted and may be hidden from the public and even within the extended family. Do not disclose same-sex relationship to family or outsiders • Extended family living is common with collective input from all members • Beneficence a normative statement to act for others' benefit may mean that the healthcare professional should not reveal grave diagnoses or outcome directly because it may cause them to give up hope. Therefore, the professional should disclose this information to the family who makes the decision to disclose the diagnosis to the individual. An alternative is to tell a story about someone else who has the condition	• Egalitarian decision-making is the norm, although there are variations. Ask who is the primary decision-maker for health-related concerns • Individual autonomy is the norm • Younger people are expected to become responsible and independent at a young age. Determine responsibilities for children and teenagers. • Children are encouraged to express themselves. Allow children to have a voice in decision-making • Each person in a group has an equal right to express an opinion • No stigma is attached for placing a family member in long-term care or substance misuse rehab • Alternative lifestyles are gaining more acceptance than in the past. Ask about same-sex relationships after a modicum of trust has been established • Nuclear family living is the norm. However, the professional must still ask who else lives in the household and what are their responsibilities • Beneficence a normative statement to act for others' benefit requires the healthcare professional to reveal grave diagnoses or outcome directly to the individual in order to make informed decisions regarding the future
High-risk health behaviors	
• Accountability is a family affair or some hierarchal authority • High-risk health behaviors are less likely to be revealed to healthcare professionals. Do not disclose substance misuse to family members	• People are accountable for their own actions • High-risk health behaviors are revealed to healthcare professionals. However, it is still best to ask about substance misuse after a modicum of trust has been established

(continued)

Table 6.1 (continued)

Collectivistic cultures	Individualistic cultures
Healthcare practices	
• Traditional practices are common as a first line of defense for minor illnesses. Specifically ask about traditional practices, including herbs • Complementary and alternative therapies are frequently preferred over allopathic practices. Specifically ask about complementary and alternative practices • Preventive practices are stressed • Rehabilitation is frequently a family responsibility. Great stigma can occur by placing a family member in a long-term care or rehab facility • Self-medication is common and expends to prescription medicines that may be obtained from overseas pharmacies and friends. Specifically ask what medicines the person is taking • Pain may be seen as atonement for past sins. Take every opportunity to dispel this myth • Mental health issues may be hidden because they carry a stigma for the family. Disclose mental health and substance misuse only to professionals who "need to know" • Advance directives that convey how the individual wants medical decisions made in the future may not be acceptable to some because this is a family, not individual, responsibility	• Traditional practices are common as a first line of defense for minor illnesses. Ask about over-the-counter medications and herbs • Complementary and alternative therapies are gaining acceptance because they are less invasive. Specifically ask the individual about their complementary and alternative practices • Curative healthcare practices have been the norm, but preventive practices and healthy living are gaining acceptance • Rehabilitation is well-integrated into allopathic care • Liberal pain medication is expected although recent research is sometimes discouraging this • Mental health issues do not usually carry a stigma for the family. However, ask the person about disclosure of substance misuse and reveal it only to those who need to know • Advance directives that convey how the individual wants medical decisions made in the future are compatible with individualism
Healthcare practitioners	
• Allopathic professionals may be seen as a first resource for major health problems, although traditional healers may be seen simultaneously. Professionals should partner with traditional healers • Spiritual leaders frequently serve as alternative practitioners for emotional concerns and substance misuse • Age of the professional may be a concern. Ask the individual if they prefer an older professional • Opposite sex healthcare provider may not be acceptable with devout Jewish and Muslim individuals. Ask the individual if a same-sex professional is required for non-life-threatening conditions	• Age of professional healthcare providers is usually not a concern • Same-sex healthcare providers are usually not required except for traditional Muslims and orthodox Jews. Specifically ask if a same-sex professional is required for non-emergent conditions

A degree of individualism and collectivism exists in every culture. Some people from an individualistic culture will, to some degree, align themselves toward the collectivistic end of the scale. Some people from a collectivist culture will, to some degree, hold values along the individualistic end of the scale. Thus, the information in this table should be seen as a guide

individual choice and personal responsibility; the concept of progress, competitiveness, shame, and guilt; help-seeking; expression of identity; and interaction/communication styles (Hofstede 2001; Hofstede and Hofstede 2005; Rothstein-Fisch et al. 2001). One should not confuse individualism from individuality. Individuality is the sense that each person has a separate and equal place in the community and where individuals who are consid-

ered "eccentrics or local characters" are tolerated (Purnell 2010; Singelis 1998; Triandis 2001).

6.2.1 Individualism

Individualism is a moral, political, or social outlook that stresses independence (Bui and Turnbull 2003; Greenfield et al. 2003; Markus and Kitayama 1991; Hofstede and Hofstede 2005; Purnell 2013; Triandis 2001). Consistent with individualism, individualistic cultures encourage self-expression. Adherents freely express personal opinions, share many personal issues, and ask personal questions of others to a degree that may be seen as offensive to those who come from a collectivistic culture. Direct, straightforward questioning with the expectation that answers will be direct is usually appreciated with individualism. Small talk before getting down to business is not always appreciated. However, the healthcare provider should take cues from the patient before this immediate, direct, and intrusive approach is initiated. Individualistic cultures usually tend to be more informal and frequently use first names. Ask the patient by what name she/he prefers to be called. Questions that require a "yes" or "no" answer are usually answered truthfully from the patient's perspective. In individualistic cultures with values on autonomy and productivity, one is expected to be a productive member of society (Purnell 2011, 2013; Singelis 1998). Some highly individualistic countries include Australia, Belgium, the United States, Great Britain, England, Canada, Finland, Germany, Ireland, Israel, Great Britain, Finland, Luxembourg, Norway, the Netherlands, postcommunist Poland, Slovakia, South Africa, Sweden, and Switzerland, to name a few (Darwish and Huber 2003).

Individualistic cultures expect all to follow the rules and hierarchical protocols, and each person is expected to do his/her own work and to work until the job is completed (Eshun and Hodge 2014). In addition, children are often expected to become responsible at a young age and have more independence and self-expression. However, in situations where the group makes decisions, each member has an equal right to express their opinions, and opinions can differ greatly, enhancing the chance the decision is better than what one person's decision would be. The expectation is that all will follow the decisions made (Eshun and Hodge 2014).

Individualistic cultures socialize (enculturate) their members to view themselves as independent, separate, distinct individuals, where the most important person in society is self. A person feels free to change alliances and is not bound by any particular group (shared identity). Although they are part of a group, they are still free to act independently within the group and less likely to engage in "groupthink."

6.2.2 Collectivism

Collectivism is a moral, political, or social outlook that stresses human interdependence—it is important to be part of a collective. The individual is defined in terms of a reference group—family, church, work, school, or some other group. Collectivism can stifle individuality and diversity leading to a common social identity (Bui and Turnbull 2003; Greenfield et al. 2003; Hofstede and Hofstede 2005; Markus and Kitayama 1991; Triandis 2001). Some collectivistic cultures include American Indian/Alaskan Native and most indigenous populations, Asian Indian, Chinese, Korean, Pakistani, Filipino, Japanese, Mexican, Spanish, and Taiwanese (Darwish and Huber 2003).

Most collectivist cultures are high context where implicit communication may be valued over explicit communication: the meaning is usually embedded in the information, and the listener must "read between the lines" (Keeskes 2016). Shame and guilt are strong, and the individual must not do anything to cause shame to self, the family, or the organization. Most believe in the hierarchal structure, and one should not stand out in the crowd (Greenfield et al. 2003; Hofstede and Hofstede 2005; Markus and Kitayama 1991; Purnell 2011). To interrupt another in a conversation is considered extremely rude. Sensitive issues that may cause a stigma to family or others are not revealed.

Time is more relaxed; punctuality is valued only in business and situations where it is essential such as in making transportation connections. Most value formality; therefore, always greet the patient and family members formally until told to do otherwise. In most traditional cultures, but not all, men have decision-making authority or are the spokesperson for the family, even if they are not the primary decision-maker. Gender roles are usually less fluid than in individualistic cultures; however, expectations upon immigration may cause significant family discord (Purnell and Pontious 2014).

6.3   Knowledge of Specific Cultures Cared for in the Practice Setting

Whereas the individualistic and collectivistic framework is a good starting point for understanding culture and a broad assessment guide, providers need to obtain an understanding of the specific cultural and subcultural groups seen in their practice. Specific content of the groups should include the overview and heritage of the group, communication practices, family roles and organization, workforce issues, biocultural ecology, high-risk health behaviors, nutrition, pregnancy and the childbearing family, death rituals, spirituality and religion, healthcare practices, and healthcare practitioners. A brief description of these concepts follows (Purnell 2013; Purnell and Fenkl 2018).

1. Overview and Heritage: Includes concepts related to the country of origin and current residence and the effects of the topography of the country of origin and the current residence on health, economics, politics, reasons for migration, educational status, and occupations.

2. Communication: Includes concepts related to the dominant language, dialects, and the contextual use of the language; paralanguage variations such as voice volume, tone, intonations, inflections, and willingness to share thoughts and feelings; nonverbal communications such as eye contact, gesturing, facial expressions, use of touch, body language, spatial distancing practices, and acceptable greetings; temporality in terms of past, present, and future orientation of worldview; clock versus social time; and the amount of formality in use of names. Differences between the language spoken by the health-

care provider and the patient, educational level, and health literacy can add to communication difficulties. Effective communication is the first and probably the most important aspect of obtaining an accurate health assessment (see this chapter).

3. Family Roles and Organization: Includes concepts related to the head of the household, gender roles (a product of biology and culture), family goals and priorities, developmental tasks of children and adolescents, roles of the aged and extended family, individual and family social status in the community, and acceptance of alternative lifestyles such as single parenting, same-sex partnerships and marriage, childless marriages, and divorce.

4. Workforce Issues: Includes concepts related to autonomy, acculturation, assimilation, gender roles, ethnic communication styles, and healthcare practices of the country of origin.

5. Biocultural Ecology: Includes physical, biological, and physiological variations among ethnic and racial groups such as skin color (the most evident) and physical differences in body habitus; genetic, hereditary, endemic, and topographical diseases; psychological makeup of individuals; and the physiological differences that affect the way drugs are metabolized by the body. In general, most diseases and illnesses can be divided into three categories: lifestyle, environment, and genetics. Lifestyle causes include cultural practices and behaviors that can generally be controlled, for example, smoking, diet, and stress. Environment causes refer to the external environment (e.g., air and water pollution) and situations over which the individual has little or no control (e.g., the presence of malarial mosquitos, exposure to chemicals and pesticides, access to care, and associated diseases and illnesses). Genetic conditions are caused by genes.

6. High-Risk Health Behaviors: Includes substance use and misuse of tobacco, alcohol, and recreational drugs; lack of physical activity; increased calorie consumption; nonuse of safety measures

such as seat belts, helmets, and safe driving practices; and not taking safety measures to prevent contracting HIV and sexually transmitted infections.

7. Nutrition: Includes the meaning of food, common foods and rituals, nutritional deficiencies and food limitations, and the use of food for health promotion and wellness and illness and disease prevention. Multiple diseases and illnesses are a consequence of this major cultural component.

8. Pregnancy and Childbearing Practices: Includes culturally sanctioned and unsanctioned fertility practices, views on pregnancy, and prescriptive, restrictive, and taboo practices related to pregnancy, birthing, and the postpartum period.

9. Death Rituals: Includes how the individual and the society view death and euthanasia, rituals to prepare for death, burial practices, and bereavement behaviors. Death rituals are slow to change.

10. Spirituality: Includes formal religious beliefs related to faith and affiliation and the use of prayer, behavioral practices that give meaning to life, and individual sources of strength.

11. Healthcare Practices: Includes the focus of healthcare (acute versus preventive); traditional, magico-religious, and biomedical beliefs and practices; individual responsibility for health; self-medicating practices; views on mental illness, chronicity, and rehabilitation; acceptance of blood and blood products; and organ donation and transplantation.

12. Healthcare Practitioners: Includes the status, use, and perceptions of traditional, magico-religious, and biomedical healthcare providers and the gender of the healthcare provider.

6.4 Cultural Theories and Models for Patient Assessment

A number of cultural theories and models for patient assessment have been developed. Some are very extensive, while others are more general in nature without a specific framework. All of these theories and models should be included in formal education programs. In practice, each organization can select the model or theory that they deem fits their needs.

Although some of these simplistic techniques can be used for collecting initial interview data, they do not work well with all ethnic and cultural groups nor are they comprehensive. Two examples are acronymic approaches: LEARN and BATHE. The LEARN approach includes the following guidelines: *listen* to your patients from their perspectives; *explain* your concerns and your reasons for asking for personal information; *acknowledge* your patients' concerns; *recommend* a course of action; and *negotiate* a plan of care that considers cultural norms and personal lifestyles (Berlin and Fowkes 1983). The BATHE acronym stands for *background*, information, *affect* [sic] the problem has on the patient, *trouble* the problem causes for the patient, *handling* of the problem by the patient, and *empathy* conveyed by the healthcare provider (McCullough et al. 1998).

The limited space available here does not permit an exhaustive description of the numerous models and theories centered on culture. A brief description of the models most commonly used in practice, education, administration, and research follows.

The Campinha-Bacote Model is a practice model focusing on the process of cultural competence in the delivery of healthcare services. This model, which is currently referred to as a volcano model, is used primarily in practice and education; it does not have an accompanying organizational framework. According to Transcultural C.A.R.E. Associates (2015), individuals, as well as organizations and institutions, begin the journey to cultural competence by first demonstrating an intrinsic motivation to engage in the process of cultural competence. The five concepts in this model are cultural awareness, cultural knowledge, cultural skill, cultural encounter, and cultural desire (Transcultural C.A.R.E. Associates 2015).

The Giger and Davidhizar Model focuses on assessment and intervention from a transcultural nursing perspective. The six areas of human diversity and variation include communication, space, social orientation, time, environmental control, and biological variations (Giger and Davidhizar 2012).

The Papadopoulos, Tilki, and Taylor Model focuses on the process of cultural competence in the delivery of healthcare services and is used in education, practice, and administration. This model does not have an assessment guide or organizing framework. The four main components of this model are cultural awareness that includes an ethnohistory, cultural knowledge, cultural competence, and cultural sensitivity. The center of the model includes compassion (Papadopoulos 2006).

Leininger's Cultural Care: Diversity and Universality Theory and Sunrise Model promote understanding of both the universally held and common understandings of care among humans and the culture-specific caring beliefs and behaviors that define any particular caring context or interaction. This theory incorporates (a) care (caring); (b) generic, folk, or indigenous care knowledge and practices; (c) professional care knowledge and practices that vary transculturally; (d) worldview, language, philosophy, religion, and spirituality; and (e) kinship, social, political, legal, educational, economic, technological, ethnohistorical, and environmental contexts of cultures. Within a cultural care diversity and universality framework, nurses may take any or all of three culturally congruent action modes: (a) cultural preservation/maintenance, (b) cultural care accommodation/negotiation, and (c) cultural care repatterning/restructuring (McFarland and Wehbe-Alamah 2015).

Spector's HEALTH Traditions Model incorporates three main theories: Estes and Zitzow's heritage consistency theory, the HEALTH Traditions Model, and Giger and Davidhizar's theory about the cultural phenomena affecting health. The HEALTH Traditions Model is based on the concept of holistic health and explores what people do to maintain, protect, or restore health. This model emphasizes the interrelationship between physical, mental, and spiritual health with personal methods of maintaining, protecting, and restoring health. Spector also provides a heritage assessment tool to determine the degree to which people or families adhere to their traditions. A traditional person observes his or her cultural traditions more closely. A more acculturated individual's practice is less observant of traditional practices (Spector 2009).

The cultural safety model includes actions which recognize and respect the cultural identities of others and safely meet their needs, expectations, and rights. Strategies that enhance the ability to be culturally safe are (a) reflecting on one's own culture, attitudes, and beliefs about "others"; (b) having clear, value-free, open, and respectful communication; (c) developing trust; (d) recognizing and avoiding stereotypical barriers; (e) being prepared to engage with others in a two-way dialogue where knowledge is shared; (f) and understanding the influence of culture shock (Cultural Connections for Learning: Cultural Safety 2013).

Cultural humility has three processes: (a) lifelong commitment to self-evaluation and self-critique, (b) a desire to fix power imbalances, and (c) aspiring to develop partnerships with people and groups who advocate for others (American Psychological Association 2013).

The Purnell Model for Cultural Competence has been classified as a holographic and complexity theory because it includes a model and organizing framework that can be used by all health disciplines. The purposes of this model are to (a) provide a framework for all healthcare providers to learn concepts and characteristics of culture; (b) define circumstances that affect a person's cultural worldview in the context of historical perspectives; (c) provide a model that links the most central relationships of culture; (d) interrelate characteristics of culture to promote congruence and to facilitate the delivery of consciously sensitive and competent healthcare; (e) provide a framework that reflects human characteristics such as motivation, intentionality, and meaning and provide a structure for analyzing cultural data; and (f) view the individual, family, or group within their unique ethnocultural environment (Purnell and Fenkl 2018) (see Appendices 1 and 2).

6.5 Interdisciplinary Practice

Cultural competence is a requisite for all professionals who have direct or indirect contact with patients. Most cultural concepts, knowledge, and practice skills are shared by all health disciplines, making cultural competence a requirement for all. For example, cross-cultural communication principles do not change for direct care professionals, auxiliary staff, or administrative personnel. Workshops and conferences should include multidisciplinary professionals where personal cultural stories can be shared.

6.6 Recommendations

Recommendations for clinical practice, administration, education, and research follow.

6.6.1 Recommendations for Clinical Practice

Staff at all levels should attend continuing education classes, in-services, conferences, and other learning experiences to maintain cross-cultural skills. Upon admission, professional staff need to use a comprehensive cultural assessment tool that can be added to as time and circumstances permit (see this chapter). The assessment should include the patient's cultural and ethnic background as well as familiar genetic and hereditary health conditions. The assessment needs to include not just current work environment but previous work as well. In addition, the work history needs to be completed for patients who are retired. Environmental living arrangements are included in an assessment.

6.6.2 Recommendations for Administration

Organizational administration has the prime responsibility to assure that culturally competent care is delivered throughout the organization. The organization's mission and philosophy must be addressed at the department level as well as each unit within a department. Administrators and managers, whether in direct or indirect care, must role model cultural competence and work with national and community organizations to ensure that patients' needs are being met. They should also seek positions and be involved on community and national boards.

Staff should be provided with unit-written resources and partner with universities for online resources that all staff can access. In addition, administration can support and host workshops and conferences as effective approaches to culturally congruent nursing practice. Hosting community health fairs with ethnic community organizations that support vulnerable populations adds value to the organization's mission.

6.6.3 Recommendations for Education

In the academic setting, all the concepts included in Chap. 2, knowledge of cultures, should be included. The preference is to have a separate course on culture that includes both cultural general as well as cultural specific information in every course and include the use of complementary and alternative practices. What might be complementary and alternative in one culture may be mainstream health care in other cultures.

The curriculum must include content on vulnerable populations, socioeconomics, and cultural general information on the populations in clinical areas that also stress the importance of individual cultural values and beliefs. Culture needs to also be integrated throughout all courses such as pathophysiology, pharmacology, and simulation labs and clinical courses. If a specific cultural course is not feasible, maintain a system that assures cultural content is included in all courses so that cultural content is not lost.

In the service setting, cultural content needs to be addressed in orientation with annual in-service training in cultural competence for all levels of staff including management, other professionals, and auxiliary staff in any department with patient contact. Classes to increase staff's cultural knowledge about the ethnically diverse patients who receive health services in the facility should be conducted and reinforced in the organization's intranet with population health beliefs and values.

Educators should mentor staff for whom the dominant language is not the same as the patient's for sociopragmatic competence specific to the medical setting (Sedgwick and Garner 2017). A variety of modalities to teach cultural competency can include workshops, conferences, online training, films, and immersion experiences whether in diverse communities, in the home environment, or in other countries. Faculty should partner with transcultural experts to provide staff with continuing education courses, consultation, and practice skills for culturally competent care.

6.6.4 Recommendations for Research

Journal clubs can be established to review current scholarly evidence-based literature on the populations served by the organization and should be instituted and offered at times that clinical staff can attend. Consultants from local university and college faculty can be employed to facilitate implementation of evidence-based cross-cultural practice. Staff wanting to conduct research can partner with local faculty for expertise in the research process and study design.

An interdisciplinary team of researchers and educators can collaborate on quality improvement projects and to apply for funding. Initial research should be on ethnic/cultural groups common to the organization. Although it might not be possible to translate satisfaction surveys in all the patients' languages served by the organization, at least they should be translated into the most common languages of patients; otherwise, only part of the data is collected. The results of satisfaction served can be used in quality improvement projects or to conduct research.

Conclusion

Cultural competence has become one of the most important initiatives worldwide for a number of reasons. Diversity has increased in many countries due to wars, political strife, world socioeconomic conditions, and migration. In addition, the last few decades have demonstrated that culturally congruent care increases patient satisfaction, improves patient care, and reduces cost. The recognition of the social determinants of health with vulnerable populations (see Chap. 1) has been a focus to help alleviate heath disparities. Therefore, a requisite is to include culturally competent education in formal health-related programs and continue the process where the organization includes cultural competence during orientation and yearly thereafter. Cultural competence education and training are for all healthcare providers, including those who encounter diverse patients and families even though they may not be direct care providers.

Formal education must include content on the various models and approaches to learn culture and provide a stand-alone course on culture if possible and then integrate culture in every theory and clinical course. If a separate stand-alone course is not possible, the education organization needs to keep a tracking system to assure that culture is included in every course. Cultural competence is required for the organization and the individual provider. The American Association of Colleges of Nursing; the Office of Minority Health in the United States, Australia, and New Zealand; Royal College of Nursing; American Medical Association; National Medical Association; International Council of Nursing; and the American Nurses Association have all recognized the importance of culturally competent education.

Appendix 1: Recommended Content for Beginning Level Cultural Competency Education

Beginning level includes vocational or practical nursing programs, associate degree and diploma programs, and continuing education and in-service programs. The cultural content can be provided in a separate course as well as integrated into existing clinical curriculum. Modules of key concepts can be developed to provide for the greatest flexibility of presentation of this material. Key concepts that need to be integrated follow.

Overall Program Objectives Related to Culture

Develop cultural assessment skills of self and others (individuals and families):

1. Identify cultural similarities and differences and potential approaches to differences.
2. Use culture-related resources available for potential problems.
3. Recognize forms of discrimination in nursing care and take action to prevent or address them.

Content Related to Culture

1. Effective communication is essential for healthcare practice at all levels. A sample communication exercise is included (see Appendix 2 Chap. 14).
2. Culturally congruent care should be integrated as a component of every clinical course.
3. Social and material determinants of health should be included in theory courses and reinforced in clinical courses.
4. Cultural patterns and values of select cultural and ethnic or subcultural groups should be included in theory courses and reinforced in clinical courses.
5. Common cultural terms should be included in theory courses and reinforced in clinical courses. Some essential terms and concepts are collectivism, individualism, and individuality; cultural awareness, sensitivity, competence, and congruency; cultural imposition, relativism, and imperialism; cultural assimilation and accommodation, ethnocentrism, and stereotyping versus generalizing; individual and organizational cultural competence; interpretation versus translation; and ethnicity and subculture.
6. Biocultural variations should be incorporated into anatomy and physiology and pathophysiology and reinforced in clinical courses.
7. Genetic and hereditary diseases should be included in pathophysiology courses and reinforced in all clinical courses.
8. Common illnesses and diseases in cultural and ethnic groups should be included in pathophysiology and reinforced in clinical courses.
9. Dietary practices that include prescriptive, restrictive, and taboo practices of specific cultural and ethnic groups should be included in all clinical courses.
10. Health belief systems and complementary and alternative practices can be incorporated in pharmacology and/or assessment and reinforced in all clinical settings.

Appendix 2: Recommended Content for Advanced-Level Cultural Competency Education

Components of culture should be integrated into courses such as health assessment, pharmacology, anatomy and physiology, and all specialty clinical courses. Communication strategies beginning with assessing the client's preferred language and health literacy along with spatial distancing, eye contact, greetings, temporality, touch, and name format are essential. Interpretation and translation that include sign languages are also essential components of communication (see Chap. 14). In a pharmacology course, the racial/cultural difference in response to drugs should be included. In physiology and pathophysiology courses, the biocultural aspects of diseases should be included as well as the biocultural variations in pain, height, weight, musculoskeletal variations, and physical appearances in general.

The following is a sample stand-alone course recommended for senior healthcare practitioners, nurse practitioners, and masters and doctoral level students. Cultural case studies should be included in all courses with content appropriate for the course. In addition, resources for teaching culture are included.

Course Description

Components of this course can be used in in-service and continuing education classes as deemed relevant or pertinent by the organization. A comprehensive course should include theories and models focused on culture, social and material determinants of health, health disparities, selected culturally specific groups commonly found in the catchment area of the school or organization, and common research methodologies used in cultural research. Evidence-based practice must be incorporated in discussions and formal scholarly papers (see Chap. 30). Students will critically reflect on their own cultural beliefs and values. Assignments should include group discussions on cultural and religious groups with an application to nursing practice. A formal team paper with four to six students is recommended because it increases learning knowledge. The team paper should be on a cultural or subcultural group different from anyone on the team.

Suggested Course Objectives

Upon completion of this course, the student will be able to:

1. Articulate the concepts that explain cultural diversity and their relevance for nursing practice
2. Examine cultural issues and trends in nursing practice
3. Analyze selected population group cultural patterns and behavioral manifestations of cultural values

4. Evaluate the socioeconomic impact of client's cultural needs upon levels of care: primary, secondary, and tertiary
5. Articulate theory, research methods, and advanced multicultural-sensitive nursing practice concepts
6. Formulate a model of care integrating culturally sensitive assessment, planning, intervention, and evaluation
7. Analyze impact of public and organizational policies on health of individuals and populations
8. Develop collaborative engagement with individuals and groups to mitigate health inequity
9. Promote engagement of individuals, groups, and organizations in health promotion for disadvantaged populations
10. Develop cross-cultural leadership to promote culturally competent care and retention of multicultural workforce

Possible Teaching Strategies

PowerPoint lectures

Live classroom or online discussions of cultural, ethnic, or subcultural groups

Required and recommended readings determined by the faculty teaching the course

Recommended Web sites

Topical Outline

A. Introduction to culture and related concepts
   1. Values and culture
   2. Vulnerability as a framework
   3. Expanding definitions of cultural groups and underserved populations
   4. Review of common cultural terms: collectivism, individualism and individuality; cultural awareness, sensitivity, competence and congruency; cultural imposition, relativism, and imperialism; cultural assimilation and accommodation, ethnocentrism, stereotyping, and generalizing; individual and organizational cultural competence; interpretation versus translation; and ethnicity and subculture.

B. Selected theoretical models for nursing practice
   1. Andrews and Boyle Assessment Guide
   2. Campinha-Bacote's Model The Process of Cultural Competence in the Delivery of Healthcare Services
   3. Giger and Davidhizar Transcultural Assessment Model
   4. Leininger's Culture Care Diversity and Universality Theory
   5. Jeffrey's Cultural Competence and Confidence (CCC) Model: Transcultural Self-Efficiency
   6. Papadopoulos, Tilki, and Taylor Model for Developing Culturally Competent and Compassionate Healthcare
   7. Purnell Model for Cultural Competence
   8. Schim, Dorenbos, Benkert, and Miller Dimensional Puzzle Model of Culturally Competent Care
C. Managing health disparities through culturally competent research
   1. Minorities, migrants, and refugees
   2. Health disparities in the catchment area where students do clinical
D. Cultural patterns and values of select cultural and ethnic, or subcultural groups: Hispanic/Latino, Arab/Muslim, Jewish, Haitian, Lesbian Gay Bisexual Transgender, Alcoholics Anonymous, and/or others. Some should come from the catchment area where the students practice and at least one that is not common among the community to give the course a global perspective.

- Biocultural ecology
- High-risk health behaviors
- Nutrition and the meaning of food
- Pregnancy and the childbearing family
- Death and dying rituals
- Spirituality and religion
- Healthcare practices including complementary and alternative practices

2. In a team paper, each team should have no more than four to six members.
3. Most references should come from the last 6 years, although classic references are acceptable.
4. Most of the references should come from the research literature. Internet sources are acceptable as long as they come from governmental organizations, universities, or professional associations and organizations. Wikipedia is not an acceptable reference because content has not been refereed. Blogs and travel sites are not acceptable.
5. Once the literature review is completed, create a list of at least four recommendations for research based on gaps in the literature. The research questions must be something that a graduate student can accomplish. For each question, identify if the research is qualitative or quantitative research, the specific methodology (phenomenology, grounded theory, correlational, quasi-experimental, etc.), and a brief description of the methods to carry out this research.
6. Identify applications to *practice*. Be specific, not something general that would be the same for any cultural group.

Scholarly Formal Paper on a Specific Cultural, Ethnic, or Subcultural Group

1. Conduct a literature review on four domains of a cultural, ethnic, or subcultural group different from your own culture. The domains for the literature review can include:
   - Heritage overview (as the introduction)
   - Communication
   - Family roles and organization
   - Workforce issues

Resources for Advanced Courses in Cultural Competency Education

- American Association of Colleges of Nursing. (2017). Essentials of Baccalaureate and Graduate Education in Nursing. Available at http://www.aacnnursing.org/. [Accessed 7 December 2017].
- Andrews, M.M., and Boyle, J.S. (2016). Transcultural concepts and nursing care (7ed.). Philadelphia, Wolters Kluwer.

- Campinha-Bacote, J. Transcultural C.A.R.E. Associates. Available at http://transcultural-care.net/the-process-of-cultural-competence-in-the-delivery-of-healthcare-services/. [Accessed 7 December 2017].
- Douglas, M. and Pacquiao, D. (2010). Core Curriculum for Transcultural Nursing and Health Care. Sage Publications. http://www.tcns.org/TCNCoreCurriculum.html. [Accessed 7 December, 2017].
- CIA World Factbook. Available at http://rubyworldfactbook.com/, [Accessed 7 December, 2017].
- Giger, J., and Davidhizar, R. (eds.) (2012). Transcultural nursing: assessment and intervention (3rd. ed.). Philadelphia, PA: Elsevier.
- Jeffreys, M.R. (2010). Teaching cultural competence in nursing and health care. NY: Springer.
- European Transcultural Nursing Society. Available at http://europeantransculturalnurses.eu/. [Accessed 7 December 2017].
- McFarland, M and Wehbe-Alamah, HB. (eds). (2015). Leininger's culture care diversity and universality: a worldwide nursing theory, (3e). Burlington, ME: Jones & Bartlett Learning.
- Papadopoulos, Tilki, and Taylor Model for Developing Culturally Competent and Compassionate Healthcare. Available at http://cultureandcompassion.com/what-is-culturally-competent-compassion-2/, [Accessed 7 December 2017].
- Purnell, L. (2013). Transcultural health care: a culturally competent approach. Philadelphia: F.A. Davis.
- Sagar, P. (2014). Transcultural nursing education strategies. NY: Springer Publishing Company.
- Schim, Dorenbos, Benkert, & Miller, (2007). Dimensional Puzzle Model of Culturally Competent Care Available at http://europepmc.org/articles/PMC3074191. [Accessed 7 December 2017].
- Transcultural Nursing Society. Available at http://www.tcns.org/. [Accessed 7 December 2017].
- United Nations Millennium Development Goals. (n.d.). Available at http://www.un.org/millenniumgoals/. [Accessed 7 December, 2017].
- U.S. Department of Health and Human Services Office of Minority Health, (n.d.). National CLAS Standards. Available at https://minorityhealth.hhs.gov/omh/browse.aspx?lvl=2&lvlid=53. [Accessed 7 December 2017].

References

American Psychological Association (2013) Reflections on cultural humility. http://www.apa.org/pi/families/resources/newsletter/2013/08/cultural-humility.aspx. Accessed 29 July 2017

Berlin EA, Fowkes WC (1983) A teaching framework for cross-cultural health care: application in family practice. West J Med 139(12):93–98

Bui Y, Turnbull A (2003) East meets west: analysis of person-centered planning in the context of Asian American values. Educ Train Ment Retard Dev Disabil 38:18–31

Cultural Connections for Learning: Cultural Safety (2013) http://www.intstudentsup.org/diversity/cultural_safety/. Accessed 29 July 2017

Darwish AFE, Huber GU (2003) Individualism vs collectivism in different cultures: a cross-cultural study. Intercult Educ 14(1):48–55

Douglas M, Rosenketter M, Pacquiao D, Clark Callister L et al (2014) Guidelines for implementing culturally competent nursing care. J Transcult Nurs 25(2):109–221

Eshun S, Hodge D (2014) Mental health assessment among ethnic minorities in the United States. In: Gurung RAR (ed) Multicultural approaches to health and wellness in America, vol 1. Praeger, Santa Barbara

George RE, Thornicroft G, Dogra N (2015) Research paper: exploration of cultural competency training in UK healthcare settings: a critical interpretive review of the literature. Divers Equal Health Care 12(3):104–115

Giger J, Davidhizar R (eds) (2012) Transcultural nursing: assessment and intervention, 3rd edn. Elsevier, Philadelphia

Greenfield P, Trunbull E, Rothstein-Fisch C (2003) Bridging cultures. Cult Psychol Bull 37:6–16

Hofstede G (ed) (2001) Culture's consequences: comparing values, behaviors, institutions, and organizations across nations, 2nd edn. Sage, Thousand Oaks

Hofstede G, Hofstede J (eds) (2005) Cultures and organizations: software of the mind, 2nd edn. McGraw-Hill, New York

Keeskes I (2016) Can intercultural pragmatics bring some new insight into pragmatic theories? In: Capone A, Mey JL (eds) Interdisciplinary studies in pragmatics, culture and society. Springer, New York

Markus HR, Kitayama S (1991) Culture and the self: implications for cognition, emotion, and motivation. Psychol Rev 98:224–253

McCullough J, Ramesar S, Peterson H (1998) Psychotherapy in primary care: the BATHE technique. Am Fam Physician 57(9):2131–2134. http://www. aafp.org/afp/980501ap/mcculloc.html. Accessed 29 July 2017

McFarland M, Wehbe-Alamah HB (eds) (2015) Leininger's culture care diversity and universality: a worldwide nursing theory, 3rd edn. Jones & Bartlett Learning, Burlington

Papadopoulos I (2006) Transcultural health and social care: development of culturally competent practitioners. Churchill Livingstone, London

Purnell L (2010) Cultural rituals in health and nursing care. In: Esterhuizen P, Kuchert A (eds) Diversiteit in de verpleeg-kunde [Diversity in nursing]. The Netherlands, Springer Utigeverij

Purnell L (2011) Application of transcultural theory to mental health-substance use in an international context. In: Cooper D (ed) Intervention in mental health-substance use. CRC Press, Boca Raton

Purnell L (ed) (2013) Transcultural health care: a culturally competent approach. F.A. Davis, Philadelphia

Purnell L, Fenkl E (eds) (2018) Guide to culturally competent health care. F.A. Davis, Philadelphia

Purnell L, Pontious S (2014) Collectivist and individualistic approaches to cultural health care. In: Gurung R (ed) Multicultural approaches to health and wellness in America, vol 1. ABC-CLIO-LLC, Santa Barbara

Rothstein-Fisch C, Greenfield P, Quiroz B (2001) Continuum of individualistic and collectivistic values. National Center on Secondary Education. http://www. ncset.org/publications/essentialtools/diversity/partIII. asp. Accessed 29 July 2017

Sagar P (2014) Transcultural concepts in adult health courses. In: Sagar P (ed) Transcultural nursing education strategies. Springer Publishing Co. LLC., Philadelphia

Sedgwick C, Garner M (2017) How appropriate are the English language test requirements for non-UK-trained nurses? A qualitative study of spoken communication in UK hospitals. Int J Nurs Stud 71:50–59. https://doi.org/10.1016/j.ijnurstu.2017.03.002

Singelis TM (1998) Teaching about culture, ethnicity, and diversity. Sage Publications, Thousand Oakes

Spector R (2009) Cultural diversity in health and illness, 7th edn. Pearson Prentice Hall, Upper Saddle River

The Joint Commission (2010) Advancing effective communication, cultural competence, and patient- and family-centered care: a roadmap for hospitals. The Joint Commission, Oakbrook Terrace. https://www. jointcommission.org/topics/health_equity.aspx. Accessed 9 Sept 2017

The Joint Commission International (2011) Patients beyond Borders. http://www.patientsbeyondborders. com/about/accreditation-agency/joint-commission-international. Accessed 29 July 2017

Transcultural C.A.R.E. Associates (2015) http://www. transculturalcare.net. Accessed 29 July 2017

Triandis H (2001) Individualism-collectivism and personality. J Pers 69(6):907–924

Case Study: Traditional Health Beliefs of Arabic Culture During Pregnancy

7

Jehad O. Halabi

Muna is 37 years old. She is 5 months pregnant and has insulin-dependent diabetes mellitus, hypertension, and anemia. She has four children; two were born by cesarean section. The household income is equivalent to US $150 per month, and she lives in a rural area with her in-laws. Muna completed her education until sixth grade and then left school because it was far from her home. She married at the age of 16 to Ali who is 50 years old and employed in a cement factory. He also has insulin-dependent diabetes mellitus and hypertension, and he is a heavy smoker. Muna is his second wife. Muna's cousin, Huda, is a nursing student. One day, Huda visited Muna and had the following discussion.

Huda: (Knocks on the door.)

Muna: "Whose there?"

Huda: "This is your cousin Huda."

Muna: (Kissing her) "Welcome, I haven't seen you for a long time. I miss you. Come in for coffee."

Huda: "Oh, are you pregnant again?"

Muna: (Laughing and saying) "Yeah. I'm 5 months pregnant because my husband likes children."

Huda: "Why did you become pregnant? You have diabetes, hypertension, and anemia. Your last baby is about 7 months old, and you can hardly afford your family's expenses."

Muna: "My husband refuses to let me use any family planning method. He wants a large family. He thought that the children might support him when he gets older. Do you want my husband to marry another woman?"

Huda: "What about Ali's diabetes and hypertension? We discussed these conditions in our class today. Is he still smoking heavily?"

Muna: "His sugar level and blood pressure are always high."

Huda: "How about your sugar and blood pressure?"

Muna: "They are high too."

Huda: "Aren't you following the treatments as you should?"

Muna: "Sometimes I do. You know it is hard to afford insulin. It is expensive. We borrow some medicine from our neighbors. They told us that it works well. We tried different kinds of herbs. My mother gave me this blue stone to put around my neck to prevent others' envy to affect my health."

Huda: "Oh Muna, this is nonsense. Yesterday I called my mother to ask about your health. I was surprised that she doesn't know that you have diabetes and high blood pressure. You said that even your husband doesn't know?"

Muna: Shouting at Huda. "Did you tell her that we both have diabetes?"

J. O. Halabi, Ph.D., R.N., T.N.S.
College of Nursing, King Saud bin Abdulaziz
University of Health Sciences—National Guard,
Al Ahsa, Kingdom of Saudi Arabia
e-mail: halabije@nga.med.sa, halabij@ksau-hs.edu.sa

© Springer International Publishing AG, part of Springer Nature 2018
M. Douglas et al. (eds.), *Global Applications of Culturally Competent Health Care: Guidelines for Practice*, https://doi.org/10.1007/978-3-319-69332-3_7

Huda: "Why are you angry? Is it a shame that anybody knows this?"

Muna: "Yes. I have a daughter, who is 14, and she is at the age of getting married. I am afraid that nobody will ask to marry her. You know people think diabetes is a hereditary disease. You forget this, but you belong to our culture."

Huda: "But you believe in Allah. You told me before that having pain, sickness, and illness is a means of guaranteeing physical and psychological peace. You said it removes your sins and helps you go to paradise. Oh God! How do I solve this conflict! Am I a bad nursing student?"

Muna: "I agree with you. I try to do what you told me, but you should ask me first if I want anybody to know that I have diabetes. Do you want to drink tea?"

(They continue their conversation while drinking tea.)

Huda: "Where do you think you will deliver the baby?"

Muna: "Maybe at home."

Huda: "I forgot to tell you that a nurse will come to visit you. I saw her at the clinic. She was asking people for directions to your house."

(The nurse knocks on the door.)

Nurse: "Good morning Muna."

Muna: "Good morning Nurse. The tea is still warm. Come in. This is my cousin Huda. She is a nursing student."

Nurse: "How are you Muna? How do you feel today?"

Muna: "Well, I'm *ok*. Don't worry about me. I can take care of myself. But how did you find my home?"

Nurse: "Muna, I asked the neighbors and people in the street about the diabetic woman who lives here. It wasn't easy to find you; it seems that they don't know you have diabetes."

Muna: "My God! Why you tell everybody? Both of you put me in trouble. What should I do? This is a disaster. My husband doesn't know I have diabetes. What if he found out? What if he left me? What if nobody marries my daughters?" Crying…

Nurse: "I came here to follow up on your treatment plan. Why did you miss your last clinic appointment? I told you about the importance of diet and exercise. Did you follow my suggestions?"

Huda: "I think she doesn't follow any of your suggestions."

Muna: "How do you expect me to follow your suggestions with this hard life? How can I cook special food for myself while I have large family, and they can see what I eat? I also can't afford it. You want me to exercise and walk around in the street where people can observe me! How can I do that? What will they say about me?"

Nurse: "I don't understand what you mean. I assume that everybody can do that if they want to. Do you follow the 2500 calorie diet that I gave you? I noted at the clinic that your weight is increasing."

Muna: "Yes I follow exactly the 2500 g you told me about."

Nurse: "Can you show me how you follow it and do the calculations?"

Muna: "Here is the scale I bought from the grocery shop. I put the food on the scale up to 2500 g, and then I eat it. I do that all the time since you told me."

Nurse: "My God, you don't understand. I said 2500 calories not grams. You are..."

Muna: "Nurse, I don't understand. You are shouting at me, and at the clinic the doctor asked me why I continue to look like a cow. What is this? I don't want your help; leave me alone."

Huda: "You know. She also borrows medications from her neighbors."

Nurse: "You borrow medication? Why?"

Muna: "Well, all medications are the same. We all share medications with one another. At the end, God controls everything, and it is in His hands. Why bother? Take it easy and forget it. I have been doing that for a long time. You never asked me about that."

Nurse: "I don't want to force you to do things. You know God's order to take care of ourselves. We will talk about it later. Can we just talk about the plan for this visit?"

Muna: "Can you tell me why you came here for this visit. What brought you here? After all, you exposed my secret to everybody. What do you want?"

Nurse: "I want to talk to you about your health. Do you have any concerns?"

Muna: "I suffer from heartburn, and somebody told me that it is due to the hair of the baby. I was told not to drink cinnamon because it initiates contractions and not to sleep with my husband because it affects the baby's development. They also told me not to take a warm bath because it affects the baby's movement. I heard that I should eat whatever I desire so that the baby will not have any birthmarks on his body. I have to avoid drinking too much water to minimize going to the bathroom often."

Nurse: "You have misinformation (misunderstanding) about certain issues, especially changes related to pregnancy. This pamphlet will give you more information. I will visit you next Monday at 10 am."

Huda: "So this is how difficult patients will be when I graduate from nursing. I am leaving now."

(The nurse and Muna continue to talk.)

Muna: "Ok nurse, please don't go now. I have things to say but I couldn't say them in Huda's presence."

Nurse: "We can talk about it next time."

Muna: "Let's visit my neighbor Sawsan. She had her first baby boy."

(Muna and the nurse knocked on Sawsan's door.)

Muna: "Hello Sawsan, I have the nurse with me (shakes her hand). I want her to see how good I am. Do you follow what I told you to do after the delivery?"

Sawsan: "Oh, I did everything you told me to do."

Nurse: "What have you told her to do?"

Muna: "She should stay in bed for 40 days and should avoid getting close to her husband till the end of 40 days, not taking a shower, not drinking lemon, and not letting anybody enter her room while she has her menses because this will affect her milk. Wait until after the third day of delivery to start breastfeeding because it isn't healthy for the baby. Don't use any family planning method because that could lead to becoming barren. Don't let anybody see her baby until she puts the blue stone around his neck (to ward off envy). I also told her she should wrap a belt around her

abdomen to let her uterus return to its normal position. She should also eat lots of meat and chicken every day. She should eat enough for two people, not just one."

Nurse: "Really! What about her baby Muna? Did you tell her anything special?"

Muna: "I told her many things! Like, she should put kuhl/kohl around his eyes to make them look bigger. And wrap him tightly with a sheet to let him grow taller and to help him sleep better. She should put salt and oil on his body and leave it on for 10 hours in order to make his skin softer. She should also put some Arabic coffee or kohl on his umbilicus to promote healing."

Nurse: "Oh Muna, how can you tell her these things? These practices are crazy and unhealthy. Here is a pamphlet with suggestions from health professionals. I should tell your doctor what you are doing so he can arrange to have an open discussion with you about these things next week."

Muna: "Nurse, you think that I can read these things! You always give me papers to read. But I can arrange with my neighbors to attend this discussion with me. They can help me understand."

Nurse: "Oh, yes. Good, you women in the countryside understand each other very well. How about if you all come to the health center and have this open discussion there with other women like yourself?"

Muna: "We will meet there if we can. We will have to ask our husbands' permission and then let you know."

Nurse: "Why ask your husband? You should make more decisions independently. Don't be 'weak' women. I don't understand you. You can't even make a small decision like this. I'm leaving now."

Muna and Sawsan: "Are we small children? I thought we are grown up women. We are nothing as you see."

Nurse: "Bye, Salam-Alaikum."

7.1   Cultural Issues

The patient is a middle-aged rural pregnant woman with limited formal education and has diabetes mellitus, hypertension, and anemia. Her illnesses were unknown to her husband, relatives, and neighbors. These diseases are disorders characterized by chronicity and predispose the person to an increased risk of complications. They have an impact on the mother and baby, resulting in a high-risk pregnancy. The risks are higher due to nonadherence with medication.

This patient is unable to afford the medications due to her low socioeconomic status. She shares and borrows medications. Like many rural women, she uses traditional herbs. This can lead to psychosocial problems or complications with prescriptive medications (Cleveland Clinic 2017).

The patient has cultural beliefs and perceptions about health and practices that could put her at risk. She hides diabetes from others because she believes that it is shameful. It could cause negative perceptions by her neighbors and lead to unacceptance. The client fears marriage insecurity and failure. She had multiple pregnancies and avoided family planning to stay secure. In addition, she used traditional treatments and amulets for protection and ward off envy. These perceptions need to be carefully assessed and considered in planning health care for this client.

The patient has misinformation about pregnancy and postpartum care. She follows several cultural practices that are based on traditional beliefs and perceptions. Women exchange these ideas through their social interactions with others, including their neighbors.

The patient indicated the necessity of asking her husband about attending the clinic and expressed that any such activities are needed to be discussed with the spouse ahead of time. She is not allowed to make a decision on her own.

The nurse, a role model, and the nursing student have their assumptions about this client. Insufficient assessment and awareness of the client's beliefs were judgmental and lacked respect. The nurse followed the medical model ideas and assumed that her scientifically based advice would be followed. She bombarded the patient with information learned in college without incorporating the patient's personal and cultural values and beliefs. Even though they both are from the same cultural background, they have

not explored the subculture and worldview of this rural patient. The nurse and the nursing student were not effective in understanding the patient's concerns. The patient tried to express her thoughts and beliefs to the nurse, assuming that they would understand her. They were not effective.

Communication with the patient was limited to providing her with written instructions in the form of a pamphlet. The assumption was that the patient would be able to figure out, on her own, the misconceptions and questionable practices. The nurse assumed that the patient could read and understand the pamphlets. She failed to assess the educational and background level of the patient to make sure she could read and benefit from such material.

The nurse criticized the patient and accused her of being crazy because she was following potentially unhealthy practices for the mother and the baby. She labeled the client by stating "rural women understand each other."

The nurse accused the patient of being a weak woman who could not make a small decision on her own. The patient felt belittled and that she was being treated like "a small child." The patient recognized that the nurse was talking to them in a condescending way (inferiorly).

7.2　Culturally Competent Strategies Recommended

Pregnant women are at an increased risk for health problems. Rural women from Arabic cultures are particularly at risk of health problems due to multiple pregnancies and increased incidence of chronic health problems such as diabetes, hypertension, and anemia. Their health beliefs and practices might be of special concern to nurses because they are disrespected or unrecognized.

Health is highly individual and influenced by everything with whom clients interact, including their internal and external environment (WHO 2006). Values are transmitted from and influenced by their sociocultural traditions and environment (Berman et al. 2016). Patients' cultural beliefs and values are reflected in their behaviors and practices. These cannot be judged as right or wrong by nurses who have differing values from that of their clients. Rather, values and beliefs need to be examined and clarified using a caring process of values clarification.

7.2.1 Individual and Family Level Recommendations

- Remain objective without conveying approval or disapproval to avoid biases and misconceptions that may lead to cultural imposition and force personal values and beliefs on other cultures and subcultures (Miller-Keane 2003).
- Promote behavioral changes through education and practice.
- Respect patients' different values and beliefs. Learn about clients' values, beliefs, norms, customs, and practices to develop culturally congruent practice.
- Search for information about the culture of patients.
- Be committed to respecting the principal values of any culture and avoid voicing disagreement with values that can create conflicting situations.
- Accept differing nonharmful values, beliefs, and perceptions among different cultures as well as within cultures (Ludwick and Silva 2000).
- Assess beliefs within a cultural context.

7.2.2 Organizational Level Interventions

- Incorporate cultural care and related concepts in the curriculum and provide learning experiences for nursing students at all levels. Incorporate role-playing and drama using real case scenarios and situations from different cultures.
- Establish continuing education programs and in-service training activities for nurses to update their cultural knowledge and competence with different cultural groups.

- Provide opportunities for nursing students to come in contact with patients from a variety of cultural and ethnic groups where possible.
- Encourage participation of nurses and nursing students in various activities that aim to increase their cultural skills such as seminars, workshops, conferences, online material, and exchange opportunities if available (Gebru and Willman 2010; Mager and Grossman 2013) and global learning experiences (Jones et al. 2010).
- Provide certified programs or certified cultural classes/courses through known cultural societies and/or experts from different cultures.
- Incorporate cultural assessment tools (Purnell 2014; Purnell and Finkl 2017) as part of health records and care plans for patients.
- Conduct research studies to assess students and nurses' cultural competence in order to plan action plans and programs.

7.2.3 Community Societal Level Recommendations

- Collect information about cultural and sociodemographic data of patients from different cultures (such as Arab and rural communities) as well as the health beliefs and norms related to health, illness, and care.
- Understand that health decisions are not necessarily made by one individual. In some cultures, patients have to include their families, relatives, community, and even society in simple decisions.
- Explore how to incorporate cultural sensitivity into nursing care. Do not assume that a non-Western (e.g., Arab) patient can have full control over health decisions as in Western culture. These decisions are usually made by somebody else, such as the head of the family or the elder person and, therefore, should be respected as part of their traditions (Berman et al. 2012).
- Recognize that even when people are from the same culture, there are diversity and variation within the group (e.g., rural vs. urban). For example, the Arab regions extend across 23

countries who share similar language and traditions; however, each region has its own specific practices (Berman et al. 2012; Muliira and Muliira 2013; Nies and McEwan 2007).

- Provide culturally sensitive care and avoid stereotyping clients and focus on differences as well as similarities (Leininger 1991, 2002).
- Recognize that the cognitive aspects of specific cultural groups can lead to stereotyping instead of identifying the unique needs of the patient (Williamsona and Harrison 2010).
- Cultural preservation and maintenance entail the use of cultural practices for health and use of herbs, as well as the cultural accommodation of clients' opinions and negotiation, helping create a linkage between the nurse's scientific framework and the cultural perspectives of patients (Berman et al. 2016; Leininger 2002).
- Collaborate with key community leaders and plan culturally congruent health campaigns aimed at health awareness and health promotion for pregnant as well as other women.
- Establish partnerships with local communities in order to disseminate information and health education programs related to women's health, especially at-risk women.
- Establish support groups and common-interest groups for women from disadvantaged areas such as rural women.
- Encourage women leaders to come forward and help other women from the same cultural background.
- Prepare health education material in a simple format consistent with the educational level of recipients.
- Train traditional midwives who work with pregnant women to provide safe and cultural competent care to women and their children.

Conclusion

Clients might have several misunderstandings and health beliefs adopted from their communities. Their educational background might limit their ability to seek and obtain information about their health as well as their pregnancy and neonatal care. This case study is further complicated by the fears related to marriage and concern for children's future. The fear of stigmatization limits patients' interactions with people and the ability to disclose health situation to others such as close family and husband.

Furthermore, financial limitations as well as knowledge deficits hinder the patient's compliance with treatment standards and evidence-based practice. An inability to make an autonomous decision is evident due to family's cultural interaction system. The nurse lacked cultural competence for assessing and planning culturally congruent interventions for the patient, even though she came from a similar cultural background. In addition, she was not a role model for the nursing student in her interaction. Cultural assumptions and impositions must be avoided in providing care to patients from diverse cultures. A recommendation is to use the Guidelines for Implementing Culturally Competent Nursing Care (Douglas et al. 2014). Different strategies and interventions are needed at different levels for the patient and her family, the organization, and as well as the wider community to enhance the best evidence-based cultural care for pregnant women from a disadvantaged environment.

References

Berman A, Erb GL, Snyder S, Abdalrahim MS, Abu-Moghli F et al (eds) (2012) Fundamentals of nursing concepts, process and practice. Arab World Edition. Pearson International, New Jersey

Berman A, Snyder SJ, Fransden G (eds) (2016) Kozier and Erb's fundamentals of nursing concepts, process and practice, 10th edn. Pearson International, New Jersey

Cleveland Clinic (2017) Herbal supplements, helpful of harmful. https://my.clevelandclinic.org/health/articles/herbal-supplements-heart-health. Accessed 28 Apr 2017

Douglas MK, Rosenkoetter M, Pacquiao D, Callister LC et al (2014) Guidelines for implementing culturally competent nursing care. J Transcult Nurs 25(2):109–121. https://doi.org/10.1177/1043659614520998

Gebru K, Willman A (2010) Education to promote culturally competent nursing care—a content analysis of student responses. Nurse Educ Today 30:54–60. https://doi.org/10.1016/j.nedt.2009.06.005

Jones ED, Ivanov LL, Wallace D, VonCannon L (2010) Global service learning project influences culturally sensitive care. Home Health Care Manag Pract 22(7):464–469. https://doi.org/10.1177/1084822310368657

Leininger M (1991) Culture care diversity and universality: a theory of nursing. National League for Nursing Press, New York

Leininger MM (2002) Culture care theory: a major contribution to advance transcultural nursing knowledge and practices. J Transcult Nurs 13(1):189–192

Ludwick R, Silva MC (2000) Ethics: nursing around the world: cultural values and ethical conflicts. Online J Issues Nurs 5(3). www.nursingworld.org/MainMenuCategories/ANAMarketplace/ANAPeriodicals/OJIN/Columns/Ethics/CulturalValuesandEthicalConflicts.aspx. Accessed 29 Apr 2017

Mager DR, Grossman S (2013) Promoting nursing students' understanding and reflection on cultural awareness with older adults in home care. Home Healthc Nurse 31(10):582–588

Miller-Keane (2003) Miller-Keane encyclopedia and dictionary of medicine, nursing, and allied health, 7th edn.

Saunders, an imprint of Elsevier, Inc. http://medical-dictionary.thefreedictionary.com/cultural+imposition. Accessed 29 Apr 2017

Muliira JK, Muliira RS (2013) Teaching culturally appropriate therapeutic touch to nursing students in the Sultanate of Oman. Holist Nurs Pract 27(1):45–48. https://doi.org/10.1097/HNP.0b013e318276fccf

Nies MA, McEwan M (eds) (2007) Community/Public health nursing: promoting the health of population, 4th edn. Saunders Elsevier, St. Louis

Purnell L (ed) (2014) Transcultural healthcare: a culturally competent approach, 4th edn. F.A. Davis, Philadelphia

Purnell L, Finkl E (eds) (2017) Guide to culturally competent health care. F.A. Davis, Philadelphia

WHO (2006) Constitution of the World Health Organization. World Health Organization, Geneva. http://www.who.int/governance/eb/who_constitution_en.pdf. Accessed 26 May 2017

Williamsona M, Harrison L (2010) Providing culturally appropriate care: a literature review. https://doi.org/10.1016/j.ijnurstu.2009.12.012. Accessed 26 May 2017

Case Study: Perceived Cultural Discord and Possible Discrimination Involving a Moroccan Truck Driver in Italy

8

Alessandro Stievano, Gennaro Rocco, and Giordano Cotichelli

Ahmed is a 40-year-old Moroccan truck driver who has been working in Italy for the last 13 years. Ahmed has a basic level of education and a sufficient conversational skill in the Italian language. Ahmed lives alone, and although is married with two children, his wife and children were left behind in Morocco. He is also financially accountable for his visually disabled younger brother who lives in Morocco. Ahmed, being the sole breadwinner, relies on his truck driving job to support himself, his immediate family, and his brother's family (Pfau-Effinger 2004).

Ahmed travels back to Morocco a couple of times year where he is often greeted with joy and gratitude for the financial support he offers. Ahmed wishes that one day, once he is financially capable, he could return to Morocco; however, as an added security option, he is also pursuing steps to acquire Italian citizenship. Given his truck driving occupation, Ahmed did not have opportunities to develop strong ties with the local Moroccan immigrant community in his town of residence in the Northern Italy. His connection to the community was through sporadic contacts with the local imam (religious clerk).

A few months ago, Ahmed started to experience and complained of severe acute back pain. Over time his pain became more frequent and more intense. One night he was obliged to rush to the accident and emergency room where he was visited by an orthopedic surgeon who advised him to have a series of examinations to rule out spondyloarthrosis. He prescribed a therapy with nonsteroidal anti-inflammatory drugs and suggested that he take time off work to rest and heal. The physician also advised him to modify his work duties and refrain from continuing as a truck driver.

8.1 Cultural Issues

As was recommended by the treating physician, Ahmed took 2 weeks off work to rest and to receive anti-inflammatory injection to relieve his pain. However, he refrained from seeking further diagnostic testing as ordered by the accident and emergency room physician. The truck company proprietor was very sympathetic with his condition and allowed Ahmed to modify his work duties by offering him an office position as an accountant. While Ahmed appreciated his boss's accommodation, he nonetheless was worried that

A. Stievano, Ph.D., M.Sc.N., R.N. (✉)
University of Tor Vergata, Rome, Italy

Center for Nursing Excellence, Ipasvi Rome Nursing Board, Rome, Italy

G. Rocco, Ph.D., R.N., FAAN
Centre of Excellence for Nursing Scholarship, Ipasvi Rome Nursing Board, Rome, Italy

G. Cotichelli, Ph.D., R.N.
Faculty of Medicine, University of Ancona, Ancona, Italy

© Springer International Publishing AG, part of Springer Nature 2018
M. Douglas et al. (eds.), *Global Applications of Culturally Competent Health Care: Guidelines for Practice*, https://doi.org/10.1007/978-3-319-69332-3_8

his income would be impacted. His very reason for being in Italy and away from his family is that they depended on his ability to generate income to sustain himself and his family.

While receiving injection therapy in a nursing-run outpatient clinic, Ahmed resisted the nurse's effort to help him adhere to the treating physician's order for further diagnostic tests. He did not engage in the nurse's therapeutic care plan, and at some point during the course of treatment, he became belligerent and argumentative. He shifted blame for not getting better on the dysfunctional bureaucratic system.

Efforts toward establishing and building a therapeutic relationship with Ahmed came to a halt when his demeanor became verbally aggressive with the nursing staff. The result of this harsh conversation was a further worsening of an already degraded relationship with the nursing staff. Ahmed, at a certain point to avoid possible debates with the healthcare team, declared that he would be better off if he received the injections from a fellow countryman who had studied medicine in Morocco. He also was against having an orthopedic consultation and possible diagnostic workup for fear that a potential orthopedic diagnosis may declare him unfit, potentially losing his truck driving job. He was also scared of losing the right to ask for Italian citizenship.

Ahmed's physical health worsened due to his excessive use of steroidal anti-inflammatory drugs—drugs for which Ahmed experienced gastric discomfort—although he was verbally informed about possible gastric complications by the orthopedic surgeon in the accident and emergency room. Despite the fact that Ahmed had an adequate command of the Italian language, during one of his visits to the outpatient department, he was not able to make himself fully understood and explain the pain he felt in direct relation to gastric symptomatology.

The attending nurse also ignored his complaints because she was convinced that it was just another excuse to keep him on the anti-inflammatory injection therapy. Ahmed perceived the nurse's lack of attention to his complaints based on prejudice and racism. He was justifying his attitude on his overall perception of narrow-mindedness against people who were coming from the Maghreb region in Morocco. However, some nurses working in the clinic had concerns and doubted that Ahmed was "another of those North Africans" who did not feel like having a burdensome and onerous job and that he longed for having the nonsteroidal anti-inflammatory drugs just to receive some more time off work.

8.2   Cultural Issues

To study the global movements of people is a health priority in the globalized world (Tschudin and Davis 2008). The mass inflow of immigrants and refugees to Italy is very complicated and goes beyond traditional migration theories of push-and-pull factors (Prescott and Nichter 2014). In fact, the interconnections of political and economic reasons that are at the ground of the migratory processes to Italy ought to be analyzed through the lens of the ever-changing global trajectories (Stievano et al. 2017). Despite the 2008 economic recession, Italy is a country that hosts a high number of immigrants: 5,200,000 (Idos Migrantes 2016). Italy is Europe's main gateway for asylum-seekers from Africa. Although most of those asylum-seekers are rescued during the journey from the North African coasts to the Southern Italy shores, a large percentage of these refugees end up being homeless in Italy and in other European nations due to the lack of supportive systems. Italy is home to immigrant from North African and Eastern European countries. Romanian immigrants form the largest group (1,131,839, 22.9%), followed by Moroccans (510,450, 13%), Albanians (490,483, 9.3%), Chinese (265,820, 5.4%), and Ukrainians (226,060, 4.6%). Other immigrants are from the Philippines 3.3%, India 3.0%, Moldova 2.8%, Bangladesh 2.4%, and Egypt 2.2% (Idos Migrantes 2016). Hence, Moroccans are the second largest immigrant community in Italy and represent one of the most important countries in the Maghreb area. Nowadays, the migration from Morocco to Italy is one of the longest and largest migrations in Europe, and Moroccans who are present in Italy in 2016 were

510,450 which is equal to 13% of the non-European residents in Italy (Ministry of Work and Social Welfare 2016).

There is no doubt that the continuous influx of immigrants is taxing the Italian systems, especially the housing and the healthcare system. The Italian society is reeling the brunt of immigrant groups who do not know or adhere to the local norms or abide the laws. Current security concerns in Italy and worldwide may heighten stereotypes and may have an impact on the nature of care that is offered or perceived. Adding to the already held negative attitude that Moroccans tend to avoid hard work, the potential for non-culturally responsive healthcare encounters is very high.

After having delineated the cultural setting where this case had taken place, some considerations must to be highlighted. Ahmed's impetus for coming to Italy is similar to those of his compatriots—the search for economic opportunities with higher pay and better working conditions (Correia et al. 2015). Ahmed came seeking work in Italy in order to provide not only for his own immediate family but also for his extended family. In the eyes of his family, he is the beacon of hope and the anchor for their survival and potential progress. This conceptual mindset is possibly the source of anxiety and uncertainty for Ahmed because, as his health is worsened, he is likely to fail in meeting the financial obligation toward his family.

Ahmed's possible avoidance of seeking further orthopedic consultation may be based on his fear of being labeled inept or disabled and as such limit his chances to continue with his truck driving job. Ahmed is also frightened to seek help from his fellow citizens and from the spiritual guide of his community, the Imam, because he fears he could be seen as a fragile man. He is also worried that his dignity and reputation as a strong man who is looked up to may be tarnished.

8.3 Culturally Competent Strategies Recommended

In healthcare settings with cross-cultural encounters such as the case of Ahmed, the knowledge and skills of the healthcare provider demand not only knowledge and skills of the client culture and the societal stigma associated with the client's background but, as in this situation, require the reflective unpacking and evaluation of the client's personnel trials and tribulation and his or her real or perceived threats of discrimination due to racism. As a strategy, healthcare providers must consider multidimensional assessment and intervention approaches.

8.3.1 Individual-/Family-Level Interventions

- Assessment must include external forces impacting the person and the available coping resources.
- Assessment and intervention strategies of the contextual variables impacting the cross-cultural health encounter include the organizational and socio-structural levels of interventions to meet the healthcare needs of persons similar to Ahmed's.
- Consideration of the geopolitical forces and their impact on the host society and on the individual immigrant is increasingly important in ensuring fair treatment.
- Offering interprofessional case studies and educational lectures/seminars to enhance healthcare providers' understanding of intersecting cross cultural variables that can potentially affect the healthcare outcomes of persons similar to Ahmed's.
- Attention should be paid to repairing and rebuilding the therapeutic relationship between Ahmed and the nursing staff through intentional and focused communication and problem-solving among the healthcare providers and through a culturally responsive care plan (Bergum and Dossetor 2005).

8.3.2 Organizational-Level Interventions

- Establish specific policies and procedures focused on the care of vulnerable and underserved immigrant populations with a special emphasis on social determinant variables such as gender, age, ethnic and religious backgrounds, and cultural beliefs and values.

- Supportive health organization's resources are required to assist healthcare providers in delivering culturally responsive healthcare.
- Offer ongoing training and education toward culturally responsive and congruent care and language and cultural interpretive services.

8.3.3 Community-/Societal-Level Interventions

- An enhanced evaluation of the influxes of immigrants is the first step to carry out a personalized cultural congruent plan of care (Douglas et al. 2014).
- Know the diverse habits of the main ethnic groups and provide information that healthcare providers should consider in order to have a stronger connection with the North African community.
- Involve social care networks to provide a better link with the North African community to assist in improving the understanding of Ahmed's social and economic concerns by healthcare providers.
- Social work professionals should strategically connect Ahmed with his community and with a religious guide to provide advice, support, and resources.

Conclusion

Ahmed's clinical case represents a common health situation in Italy where the culture, organizations, and professionals intersect to produce unwarranted negative health encounters for both the patient and the healthcare provider. Offering quality, cost-effective, and culturally responsive healthcare outcomes requires knowledge and skills on the part of healthcare providers, supportive resources on the part of the healthcare organizations, and culturally responsive community resources.

Acknowledgments The authors of this case study would like to acknowledge the assistance of Marianne Hattar-Pollara, PhD, RN, FAAN in editing this case study. Dr. Hattar-Pollara is the Chair of the Department of Nursing at California State University, Northridge. Her email is marianne.hattar@csun.edu.

References

Bergum V, Dossetor J (2005) Relational ethics: the full meaning of respect. University Publishing Group, Hagerstown

Correia T, Dussault G, Pontes C (2015) The impact of the financial crisis on human resources for health policies in three southern-Europe countries. Health Policy 119:1600–1605

Douglas MK, Rosenkoetter M, Pacquiao DF, Callister LC, Hattar-Pollara M, Lauderdale J, Purnell L (2014) Guidelines for implementing culturally competent nursing care. J Transcult Nurs 25(2):109–121. https://doi.org/10.1177/1043659614520998

Idos Migrantes (2016) Statistic immigration report 2016. Imprinting Publishing, Rome

Ministry of Work and Social Welfare (2016) The Moroccan community in Italy. Annual report on the presence of migrants. Anpal Servizi, Rome

Pfau-Effinger B (2004) Socio-historical paths of the male breadwinner model—an explanation of cross-national differences. Br J Sociol 55(3):377–399

Prescott M, Nichter M (2014) Transnational nurse migration: future directions for medical anthropological research. Soc Sci Med 107:113–123

Stievano A, Olsen D, Tolentino Diaz Y, Sabatino L, Rocco G (2017) Indian nurses in Italy: a qualitative study of their professional and social integration. J Clin Nurs 26(23–24):4234–4245. https://doi.org/10.1111/jocn.13746

Tschudin V, Davis AJ (2008) The globalisation of nursing. Radcliffe Publishing, Abingdon

Case Study: A Multiracial Man Seeks Care in the Emergency Department

Marianne R. Jeffreys

Franklin is a 58-year-old multiethnic, multiracial man of African-American, Cherokee, and Scottish background who views all aspects of his heritage as important. He also considers being multiracial as a unique cultural experience. He grew up in a multi-generation household consisting of his paternal grandmother (Cherokee), mother (third-generation Scottish-American), father (African-American and Cherokee), and his three brothers and two sisters. Unable to marry in their home state due to miscegenation laws, Franklin's parents married in a US state that permitted interracial marriages where they then settled to start a new life and family together. The opening of a factory with employee housing provided steady employment that led to a factory-sponsored mortgage to purchase a family home in a new housing development bordering the factory. Although federal laws purported "equal opportunities" in employment, education, and housing, the reality was that overt and covert discrimination existed, so factory work and company housing were greatly welcomed.

With both high school-educated parents working many overtime shifts, Franklin and his siblings were raised by his grandmother who shared many Cherokee traditions through storytelling, cooking, and everyday activities. Although never

M. R. Jeffreys, Ed.D., R.N.
Graduate College and College of Staten Island, The City University of New York (CUNY),
New York, NY, USA

able to quit smoking, she strongly insisted that her grandchildren would never become smokers and advocated a diet of fresh vegetables, poultry, and fish, outdoor exercise, and post-secondary trade school or college education. The family's diet consisted of many fresh vegetables grown in their backyard, fish and crabs caught in the adjacent river, and eggs and chickens from a nearby farm.

The factory has long been closed, with the dilapidated property now declared a superfund site that is yet to be cleaned and proclaimed environmentally safe. The nearby farm, frequently sprayed with pesticides during the 1960s and 1970s, had been recently transformed from a remediated superfund site to a crowded low-income housing complex. Signs along the riverbank display warnings against eating more than one fish or crab per month, noting extra cautions for pregnant women and young children. Franklin's grandmother, a lifelong smoker, died 2 decades ago from a stroke, but his parents still reside in the family homestead, fondly reminiscing about times gone past, still in love and unable to imagine living anywhere else but "home." Since completing college on a baseball scholarship and graduate school at age 25, Franklin has been working as a high school teacher and baseball coach in a suburban town where he currently lives with his Argentinian-born wife (also a high school teacher) and their two children. On the way to his weekly visit to assist his elderly parents, Franklin stops at the one remaining local store (deli-liquor-drugstore) to pick up their prescriptions and unknowingly startles two armed men in the midst of a robbery. When Franklin flings himself in front of a pregnant teenager to protect her, he suffers a gunshot wound to the right side of the abdomen yet manages to divert other gunshots by forcefully pitching several cans of prominently displayed spam that knock out one robber and disarm and injure the other.

A work-up at the emergency room reveals that Franklin's general health is excellent; however, the doctor tells him that the abdominal scan shows a right colon mass. During emergency abdominal surgery, the surgeon removes the bullet and mass and suspects that the biopsy will confirm colon cancer. While lying semi-awake in the recovery room, Franklin overhears someone say "You would think that a black man who survived this long would know better than to still be involved in gangs and crime in that horrible neighborhood. They must have been after drugs or drug money. We better make sure he doesn't get too much narcotics. We taxpayers will end up paying for his cancer treatment one way or the other through Medicaid or the prison system. It just isn't fair."

Franklin feels angry, hurt, invisible, mislabeled, profiled, alone, sad, anxious, mistreated, and vulnerable. Vital signs on his monitor show an immediate jump of 30 beats/min and BP jumps from 124/76 to 152/92. More alert now and fighting anesthesia drowsiness, Franklin feels severe pain but hesitates to request medicine. Fatigued from his immediate response to discrimination-related stress, post-traumatic stress (crime victim), and postoperative stress, he falls into an exhausted sleep. Later, excruciating pain jolts him awake.

9.1   Cultural Issues

"Multiple heritage identity can include simultaneous membership with two or more distinct groups, membership within one select group, synthesis of cultures, and/or fluid identities that change with time, circumstances, and setting.

Many multiple heritage individuals acknowledge being multiracial or multiethnic as a separate and unique culture" (Root 1992, 1997; Jeffreys and Zoucha 2001, 2017a, b, c: 81). Individuals within multiracial families may also self-identify with groups different than their siblings or other family members (Root 1993; Tutwiler 2016).

Despite multidisciplinary literature documenting disparities in past and present-day life experiences of multiracial individuals (Remedios and Chasteen 2013; Tran et al. 2016), they lack visibility in the nursing and healthcare literature (Jeffreys and Zoucha 2017a, b). Additionally, anti-discrimination policies are frequently directed at individuals who identify with a single race (minority group), keeping multiracial individuals "invisible" and marginalized. In an effort to make this invisible group "visible," Tutwiler (2016) introduced the term "fifth minority."

While also noting that much diversity and varied experiences exist for mixed-race individuals within families, schools, communities, and society, mixed-race individuals more frequently have their heritage and identity questioned, challenged, ignored, and/or pressured to select one choice over others (Tutwiler 2016). Forced-choice dilemmas such as presenting a demographic form stating "select one" restrict identity autonomy and contribute to psychological stress (Sanchez 2010). Furthermore, forced-choice dilemmas may foster beliefs that multiracial identity is unacceptable, stigmatized, undesirable, and devalued by society. Sanchez's (2010) study suggests that multiracial people with black heritage encounter the most forced-choice dilemmas. Such experiences can result in cultural pain and adversely affect quality of everyday life and health (Jeffreys and Zoucha 2017a, b, c).

9.2   Social Structural Factors

Almost every time the US Census has been administered, it has contained different categories, and it continues to change. It was not until 1960 that Americans could choose their own race. Forty years later, Americans were permitted to select more than one option. In 2010, approximately nine million Americans selected more than one race, with Latino-white being the highest combination (Davenport 2016; Pew Commission 2015). By 2050, it is predicted that one in five Americans will claim multiracial heritage (Farley 2001; Jackson and Samuels 2011).

At one time or another until 1967, miscegenation laws in 41 US states or colonies prevented marriages, relationships, sexual intercourse, or unions between whites and 1 or more of the following groups: African-Americans, American Indians, Chinese, Filipinos, Hindus, Japanese, Koreans, Malays, and Mongolians. Of the 227 court of appeals cases concerning miscegenation (1850 to 1970), 95 were recorded as criminal (Pascoe 1996; Jeffreys and Zoucha 2001, 2017b). Children born of such unions often suffered social and economic disadvantages of illegitimacy, were stigmatized, and were assigned the racial status low on the hierarchy with "white" being highest in a society of white versus nonwhite and the hypodescent rule (one drop rule) putting blacks in the lowest status. Such disadvantages impacted opportunities for education, jobs, housing, environment, food security, and access to quality healthcare and services. In contemporary society, both conscious and unconscious biases toward minorities and multiracial children and families contribute to disparities (DeJesus et al. 2016).

9.3 Culturally Competent Strategies Recommended

Many past and present social structural factors have impacted Franklin's health and illness experience. In addition to actions specific to assist Franklin, education for all staff members is required, and reaching out to community is essential.

9.3.1 Individual-/Family-Level Interventions

- On admission (after explaining rationale for cultural background and identity questions), conduct an in-depth assessment of the person's cultural background, self-identity, values, beliefs, and healthcare practices.
- Proactively initiate culturally congruent education and screening based on the person's background (genetics), family history, lifestyle, and environmental risk factors.
- Be aware of past and current ethnohistorical, political, social, economic, and environmental factors that influence the lifestyle, health, and opportunities of multiracial, multiethnic individuals.
- Respect that multiracial people have the right to self-identify with one or more cultural identities, change self-identification over time or circumstance, embrace all identities in varying degrees, consider being multiracial as a unique identity, and change any of the above without explanation (Root 1993).
- Proactively assess and manage pain.
- Provide culturally congruent pain management education.
- Apologize for cultural mistakes and make concerted efforts to prevent future cultural mistakes.
- Provide education on colon cancer treatment, prognosis, and holistic care that incorporates culturally congruent approaches and family heritage (risk factors) without emphasizing disparities (Landrine and Corral 2015; May et al. 2015; Rice et al. 2015).
- Recognize the potential cognitive, affective, and behavioral responses to environmental stigma that may be associated with living in or near areas of pollution, high crime rates, dilapidated buildings, or other undesirable qualities (Zhuang et al. 2016).

9.3.2 Organizational-Level Interventions

- Conduct a staff meeting to address the cultural bias, pain, discrimination, and disparities Franklin experienced.
- Using a cultural competence education framework, design, implement, and evaluate organization-wide cultural competence

education for all employees concerning multi-racial, multiple heritage individuals as consumers and co-workers (Jeffreys 2005, 2016).

- Revise hospital demographic forms to include "multiracial" and permit selection of more than one option.
- Publicize/post the Bill of Rights for People of Mixed Heritage (Root 1993), incorporating in all organizational cultural competence literature with photos of multiple heritage families.
- Train peers from the community as patient navigators for proactive cancer screening, incorporating culturally congruent strategies and coordinating with available transportation, mobile units, and organizational culture (Sly et al. 2012).
- Encourage proactive cancer screening among vulnerable populations, such as low test copayments, low-cost and convenient follow-up, and incentives (Pignone et al. 2014).
- Educate healthcare providers concerning pain management, noting ethnic and racial disparities, pharmacogenetics, and current literature recommendations (Shah et al. 2015).

9.3.3 Community-/Societal-Level Interventions

- Lobby governmental officials and agencies concerning environmental cleanup.
- Coordinate community-based and culturally congruent health teaching for the promotion of healthy lifestyles and neighborhoods.
- Network with farmers and others to bring responsibly grown, healthy foods and responsibly raised or hunted animals and fish to the local community in conjunction with a cooperative business alliance with the local store.
- Negotiate strategies with storeowners to prominently display economical healthy food choices and offer incentives for their selection over less healthy choices.
- Reach out to current and past community members for screening past and current exposure to toxins and/or incidence of cancer and other diseases associated with environmental hazards.

- Create collaborative partnerships between new and old community residents for eldercare support, prescription and food delivery, teen pregnancy prevention, and childcare.
- Establish community neighborhood watch and auxiliary police force to combat crime and foster a sense of community connectedness and safety.
- Collect demographic, socioeconomic, and statistical data including morbidity and mortality rates disaggregated by ethnic and racial categories that encourage identification of multiple races and ethnicities and trend data accordingly.
- Develop a community-based participatory approach to risk reduction in at-risk communities through interprofessional collaboration, advisory boards, and ad hoc resident advisory partnerships (Derrick et al. 2008).
- Collaborate with community members, government organizations, academic institutions, other organizations, and key stakeholders to address environmental and health-related issues proactively through screening, treatment, education, and follow-up (United States Environmental Protection Agency 2016).

Conclusion

Past and present policies, politics, myths, stereotypes, and societal attitudes influence the lived experience of multiracial individuals, often resulting in marginalization, disparities, invisibility, cultural pain, and/or unmet needs (Jeffreys and Zoucha 2017a). Acknowledging the uniqueness of multiple heritage individuals without attaching pity, stigmatization, alienation, marginalization, forced-choice pressures, or lowered social status is an important first step in making this "culture" truly visible and fully appreciated (Jeffreys and Zoucha 2001, 2017b).

Creating a culturally safe environment visibly inclusive of multiracial/multiple heritage individuals is an ethical, legal, and interprofessional expectation. Without it, social justice, environmental justice, and quality healthcare cannot be achieved. The Bill of Rights for People of Mixed Heritage (Root

1993) succinctly captures the cultural, lived experience of mixed-heritage people, providing a valuable guide for everyday contemplation, advocacy, and action.

References

Davenport LD (2016) The role of gender, class, and religion in biracial Americans' racial labeling decisions. Am Sociol Rev 81(1):57–84

DeJesus A, Hogan J, Martinez R, Adams J, Lacy TH (2016) Putting racism on the table: the implementation and evaluation of a novel racial equity and cultural competency training/consultation model in New York City. J Ethn Cult Divers Soc Work 25(4): 300–319

Derrick CG, Miller JSA, Andrews JM (2008) A fish consumption study of anglers in an at-risk community: a community-based participatory approach to risk reduction. Public Health Nurs 25(4):312–318

Farley R (2001) Identifying with multiple races. Report 01-491. University of Michigan, Population Studies Center, Ann Arbor. As cited in Shih M, Sanchez DT (2009) When race becomes even more complex: toward understanding the landscape of multiracial identity and experiences. J Soc Issues 65(1):2

Jackson KF, Samuels GM (2011) Multiracial competence in social work: recommendations for culturally attuned work with multiracial people. Soc Work 56(3):235–245

Jeffreys MR (2005) Clinical nurse specialists as cultural brokers, change agents, and partners in meeting the needs of culturally diverse populations. J Multicult Nurs Health 11(2):41–48

Jeffreys MR (2016) Teaching cultural competence in nursing and health care: inquiry, action, and innovation, 3rd edn. Springer, New York

Jeffreys MR, Zoucha R (2001) The invisible culture of the multiracial, multiethnic individual: a transcultural imperative. J Cult Divers 8(3):79–83

Jeffreys MR, Zoucha R (2017a) Revisiting "the invisible culture of the multiracial, multicultural individual: a transcultural imperative". J Cult Divers 24(1):3–5

Jeffreys MR, Zoucha R (2017b) The invisible culture of the multiracial, multicultural individual: a transcultural imperative: a reprint from 2001. J Cult Divers 24(1):6–10

Jeffreys MR, Zoucha R (2017c) Book review: mixed-race youth and schooling: the fifth minority. J Cult Divers 24(1):11–12

Landrine H, Corral I (2015) Targeting cancer information to African Americans: the trouble with talking about disparities. J Health Commun 20:196–203

May FP, Almiro C, Ponce N, Brennen MR, Spiegel BMR (2015) Racial minorities are more likely than whites to report lack of provider recommendation for colon cancer screening. Am J Gastroenterol 110:1388–1394

Pascoe P (1996) Miscegenation law, court cases, and ideologies of "race" in twentieth-century America. J Am Hist 83(1):44–69

Pew Commission (2015) http://www.pewsocialtrends.org/2015/06/11/chapter-1-race-and-multiracial-americans-in-the-u-s-census/. Accessed 18 Sept 2017

Pignone MP, Crutchfield TM, Brown PM, Hawkey S, Laping JL, Lewis CL, Lich KH, Richardson LC, Tangka FKL, Wheeler SB (2014) Using a discrete choice experiment to inform the design of programs to promote colon cancer screening for vulnerable populations in North Carolina. BMC Health Serv Res 14:611. https://doi.org/10.1186/s12913-014-0611-4

Remedios JD, Chasteen AL (2013) Finally, someone who "gets" me! Multiracial people value others' accuracy about their race. Cult Divers Ethn Minor Psychol 19(4):453–460

Rice LJ, Brandt HM, Hardin JW, Annang Ingram L et al (2015) Exploring perceptions of cancer risk, neighborhood environmental risks and health behaviors of blacks. J Community Health 40:419–430. https://doi.org/10.1007/s10900-014-9952-5

Root MPP (1992) Racially mixed people in America. Sage, Newbury Park

Root MPP (1993) Bill of rights for people of mixed heritage. Online. http://www.drmariaroot.com/doc/BillOfRights.pdf

Root MPP (1997) Multiracial Asians: models of ethnic identity. Amerasia J 23(1):29–41

Sanchez DT (2010) How do forced-choice dilemmas affect multiracial people? The role of identity autonomy and public regard in depressive symptoms. J Appl Soc Psychol 40(7):1657–1677

Shah AA, Zogg CK, Zafar SN, Schneider EB, Cooper LA et al (2015) Analgesic access for acute abdominal pain in the emergency department among racial/ethnic minority patients: a nationwide examination. Med Care 53(12):1000–1009

Sly JR, Jandorf L, Dhulkifl R, Hall D et al (2012) Challenges to replicating evidence-based research in real-world settings: training African-American peers as patient navigators for colon cancer screening. J Cancer Educ 27:680–686

Tran AGTT, Miyake ER, Csizmadia A, Martinez-Morales V (2016) "What are you?" multiracial individuals' responses to racial identification inquiries. Cult Divers Ethn Minor Psychol 22(1):26–37

Tutwiler SW (2016) Mixed-race youth and schooling: the fifth minority. Routledge, New York

United States Environmental Protection Agency (2016) EJ 2020 action agenda: the US EPA's environmental justice strategic plan for 2016-2020. Author, Washington, DC

Zhuang GJ, Cox J, Cruz S, Dearing JW et al (2016) Environmental stigma: resident responses to living in a contaminated area. Am Behav Sci 60(11):1322–1341

Critical Reflection

10

Larry Purnell

Guideline: *Nurses shall engage in critical reflection of their own values, beliefs, and cultural heritage in order to have an awareness of how these qualities and issues can impact culturally congruent care.*

Douglas et al. (2014: 110)

10.1   Introduction

An understanding of one's own cultural values and beliefs as well as the culture of others is essential if healthcare providers are to deliver culturally congruent care to patients, families, the community, and organizations where healthcare is delivered. Personal cultural reflectivity can help assure that the healthcare provider does not engage in cultural imposition or cultural imperialism and make a concerted attempt at cultural relativism (see Chap. 2). Moreover, in critical reflection, the healthcare provider analyzes his or her personal cultural beliefs, values, and worldview, therefore, challenging personal beliefs and assumptions to improve professional practice (Timmins 2006). Reflective thinking includes actions, analysis, and evaluation which can further increase personal cultural awareness (Canadian Nurses Association 2010). Critical reflection is more than just "thinking about" or "thoughtful" practice. It is a way of "critiquing" our practice in a systematic and rigorous way.

Although there is no one agreed-upon definition of critical reflection, a few have been consistently been recognized over time. Adapted from

L. Purnell, Ph.D., R.N., FAAN
School of Nursing, University of Delaware, Newark, DE, USA

Florida International University, Miami, FL, USA

Excelsior College, Albany, NY, USA
e-mail: lpurnell@udel.edu

Dewey, critical reflection is an active, persistent, and careful consideration of any belief or supposed form of knowledge in light of the grounds that support it. Moreover, it includes a conscious and voluntary effort to establish a belief upon a firm basis of evidence and rationality (Dewey 1933).

According to Mezirow (1990), critical reflection is a process: testing the justification of validity of premises that have been taken for granted. One consistency on definition of critical reflection is that it is a process of questioning one's beliefs, values, and behaviors to justify things we do in contrast with others' beliefs, values, and behaviors. Regardless of the different definitions on critical reflection, four criteria include the following: (a) reflection moves the learner from one experience into the next with deeper understanding of relationships and connections with other experiences and ideas; (b) reflection is a systematic, rigorous, and disciplined way of thinking with its roots in scientific inquiry; (c) reflection needs to occur in the community and in interaction with others; and (d) reflection requires attitudes that value personal and intellectual growth of oneself and of others. Accordingly, critical reflection is a process of reconstructing and reorganizing experiences that adds meaning to the experience (Rogers 2002).

A variety of methods exist that healthcare providers, educators, and administrators can use to teach and learn how to reflect critically: journal writing, case studies, action research, practical experience (especially with diverse groups), autobiographical stories, action learning groups, and immersion in diverse cultures. Each of these activities involves recognizing assumptions that underlie one's beliefs and behaviors and helps avoid egocentrism and seeing things from different perspectives.

A number of tools exist to help practitioners assess their views and values related to bias. Three tools are included in the following appendices:

- Appendix 1—Promoting Cultural and Linguistic Competency: Self-Assessment Checklist for Personnel Providing Primary Healthcare Services
- Appendix 2—Promoting Cultural and Linguistic Competency: Self-Assessment Checklist for Personnel Providing Services and Supports in Early Intervention and Early Childhood Settings
- Appendix 3—Personal Self-Assessment of Antibias Behavior

10.2   Personal Responsibility: Critical Reflection

Critical cultural reflection is not a casual but rather a personal responsibility and a standard to which all healthcare practitioners should strive. It begins with the novice student and continues throughout one's professional life. Respect for all cultures is fundamental (ICN Code of Ethics for Nurses 2012). To critically reflect and become culturally competent, one must do a number of things:

1. Recognize that your own culture is a product of your environment whose basis is socially constructed beginning with child-rearing practices.
2. Appreciate your own multiple identities.
3. Acknowledge assumptions, biases, and prejudices.
4. Accept responsibility and tolerate ambiguity.
5. Recognize the limits of your competence.
6. Have the capacity for introspection.
7. Work to eliminate native prejudicial tendencies.
8. Know your attitudes toward disabilities, ageism, sexism, classism, racism, and heterosexism.

10.2.1 Models of Critical Thinking

A number of models exist that healthcare providers can use in their personal critical cultural reflection. The following describes a few of the more popular models.

10.2.1.1   Ways of Knowing

Carper's (1978) seminal work in the ways of knowing identified four fundamental patterns of knowing to form a conceptual structure of nursing knowledge: personal, empirical, ethical, and aesthetic knowing. Since that time, her work has been expanded by others.

Personal knowing is what we have seen and experienced and comes through a process of observation, reflection, and self-actualization. Knowledge of self establishes professional, therapeutic relationships and propels the learner toward wholeness and integrity (Chinn 2018; Chinn and Kramer 2015). Placing oneself in situations to be challenged and taught by teachers and mentors is helpful in gaining a personal way of knowing and critically reflecting (Sullivan-Marx 2013). Carper's (1978) sense of personal knowing is engagement with others and using knowledge of self to commit, encounter, and risk commitment (Sullivan-Marx 2013). Personal knowing is introspective and consciously dissecting our own thoughts and beliefs, including personal beliefs about social justice and vulnerable populations. One needs to critically reflect on how and why assumptions are made. Ask yourself "What can I do to better the situation?"

Empirical knowing comes from research and objectivity and is systematically organized into general laws and theories. This knowledge is applied through applying evidence-based practice (see Chap. 39) and is referred to as the science of nursing (Chinn 2018; Chinn and Kramer 2015). Empirics require constantly attending to self through evidence-based learning (Sullivan-Marx 2013).

Ethical knowing is developed through the healthcare provider's moral code: a sense of knowing what is right and what is wrong. Personal ethics is based on an obligation to protect and respect human life, being true to self, and doing what ought to be done. Empirics require constantly attending to self through evidence-based learning (Sullivan-Marx 2013), especially when it comes to social justice and vulnerable populations. The *Code of Ethics for Nurses* (American Nurses Association 2015) guides professionals in developing and refining their moral code. At a minimum, question your beliefs, values, and behaviors to justify what needs to be done to create social justice. Maintain open-mindedness.

The fourth way of knowing is aesthetic knowing and is commonly known as the art of nursing. Aesthetic knowing is an "aha" moment when something new is uncovered providing the provider with new perspectives (Chinn 2018; Chinn and Kramer 2015). Aesthetics also highlights empathy as essential to understanding others (Sullivan-Marx 2013).

The practice of nursing is a holistic, human discipline. The ways of knowing allow us to understand ourselves and nursing practice at a much deeper level, to appreciate nursing as both an art and a science. Consider how the ways of knowing can assist you in being a better person, a better student, and a better nurse (Johns 1995).

In addition to Carper's ways of knowing, eight additional ways of knowing have been added to the literature: emotion, faith, imagination, intuition, language, memory, reason, and sense perception. These require balancing and blocking out unreliable knowledge and remaining receptive toward knowledge that provides genuine insight. Using all the ways of knowing will increase the healthcare provider's ability to engage in critical cultural reflection (Ways of Knowing: Theory of Knowledge.net 2017).

Emotion can act as a catalyst for reflection, be it a source of reflection or a by-product. Goleman (2005) identifies self-awareness, self-management, social awareness, and relationship skills as emotional literacy. Emotional literacy is a self-conscious awareness: an awareness of the assumptions, reasoning, evidence, and justification that underpin one's values and beliefs. Emotional intelligence is defined by a person's ability to recognize emotions and emotional states and to name them (Akers and Grover 2017; Goleman 2005). It also includes the ability to control emotions "appropriately" (a manner that is suitable or proper in the circumstances),

to recognize them in others, and to make interventions such as calming or redirecting them in useful ways (Goleman 2005). A pivotal characteristic of affective feelings is that they are informative enhancing the process and impact of critical reflection on learning, leading one to deeper and richer understanding of values and beliefs. Critical reflection undertaken by someone who has a high-level emotional literacy will have greater consciousness or awareness of their emotions, other peoples' emotions, and the interaction and impact of each (Goleman 2005; Akers and Grover 2017).

The following is an example of how one can learn from emotions, emotional literacy, and emotional intelligence. A nurse examined a 5-year-old Vietnamese child and found multiple scratch marks on his back. Shocked at the marks, she became angry and loudly asked the parents "with what did they hit the child?" She was accusing them of abusing the child. Out of fear, the parents yelled "no, no" and started to take the child home. Hearing loud voices from the examining room, another nurse entered the patient's room, examined the child, and recognized the marks as *cao gio* (coining), a recognized and common dermabrasion procedure used by the Vietnamese (and other groups) for fever, cough, and colds. The nurse in this instance was unable to control her emotions in a professional manner. As a result, the nurse was directed to learn about emotional intelligence that could lead to the ability to control her emotions.

Faith is arguably one of the more disputed ways of knowing and depends on its interpretation by the knower. It may or not may have religious connotations. One's faith is highly dependent on culture and the knowledge of the community in which one belongs. Faith refers to the notions of trust, commitment, and the acceptance of assumptions; it may fulfill a psychological need (Ways of Knowing: Faith 2017). Providers who have faith in their practice arc in a better position to critically reflect on their cultural abilities. Faith as a way of knowing is a belief without empirical evidence, a foundational truth upon which other knowledge claims are based or derived. This foundational truth can be metaphysical in nature such as a belief in a supreme being or moral in nature such as a belief in goodness (Faith as a

Way of Knowing 2017) as in seeking social justice for vulnerable populations.

A fundamental faith concept is "is there life after death." Whereas no scientific evidence exists to support this belief, many people believe this is true and encourages them to go on. In this belief, faith is mainly derived through prayer and by no other means in life. It can offer deep contemplation to self-evaluate actions (Faith as a Way of Knowing 2017).

Imagination, forming new ideas or concepts, includes the ability to be creative or resourceful. It is a way of developing knowledge without the help of our senses and allows an extra scope in understanding concepts, ideas, or phenomena. The ability to make a leap of understanding without necessarily knowing how and why is included. Healthcare providers who work in resource-poor environments frequently use their imagination in providing care.

Intuition is the ability to understand something instinctively without the need for conscious reasoning. Intuition is associated with innate knowledge and is linked to ethics and knowing instinctively the "right" and the "wrong" way and is a combination of memory, emotion, and sense perception (Cholle 2011).

Language is a system of verbal and nonverbal communication (see Chap. 2) used by each community or country. Idioms and colloquialisms that might be understood in one community may not be understood by outsiders; therefore, the healthcare provider must take caution and not use colloquialisms and idioms with patients. Patients also use colloquialisms and idioms; the onus is on the provider to get clarification of their meaning.

Memory is not a primary way of knowing. However, it provides us with initial knowledge and only afterward employs memory to modify and enhance that knowledge. Cultural knowledge increases as one works with diverse staff and vulnerable groups. Because memory is notoriously unreliable, it must be treated with care if one is to build upon objective cultural knowledge.

Reason, the way in which we try to make sense of the world, uses logic, rationality, comparison, judgment, and experience; all of these are requisites for critical reflection. Most of the time reasoning is instinctive, depends on previous experiences, and is a requisite in critical cultural reflection and self-awareness.

Sense perception, such as sight, smell, hearing, taste, and touch, is an external stimulus that is used by healthcare providers in providing care. It also includes internal perception such as a feeling, an awareness or sensitivity to attitudes or a situation, and the meaning of a word or expression or the way in which a word or expression can be interpreted. Although sensing is a valid way of knowing, to what extent can we trust our senses (Theory of Knowledge.net 2014)?

10.2.1.2 Dewey's Model of Reflective Learning

Dewey's model of reflective learning (Miettinen 2000; Rogers 2002) has four criteria. The process of reflection moves the learner from one experience to another, leading to a deeper understanding, and ensures an individual's progress and ultimately society. Reflection is systematic and disciplined and has its roots in scientific inquiry (Schon 2014). Reflection occurs within the individual, in the community, and in interactions, in this incidence with vulnerable population leading to culturally competent and congruent care. It also requires attitudes that value diversity and social justice among individuals and groups, requisites for culturally congruent care. Given Dewey's four criteria, the healthcare provider who applies these criteria is in a better cognitive situation to provide culturally competent and congruent care with vulnerable populations and have a better understanding of the social determinants of health (see Chap. 1). Interactive experiences between oneself and the world change healthcare providers' worldview (How We Think: John Dewey on the Art of Reflection and Fruitful Curiosity in an Age of Instant Opinions and Information Overload n.d.) and assist them in delivering culturally competent assessment and culturally competent care (Rogers 2002).

10.2.1.3 Habermas's Model of Critical Reflection

The critical theory of Habermas differentiates three generic cognitive areas in which to generate knowledge: work knowledge, practical knowledge, and emancipatory knowledge; they are grounded in different aspects of social existence—work, interaction, and power (The Critical Theory of Jurgen Habermas n.d.). Work knowledge is the way we control and manipulate the environment where knowledge is based upon empirical investigation and governed by technical rules. Effective control of reality directs appropriate actions. Much of what we consider "scientific" research such as physics, chemistry, and biology (shall we include nursing and medicine) belong to the work domain.

Practical knowledge, human social interaction, is governed by consensual norms and expectations of behavior between individuals. The validity of social norms is grounded in the intersubjectivity of the mutual understanding of intentions and determines what appropriate actions are. Descriptive social science, history, aesthetics, legal, and ethnographic literary belong to the domain of the practical domain.

Emancipatory knowledge identifies self-knowledge or self-reflection and is the way one sees oneself, one's roles, and social expectations. Emancipation limits our options and rational control over our lives but has been taken for granted as beyond human control. Insights gained through critical self-awareness are emancipatory in the sense that at least one can recognize and probe for underlying circumstances that shape inequality and injustice. Self-emancipation through reflection leading to a transformed consciousness includes such sciences as feminist theory, psychoanalysis, and the critique of ideology (Chinn 2018; The Critical Theory of Jurgen Habermas n.d.).

10.2.2 Kolb's Model of Experiential Learning

Kolb's model of experiential learning has six components (Kolb and Kolb 2005):

1. Learning is conceived as a process with continuing reconstruction of an experience.
2. All learning is relearning and is best facilitated by drawing out a person's beliefs and ideas about a topic (in this case culture), so they can

be examined and integrated with new, more refined ideas.
3. Learning requires resolving conflicts between opposed adaptations to the world, again in this case opposing cultures between the patient and the healthcare provider.
4. Learning is a holistic process of adapting to the world and involves integrated functioning of the whole person—thinking, feeling, perceiving, and behaving.
5. Learning results from synergetic transaction between the person and the environment through processes assimilating new experiences into existing concepts and accommodating these concepts to new experiences.
6. Learning creates knowledge where social knowledge is recreated in the personal knowledge of the learner.

10.2.2.1 Feminist Theory

Feminist theory seeks justice for women and the end of sexism in all forms and is driven by the quest for social justice and includes vulnerable populations. Currently, feminist theory has expanded to address a wide range of perspectives on social, cultural, and political phenomena and includes class and work, disability, the family, globalization, human rights, race and racism, discrimination of all types, reproduction, and sexuality. Feminist theory does not require a particular methodology but rather addresses topics of concern for social justice. Feminist theory has been divided into liberal and radical feminism.

Liberal feminism, although considered passé by some, is most aligned with the National Organization for Women (NOW). However, many disagree that liberal feminism, although considered passé because the 1967 Women's Bill of Rights that have yet to be fully implemented, in less developed and in more developed countries (Tong 2018).

Radical feminists claim that women's fundamental strength rests in their differences from men. They do not think it is in women's best interests to be part of a system that devalues caregiving practices and occupations. Women should reject this system because its values of power, dominance, hierarchy, and competition breed injustice.

10.2.2.2   Summary Ways of Knowing

Nursing and other healthcare professionals have explored and struggled with critical reflection, thinking, and reasoning. No consensus has been agreed upon as to what is the best approach. Some ways of knowing have scientific rigor, whereas others have no scientific basis and probably never will. However, there is some agreement that the nonscientific-based ways of knowing still have merit for many. Health professionals should use more than one way of knowing and expand their critical thinking and reasoning skills and engage in self-reflection and awareness when caring for patients from different cultures.

Chinn (2018) summarized emancipatory ways of knowing and critical reflection theories based on the American Association of Colleges of Nursing's document Essentials of Doctoral Education in Advanced Practice Nursing (2006). In their entirety, these essentials address competencies for advanced practice nursing for social justice and advocacy for vulnerable populations. These essentials are:

- Scientific underpinnings for practice and how they account for social and political contexts for whom care is provided
- Organizational and systems leadership for quality improvement and systems thinking with a global, social, and political systems approach
- Clinical scholarship and analytical methods for evidence-based practice by asking questions such as who will be disadvantaged or stereotyped
- Information systems/technology and patient care technology for the improvement and transformations of healthcare for disadvantaged and vulnerable populations
- Healthcare policy for advocacy in healthcare for the disadvantaged as well as all members of the community
- Interprofessional collaboration for improving patient and population health outcomes
- Clinical prevention and population health for improving a nation's health by looking at what is creating patterns of injustice, disadvantage, and discrimination

10.2.3   Recommendations

Recommendations for clinical practice, education, and research follow.

10.2.3.1   Recommendations for Clinical Practice

Nurses, and all healthcare professionals, must develop an awareness of their own existence, sensations, thoughts, and environment without letting then have an undue influence on those from other backgrounds. One must strive to learn the health beliefs, values, and cultural care practices of patients to whom care is provided. Inherent in learning patients cultures the provider must accept and respect cultural differences in a manner that facilitates the patient's and the family's abilities to make decisions to meet their needs and beliefs.

One must accept and recognize that the healthcare provider's beliefs and values may not be the same as the patient's being open to new cultural encounters and must resist judgmental attitudes such as "different is not as good." Moreover, recognize that the variant cultural characteristics determine the degree to which patients adhere to the beliefs, values, and practices of their dominant culture (see Chap. 3). To learn cultural attributes of diverse populations, make contact with and have experiences with the communities from which patients come.

As professionals, nurses must accept responsibility for their own education in cultural competence by attending conferences, reading cultural literature, and observing cultural practices. In addition, they must develop an attitude of open-mindedness, respect for individuals, and discourage racial and ethnic slurs among coworkers. Participating in cultural events provides knowledge about the primary characteristics of culture for that population and helps develop respect from for them.

Additional activities can incorporate a journal to record thoughts, experiences, and observations with culturally diverse encounters. Learning a second or third language helps increase tolerance for ambiguity and helps develop rapport with patients. Taking a self-administered tool helps determine one's biases and prejudices (see Appendices 1–3).

10.2.3.2 Recommendations for Administration

Administration must integrate diversity and inclusivity statements in the organization's mission and philosophy along with creating policies that address bias, discrimination, and racial and ethnic slurs These policies should be incorporated into performance evaluations of all staff, mangers, and administrators. Administration must also provide a budget for staff and managers to attend cultural competence courses and conferences.

Developing patient satisfaction surveys in languages spoken by the organization's patient population and specifically asking questions on bias, discrimination, and ethnic and racial slurs will help assure language-diverse populations being able to complete them. More complete data assists with questioning routines that do not meet the need of multicultural staff and patients.

Actively participating providers in community activities and organizations enhances visibility and trust in the community. Engaging city policymakers and planners in discussions on vulnerable population can help alleviate health disparities of vulnerable populations. Other activities are partnering with community churches and social service agencies to address the social and structural determinants of health in the community.

10.2.3.3 Recommendations for Education and Training

Educational leaders can organize cultural awareness activities and promote critical reflection through team meetings by discussing published case studies as well as encouraging staff to talk about cases in which they have provided care. Classes that address bias, discrimination, and racial and ethnic slurs should be included; some staff are not aware that they make racial slurs or use terminology/words that are seen as offensive to others. This will help assist staff to recognize biases and stereotyping and devise a plan to overcome them.

The education department can host programs and workshops for staff that encourage critical reflection and self-awareness of cultural values and beliefs and offer them to other area organizations that might have a different patient population.

In college settings, faculty can engage students in cultural immersion and exchange programs, especially with populations seen in the catchment area of the facility. Cultural immersions can also occur in foreign countries and in other parts of a country, especially in such large countries as the United States, China, and India as examples.

10.2.3.4 Recommendations for Research

Establish journal clubs to review current literature on critical reflection and self-awareness of staff's beliefs and values related to practice. Evidence-based publications are a requisite, although the gray literature can be used if no research publication can be found on the specific patient population. Obtaining experienced researchers can assist staff and managers to conduct research and quality improvement projects on cultural competence and critical reflection.

Conclusion

Although the literature provides numerous definitions of cultural self-awareness and cultural critical reflection, research integrating the concept of self-awareness with multicultural competence is minimal. Many theorists and diversity trainers imply that self-examination or awareness of personal prejudices and biases is an important step in the cognitive process of developing cultural competence (Andrews and Boyle 2016; Calvillo et al. 2009; Hickson 2011). Given that all healthcare providers have conscious and unconscious biases, concerted effort must be taken to recognize them and not let them affect care (Cuellar 2017). Conscious and unconscious biases can include race, ethnicity, color, socioeconomic class, gender, alternative life styles, religion, and a host of other "differences (Ghoshal et al. 2013). Introspective critical reflection requires constantly reviewing one's own thoughts, feelings, and beliefs concerning social justice and vulnerable populations. Academic literature on emotional feelings elicited by this cognitive awareness is somewhat limited regarding the potential impact of emotions and conscious feelings on behavioral outcomes. Management and administration must make a concerted effort to assist staff to recognize their conscious and unconscious bias.

Cultural critical reflection is a deliberate and conscious cognitive and emotional process of getting to know yourself: your personality, your values, your beliefs, your professional knowledge standards, your ethics, and the impact of these factors on the various roles you play when interacting with individuals different from yourself (Purnell and Salmond 2013). Critically analyzing our own values and beliefs in terms of how we see differences enables us to be less fearful of others whose values and beliefs are different from our own (Calvillo et al. 2009; Hickson 2011). The ability to understand oneself sets the stage for integrating new knowledge related to cultural differences into the healthcare provider's knowledge base, perceptions of health, interventions, and the impact these factors have on the various roles of professionals when interacting with multicultural patients. Critical reflection is a key activity in creating caring cultures because it can enable individuals to develop greater self-awareness by helping them to develop new understanding that informs actions.

Every patient and caregiver has the right to be treated without prejudice; people should not be discriminated against because of religion, ethnicity, race, socioeconomic status, or physical or mental disability. Feminist theory emphasizes social and ethical issues, as well as political and personal perspectives.

Appendix 1: Promoting Cultural and Linguistic Competency

Self-Assessment Checklist for Personnel Providing Primary Healthcare Services

Please select A, B, or C for each item listed below.

A = Things I do frequently, or statement applies to me to a great degree

B = Things I do occasionally, or statement applies to me to a moderate degree

C = Things I do rarely or never, or statement applies to me to minimal degree or not at all

Physical Environment, Materials, and Resources

_____ 1. I display pictures, posters, artworks, and other decors that reflect the cultures and ethnic backgrounds of clients served by my program or agency.

_____ 2. I ensure that magazines, brochures, and other printed materials in reception areas are of interest to and reflect the different cultures and languages of individuals and families served by my program or agency.

_____ 3. When using videos, films, or other media resources for health education, treatment, or other interventions, I ensure that they reflect the culture and ethnic backgrounds of individuals and families served by my program or agency.

_____ 4. I ensure that printed information disseminated by my agency or program takes into consideration accuracy and without bias.

Communication Styles

_____ 5. When interacting with individuals and families who have limited English proficiency, I always keep in mind that:
  * Limitations in English proficiency are in no way a reflection of their level of intellectual functioning.
    * Their limited ability to speak the language of the dominant culture has no bearing on their ability to communicate effectively in their language of origin.
  * They may neither be literate in their language of origin nor in English.

_____ 6. I use bilingual/bicultural or multilingual/multicultural staff and/or personnel and volunteers who are skilled or certified in the provision of medical interpretation services during treatment, interventions, meetings, or other events for individuals and families who need or prefer this level of assistance.

_____ 7. For individuals and families who speak languages or dialects other than English, I attempt to learn and use key words so that I am better able to communicate with them during assessment, treatment, or other interventions.

_____ 8. I attempt to determine any familial colloquialisms used by individuals or families that may impact on assessment, treatment, health promotion and education, or other interventions.

_____ 9. For those who request or need this service, I ensure that all notices and communiqués to individuals and families are written in their language of origin.

_____ 10. I understand that it may be necessary to use alternatives to written communications for some individuals and families, as word of mouth may be a preferred method of receiving information.

_____ 11. I understand the principles and practices of linguistic competency and:
* Apply them within my program or agency
* Advocate for them within my program or agency

_____ 12. I understand the implications of health literacy within the context of my roles and responsibilities.

_____ 13. I use alternative formats and varied approaches to communicate and share information with individuals and/or their family members who experience disability.

Values and Attitudes

_____ 14. I avoid imposing values that may conflict or be inconsistent with those of cultures or ethnic groups other than my own.

_____ 15. I screen books, movies, and other media resources for negative cultural, ethnic, or racial stereotypes before sharing them with individuals and families served by my program or agency.

_____ 16. I intervene in an appropriate manner when I observe other staff or clients within my program or agency engaging in behaviors that show cultural insensitivity, racial biases, and prejudice.

_____ 17. I recognize and accept that individuals from culturally diverse backgrounds may desire varying degrees of acculturation into the dominant culture.

_____ 18. I understand and accept that family is defined differently by different cultures (e.g., extended family members, fictive kin, godparents).

_____ 19. I accept and respect that male-female roles may vary significantly among different cultures (e.g., who makes major decisions for the family).

_____ 20. I understand that age and life cycle factors must be considered in interactions with individuals and families (e.g., high value placed on the decision of elders, the role of eldest male or female in families, or roles and expectation of children within the family).

_____ 21. Even though my professional or moral viewpoints may differ, I accept individuals and families as the ultimate decision-makers for services and supports impacting their lives.

_____ 22. I recognize that the meaning or value of medical treatment and health education may vary greatly among cultures.

_____ 23. I accept that religion and other beliefs may influence how individuals and families respond to illnesses, disease, and death.

_____ 24. I understand that the perception of health, wellness, and preventive health services has different meanings to different cultural groups.

_____ 25. I recognize and understand that beliefs and concepts of emotional well-being vary significantly from culture to culture.

_____ 26. I understand that beliefs about mental illness and emotional disability are culturally based. I accept that responses to these conditions and related treatments/interventions are heavily influenced by culture.

_____ 27. I recognize and accept that folk and religious beliefs may influence an individual's or family's reaction and approach to a child born with a disability or later diagnosed with a disability, genetic disorder, or special healthcare needs.

_____ 28. I understand that grief and bereavement are influenced by culture.

_____ 29. I accept and respect that customs and beliefs about food, its value, preparation, and use are different from culture to culture.

_____ 30. I seek information from individuals, families, or other key community informants that will assist in service adaptation to respond to the needs and preferences of culturally and ethnically diverse groups served by my program or agency.

_____ 31. Before visiting or providing services in the home setting, I seek information on acceptable behaviors, courtesies, customs, and expectations that are unique to the culturally diverse groups served by my program or agency.

_____ 32. I keep abreast of the major health and mental health concerns and issues for ethnically and racially diverse client populations residing in the geographic locale served by my program or agency.

_____ 33. I am aware of specific health and mental health disparities and their prevalence within the communities served by my program or agency.

_____ 34. I am aware of the socioeconomic and environmental risk factors that con-

tribute to health and mental health disparities or other major health problems of culturally and linguistically diverse populations served by my program or agency.

_____ 35. I am well versed in the most current and proven practices, treatments, and interventions for the delivery of health and mental healthcare to specific racial, ethnic, cultural, and linguistic groups within the geographic locale served by my agency or program.

_____ 36. I avail myself to professional development and training to enhance my knowledge and skills in the provision of services and supports to culturally and linguistically diverse groups.

_____ 37. I advocate for the review of my program's or agency's mission statement, goals, policies, and procedures to ensure that they incorporate principles and practices that promote cultural and linguistic competence.

Reprinted with Permission: Tawara D. Goode • National Center for Cultural Competence • Georgetown University Center for Child & Human Development • University Center for Excellence in Developmental Disabilities, Education, Research & Service • Adapted Promoting Cultural Competence and Cultural Diversity for Personnel Providing Services and Supports to Children with Special Health Care Needs and their Families • June 1989 (Revised 2009).

SCORING: This checklist is intended to heighten the awareness and sensitivity of personnel to the importance of cultural and linguistic cultural competence in health, mental health, and human service settings. It provides concrete examples of the kinds of beliefs, attitudes, values, and practices which foster cultural and linguistic competence at the individual or practitioner level. There is no answer key with correct responses. However, if you frequently responded "C," you may not necessarily demonstrate beliefs, attitudes, values, and practices that promote cultural and linguistic competence within health and mental healthcare delivery programs.

Appendix 2: Promoting Cultural and Linguistic Competency

Self-Assessment Checklist for Personnel Providing Services and Supports in Early Intervention and Early Childhood Settings

Directions: Please select A, B, or C for each item listed below.

A = Things I do frequently, or statement applies to me to a great degree
B = Things I do occasionally, or statement applies to me to a moderate degree
C = Things I do rarely or never, or statement applies to me to minimal degree or not at all

Physical Environment, Materials, and Resources

_____ 1. I display pictures, posters, and other materials that reflect the cultures and ethnic backgrounds of children and families served in my early childhood program or setting.

_____ 2. I select props for the dramatic play/housekeeping area that are culturally diverse (e.g., dolls, clothing, cooking utensils, household articles, furniture).

_____ 3. I ensure that the book/literacy area has pictures and storybooks that reflect the different cultures of children and families served in my early childhood program or setting.

_____ 4. I ensure that tabletop toys and other play accessories (that depict people) are representative of the various cultural and ethnic groups both within my community and the society in general.

_____ 5. I read a variety of books exposing children in my early childhood program or setting to various life experiences of cultures and ethnic groups other than their own.

_____ 6. When such books are not available, I provide opportunities for children

and their families to create their own books and include them among the resources and materials in my early childhood program or setting.

_____ 7. I adapt the above referenced approaches when providing services, supports, and other interventions in the home setting.

_____ 8. I encourage and provide opportunities for children and their families to share experiences through storytelling, puppets, marionettes, or other props to support the "oral tradition" common among many cultures.

_____ 9. I plan trips and community outings to places where children and their families can learn about their own cultural or ethnic history as well as the history of others.

_____ 10. I select videos, films, or other media resources reflective of diverse cultures to share with children and families served in my early childhood program or setting.

_____ 11. I play a variety of music and introduce musical instruments from many cultures.

_____ 12. I ensure that meals provided include foods that are unique to the cultural and ethnic backgrounds of children and families served in my early childhood program or setting.

_____ 13. I provide opportunities for children to cook or sample a variety of foods typically served by different cultural and ethnic groups other than their own.

_____ 14. If my early childhood program or setting consists entirely of children and families from the same cultural or ethnic group, I feel it is important to plan an environment and implement activities that reflect the cultural diversity within the society at large.

_____ 15. I am cognizant of and ensure that curricula I use include traditional holidays celebrated by the majority culture, as well as those holidays that are unique to the culturally diverse children and families served in my early childhood program or setting.

Communication Styles

_____ 16. For children who speak languages or dialects other than English, I attempt to learn and use key words in their language so that I am better able to communicate with them.

_____ 17. I attempt to determine any familial colloquialisms used by children and families that will assist and/or enhance the delivery of services and supports.

_____ 18. I use visual aids, gestures, and physical prompts in my interactions with children who have limited English proficiency.

_____ 19. When interacting with parents and other family members who have limited English proficiency, I always keep in mind that:

    _____ (a) Limitation in English proficiency is in no way a reflection of their level of intellectual functioning.

    _____ (b) Their limited ability to speak the language of the dominant culture has no bearing on their ability to communicate effectively in their language of origin.

    _____ (c) They may neither be literate in their language of original English.

_____ 20. I ensure that all notices and communiqués to parents are written in their language of origin.

_____ 21. I understand that it may be necessary to use alternatives to written communications for some families, as word of mouth may be a preferred method of receiving information.

_____ 22. I understand the principles and practices of linguistic competency and:

    (a) Apply them within my early childhood program or setting

    (b) Advocate for them within my program or agency

_____ 23. I use bilingual or multilingual staff and/or trained/certified foreign language interpreters for meetings, conferences, or other events for parents and family members who may require this level of assistance.

_____ 24. I encourage and invite parents and family members to volunteer and assist with activities regardless of their ability to speak English.

_____ 25. I use alternative formats and varied approaches to communicate with children and/or their family members who experience disability.

_____ 26. I arrange accommodations for parents and family members who may require communication assistance to ensure their full participation in all aspects of the early childhood program (e.g., hearing impaired, physical disability, visually impaired, not literate or low literacy, etc.).

_____ 27. I accept and recognize that there are often differences between language used in early childhood/early intervention settings, or at "school," and in the home setting.

Values and Attitudes

_____ 28. I avoid imposing values that may conflict or be inconsistent with those of cultures or ethnic groups other than my own.

_____ 29. I discourage children from using racial and ethnic slurs by helping them understand that certain words can hurt others.

_____ 30. I screen books, movies, and other media resources for negative cultural, ethnic, racial, or religious stereotypes before sharing them with children and their families served in my early childhood program or setting.

_____ 31. I provide activities to help children learn about and accept the differences and similarities in all people as an ongoing component of program curricula.

_____ 32. I intervene in an appropriate manner when I observe other staff or parents within my program or agency engaging in behaviors that show cultural insensitivity, bias, or prejudice.

_____ 33. I recognize and accept that individuals from culturally diverse backgrounds may desire varying degrees of acculturation into the dominant culture.

_____ 34. I understand and accept that family is defined differently by different cultures (e.g., extended family members, fictive kin, godparents).

_____ 35. I accept and respect that male-female roles in families may vary significantly among different cultures (e.g., who makes major decisions for the family, play and social interactions expected of male and female children).

_____ 36. I understand that age and life cycle factors must be considered in interactions with families (e.g., high value placed on the decisions or child-rearing practices of elders or the role of the eldest female in the family).

_____ 37. Even though my professional or moral viewpoints may differ, I accept the family/parents as the ultimate decision-makers for services and supports for their children.

_____ 38. I accept that religion, spirituality, and other beliefs may influence how families respond to illness, disease, and death.

_____ 39. I recognize and understand that beliefs and concepts of mental health or emotional well-being, particularly for infants and young children, vary significantly from culture to culture.

_____ 40. I recognize and accept that familial folklore, religious, or spiritual beliefs may influence a family's reaction and approach to a child born with a disability or later diagnosed with a disability or special healthcare needs.

_____ 41. I understand that beliefs about mental illness and emotional disability are culturally based. I accept that responses to these conditions and related treatments/interventions are heavily influenced by culture.

_____ 42. I understand that the healthcare practices of families served in my early childhood program or setting may be rooted in cultural traditions.

_____ 43. I recognize that the meaning or value of early childhood education or early intervention may vary greatly among cultures.

_____ 44. I understand that traditional approaches to disciplining children are influenced by culture.

_____ 45. I understand that families from different cultures will have different expectations of their children for acquiring toileting, dressing, feeding, and other self-help skills.

_____ 46. I accept and respect that customs and beliefs about food, its value, preparation, and use are different from culture to culture.

_____ 47. Before visiting or providing services in the home setting, I seek information on acceptable behaviors, courtesies, customs, and expectations that are unique to families of specific cultural groups served in my early childhood program or setting.

_____ 48. I advocate for the review of my program's or agency's mission statement, goals, policies, and procedures to ensure that they incorporate principles and practices that promote cultural diversity, cultural competence, and linguistic competence.

_____ 49. I seek information from family members or other key community informants that will assist me to respond effectively to the needs and preferences of culturally and linguistically diverse children and families served in my early childhood program or setting.

Reprinted with Permission: Tawara D. Goode
• National Center for Cultural Competence
• Georgetown University Center for Child &
Human Development • University Center for
Excellence in Developmental Disabilities, Edu-
cation, Research & Service • Adapted Promoting
Cultural Competence and Cultural Diversity for
Personnel Providing Services and Supports to
Children with Special Health Care Needs and their
Families • June 1989 (Revised 2009).

SCORING: This checklist is intended to
heighten the awareness and sensitivity of personnel to the importance of cultural diversity,
cultural competence, and linguistic competence in early childhood settings. It provides
concrete examples of the kinds of practices
that foster such an environment. There is no
answer key with correct responses. However,
if you frequently responded "C," you may not
necessarily demonstrate practices that promote a culturally diverse and culturally competent learning environment for children and
families within your classroom, program, or
agency.

Appendix 3: Personal Self-Assessment of Antibias Behavior

Directions: Using the rating scale of NEVER to
ALWAYS, assess yourself for each item by placing an "X" on the appropriate place along each
continuum. When you have completed the checklist, review your responses to identify areas in
need of improvement. Create specific goals to
address the areas in which you would like to
improve.

1. I educate myself about the culture and experiences of other racial, religious, ethnic and
   socioeconomic groups by reading and
   attending classes, workshops, cultural
   events, etc.
   Never _____**Always**
2. I spend time reflecting on my own upbring-
   ing and childhood to better understand my
   own biases and the ways I may have internalized the prejudicial messages I received.
   Never _____**Always**

3. I look at my own attitudes and behaviors as
   an adult to determine the ways they may be
   contributing to or combating prejudice in
   society.
   Never _____**Always**
4. I evaluate my use of language to avoid terms
   or phrases that may be degrading or hurtful
   to other groups.
   Never _____**Always**
5. I avoid stereotyping and generalizing other
   people based on their group identity.
   Never _____**Always**
6. I value cultural differences and avoid statements such as "I never think of you
   as_____," which discredits
   differences.
   Never _____**Always**
7. I am comfortable discussing issues of racism, anti-Semitism and other forms of prejudice with others.
   Never _____**Always**
8. I am open to other people's feedback about
   ways in which my behavior may be culturally insensitive or offensive to others.
   Never _____**Always**
9. I give equal attention to other people regardless of race, religion, gender, socioeconomic
   class or other difference.
   Never _____**Always**
10. I am comfortable giving constructive feed-
    back to someone of another race, gender, age
    or physical ability.
    Never _____**Always**
11. The value of diversity is reflected in my
    work, which includes a wide range of racial,
    religious, ethnic and socioeconomic groups,
    even when these groups are not personally
    represented in my community.
    Never _____**Always**
12. I work intentionally to develop inclusive
    practices, such as considering how the time,
    location and cost of scheduled meetings and
    programs might inadvertently exclude cer-
    tain groups.
    Never _____**Always**
13. I work to increase my awareness of biased
    content in television programs, newspapers
    and advertising.
    Never _____**Always**

14. I take time to notice the environment of my home, office, house of worship and children's school, to ensure that visual media represent diverse groups, and I advocate for the addition of such materials if they are lacking.

   Never _____ **Always**

15. When other people use biased language and behavior, I feel comfortable speaking up, asking them to refrain and stating my reasons.

   Never _____**Always**

16. I contribute to my organization's achievement of its diversity goals through programming and by advocating for hiring practices that contribute to a diverse workforce.

   Never _____**Always**

17. I demonstrate my commitment to social justice in my personal life by engaging in activities to achieve equity.

   Never _____**Always**

This activity was adapted from "Commitment to Combat Racism" by Dr. Beverly Tatum & Andrea Ayvazian in White Awareness: Handbook for Anti-Racism Training by Judy H. Katz. ©1978 by the University of Oklahoma Press, Norman. Reprinted by permission of the publisher. All rights reserved.

Permission was also granted from the Anti-Defamation League, Education Division, A WORLD OF DIFFERENCE® Institute © 2007 Anti-Defamation League: www.adl.org/education; email: education@adl.org.

References

Akers M, Grover P (2017) What is emotional intelligence? Psych Central. https://psychcentral.com/lib/what-is-emotional-intelligence-eq/. Accessed 2 June 2017

American Association of Colleges of Nursing (2006) Essentials of doctoral education in advanced practice nursing. http://www.aacn.nche.edu/publications/position/DNPEssentials.pdf. Accessed 5 June 2017

American Nurses Association (2015) Code of ethics for nurses with interpretive statements. Author, Silver Spring

Andrews MM, Boyle JS (eds) (2016) Transcultural concepts and nursing care, 7th edn. Wolters Kluwer, Philadelphia

Calvillo E, Clark L, Purnell L, Pacquiao D, Ballantyne J, Villaruel S (2009) Cultural competencies in health care: emerging changes in baccalaureate nursing education. J Transcult Nurs 20(2):137–145

Canadian Nurses Association (2010) Position statement: promoting cultural competence in nursing. https://www.cna-aiic.ca/~/media/cna/page-content/pdf-en/ps114_cultural_competence_2010_e.pdf?la=en. Accessed 2 June 2017

Carper BA (1978) Fundamental patterns of knowing in nursing. Adv Nurs Sci 1(1):13–23

Chinn P (2018) Critical theory and emancipatory knowing. In: Butts JB, Rich KL (eds) Philosophies and theories for advanced nursing practice. Jones & Bartlett Learning

Chinn PL, Kramer MK (2015) Knowledge development in nursing theory and process, 9th edn. Elsevier, St. Louis

Cholle FP (2011) What is intuition, and how do we use it? https://www.psychologytoday.com/blog/the-intuitive-compass/201108/what-is-intuition-and-how-do-we-use-it. Accessed 2 June 2017

Cuellar N (2017) Unconscious bias. What is yours? J Transcult Nurs 28(4):333

Dewey J (1933) How we think: a restatement on the relation of reflective thinking to the educative process. D.C. Health, New York

Douglas M, Rosenketter M, Pacquiao D, Clark Callister L et al (2014) Guidelines for implementing culturally competent nursing care. J Transcult Nurs 25(2):109–221

Faith as a Way of Knowing. http://www.agakhanacademies.org/sites/default/files/AKA%20Faith%20Booklet%20for%20IB%20TOK.pdf. Accessed 3 June 2017

Ghoshal RA, Lippard C, Ribas V, Muir K (2013) Beyond bigotry: teaching about unconscious prejudice. Teach Sociol 41(2):130–143. http://vlib.excelsior.edu/login?url=http://search.ebscohost.com/login.aspx?direct=true&db=sih&AN=86187613&site=eds-live&scope=site. Accessed 11 July 2017

Goleman D (2005) Emotional intelligence: why it can matter more than IQ. Bloomsbury Publishing, London

Hickson H (2011) Critical reflection: reflecting on learning to be reflective. Reflect Pract Interprof Multidiscip Perspect 12(6):829–839

How We Think: John Dewey on the Art of Reflection and Fruitful Curiosity in an Age of Instant Opinions and Information Overload (n.d.) https://www.brainpickings.org/2014/08/18/how-we-think-john-dewey/. Accessed 2 June 2017

ICN Code of Ethics for Nurses (2012) http://www.icn.ch/who-we-are/code-of-ethics-for-nurses/. Accessed 2 June 2017

Johns C (1995) Framing learning through reflection within Carper's fundamental ways of knowing in nursing. J Adv Nurs 22:226–234

Kolb AY, Kolb DA (2005) Kolb learning style inventory. Experience Based Learning Systems, Inc. https://search.yahoo.com/yhs/search;_ylt=A0LEViOkBIFYzecABzonnIlQ;_ylu=X3oDMTEwcTc4aWkwBGNvbG8DYmYxBHBvcwMxBHZ0aWQDBHNlYwNxc3MtcXJ3XJ3?ei=UTF-8&hspart=mozilla&hsimp=yhs-002&fr=yhs-mozilla-002&p=Kolb%2C+%26+Kolb%2C+D.A.+%282005%29.+Kolb+Learning+Style+Inventory.+Experience+Based+Learning+Systems%2C+Inc.&fr2=12642. Accessed 2 June 2017

Mezirow J (1990) Fostering critical reflection in adulthood. Jossey-Bass, San Francisco

Miettinen R (2000) The concept of experiential learning and John Dewey's theory of reflective thought and action. Int J Lifelong Educ 19(1):54–72. https://doi.org/10.1080/026013700293458. Accessed 7 June 2017

Purnell L, Salmond S (2013) Individual cultural competence and evidence-based practice. In: Purnell L (ed) Transcultural health care: a culturally competent approach, 4th edn. F.A. Davis, Philadelphia

Rogers C (2002) Dewey's model of reflective learning. Teach Coll Rec 104(4):842–866. file:///D:/dewey.pdf. Accessed 2 June 2017

Schon DA (2014) The theory of inquiry: Dewey's legacy to education. Curric Inq 22(2):119–139. http://www.tandfonline.com/doi/abs/10.1080/03626784.1992.11076093?src=recsys. Accessed 2 June 2017

Sullivan-Marx EM (2013) The bear and the canyon: toward an understanding of personal leadership. Nurs Sci Q 26(4):373–375

The Critical Theory of Jurgen Habermas (n.d.) http://physicsed.buffalostate.edu/danowner/habcritthy.html. Accessed 4 June 2017

Theory of Nursing Knowldege. http://www.theoryofknowledge.net/. Accessed March 10, 2018

Timmins F (2006) Critical practice in nursing care: analysis, action and reflexivity. Nurs Stand 20:49–54

Tong R (2018) Feminist ethics: some applicable thought for advance practice nurses. In: Butts JB, Rich KL (eds) Philosophies and theories for advanced nursing practice. Jones & Bartlett Learning

Ways of Knowing: Faith (2017) http://sohowdoweknow.weebly.com/faith.html. Accessed 3 June 2017

Ways of Knowing: Theory of Knowledge.net (2017) http://www.theoryofknowledge.net/ways-of-knowing/. Accessed 2 June 2017

Case Study: Human Trafficking in Guatemala

11

Joyceen S. Boyle

Maria Luisa, a 16-year-old young woman from Escuintla, Guatemala, fled to the United States and is currently living in Connecticut. She fled Guatemala by herself and after a very arduous and dangerous journey through Mexico entered the United States at Brownsville, Texas. She voluntarily turned herself into US immigration authorities and asked for asylum, telling them that she feared for her life if she were returned to Guatemala. Maria Luisa was very nearly a victim of trafficking for sexual exploitation in Guatemala. According to the analysis of the International Commission against Impunity in Guatemala (CICIG) and the United Nations Children's Fund (UNICEF), there are an estimated 48,500 direct victims of trafficking for the purpose of sexual exploitation in Guatemala. The illegal profits produced by this offense amount to 12.3 billion quetzals (1.75 billion US dollars), equivalent to 2.7% of the gross domestic product (GDP), more than the total budget that Guatemala spends to educate children and adolescents (CICIG and UNICEF 2016, p. 7).

In Guatemala, Maria Luisa lived with her mother, her stepfather, her siblings, and her maternal grandmother. She never met her bio-

logical father as she was abandoned by him at a very young age. Maria Luisa's family is very poor. She managed to attend school although she often did not have sufficient money to ride the bus or to purchase clothes or school supplies. She met an older boy named Geraldo at school who noticed that she often walked to school and frequently did not do the school assignment as she did not have money to purchase supplies for the project. Maria Luisa's mother expected Maria Luisa to care for the three younger children; those responsibilities also interfered with her school activities. Geraldo talked to Maria Luisa about how good his mother was to him and invited her to his home to meet his mother, Regina. Regina would cook for Maria Luisa who often went hungry and promised that if Maria Luisa moved in with her, she would take care of her; she would never have to go without anything again. Since the situation at home was not good and it seemed to Maria Luisa to be getting worse, she moved in with Regina and Geraldo.

The first day in her new home, Regina took her to buy much-needed new clothes. She then told Maria Luisa that she needed to go to work with her in a bar at night to help her out. When Regina took Maria Luisa's phone away from her, she suspected something was wrong, but she was afraid to ask. While Maria Luisa was at the bar wiping up a table, a man approached and whispered to her. He asked if she was related to Regina and Maria Luisa answered no.

J. S. Boyle, Ph.D., R.N., M.P.H., FAAN
College of Nursing, University of Arizona, Tucson, AZ, USA

College of Nursing, Augusta State University, Augusta, GA, USA
e-mail: jboyle@nursing.arizona.edu

© Springer International Publishing AG, part of Springer Nature 2018
M. Douglas et al. (eds.), *Global Applications of Culturally Competent Health Care: Guidelines for Practice*, https://doi.org/10.1007/978-3-319-69332-3_11

113

He then told her that Regina (with Geraldo's help) was going to force her into prostitution with male clients at the bar. He urged her to call her mother and he slipped her his cell phone. Maria Luisa called her mother and begged her to come and get her. The next day, Regina locked Maria Luisa in the house and would not let her out. Her mother came looking for her, but Regina refused to let Maria Luisa return to her mother's home saying that "Maria Luisa wanted to live with her and Geraldo." Maria Luisa's mother managed to file a complaint with the local police who insisted that Regina let Maria Luisa return to her mother.

For several months after this incident, Geraldo kept looking for Maria Luisa, stalking and harassing her. He threatened to take her back to his mother. Maria Luisa obtained a restraining order against Geraldo, but he said that his uncle was a police officer and he (Geraldo) did not need to pay attention to the restraining order. Maria Luisa was very frightened; she transferred to a new school, but Geraldo found her there. Geraldo would drive by her house with other boys on motorcycles, stopping to tell her that one day he would find her alone and force her back to Regina's house. For 10 months, Maria Luisa lived in fear and finally decided to leave. Even now that she is living in the United States, her former classmates in Guatemala tell her that Geraldo texts them asking about Maria Luisa's whereabouts. Maria Luisa is afraid that if she is returned to Guatemala, Regina and Geraldo will kidnap her, perhaps even kill her or force her into prostitution.

11.1   Cultural Issues

CICIG and UNICEF (2016, p. 72) report that the patriarchal culture is the most important factor for the existence of trafficking in Guatemala. Sexual violence is a constant occurrence in many Guatemalan homes, where the father, the stepfather, or other close relatives rape boys and girls at an early age. Forty-five percent of the victims of sexual or gender violence in Guatemala are under 14 years of age (CICIG and UNICEF

2016, p. 73). Gender-related violence in Guatemala is consistent with a culture of patriarchy as well as machismo and other widespread dominant expressions of masculinity that structure and reinforce the notion that men "own" women and that women should be controlled by them. At the present time, gender-based violence, including rape, sexual abuse, beatings, and killings, are often inflicted by a woman's family members, a friend, an acquaintance, a partner, a spouse, or a former spouse. Family members often reinforce behavior related to machismo by telling the abused woman that gender subordination is "normal" or that the woman did something to encourage or deserve the violence she has suffered.

The most common type of exploitation may be perpetrated by close relatives of the victim—the trafficker may be the brother, the father, an uncle, or a teacher. Many times mothers allow the abuse to continue in order not to lose income from their spouse or because they themselves are victims of domestic violence. In such a context, sexual abuse and gender violence are reproduced generationally, always against the weakest and most vulnerable. UNICEF (2014, p. 20) has noted that girls who have experienced physical, sexual, or psychological violence often have mothers who were also victims of abuse. These mothers have difficulty managing situations of sexual violence; they end up ignoring it and accepting what happened as normal.

11.2   Social Structure Factors

Because of its geographical location, Guatemala is particularly vulnerable to human trafficking. Intensified migration flows have turned it into a country of origin, transit, and destination of transnational trafficking. Hondurans and Salvadorans must cross Guatemala to reach Mexico and then the United States. Guatemala has become an important sexual destination; tourism packages promote these activities, particularly around the larger cities. However, trafficking does not stand alone as organized crimes involving drug cartels, gang violence, and particularly human trafficking are criminal activities that can only take place with the active or passive participation of state authorities. The Policia Nacional Civil (PNC), the security force responsible for civilian safety, has a long history of ignoring human rights abuses, including human trafficking for sexual exploitation. In addition, a weak judiciary system that fails to investigate, judge, and punish perpetuators of criminal activities only promotes strong criminal structures. A justice system that exhibits sexist and discriminatory behaviors that reinforce the social ideology that a victim causes or is guilty of initiating the crime (provocative dress or behaviors) excuses the behavior of the aggressor.

Victims of exploitation and trafficking have reported that municipal officials and employees are users of sexual services of girls and adolescents. According to CICIG and UNICEF (2016, p. 82), the most frequent customers are drug traffickers who pay large sums of money for sexual services. As customers, drug traffickers are extremely violent and demanding; they unmercifully abuse the victims who are treated as merchandise and may be given over to bodyguards or to other drug traffickers. The patriarchal culture also results in fewer opportunities for women. Education for boys is valued more than education for girls. Fewer girls have opportunities to break the cycle of poverty through school, and they are always in a position of social vulnerability that is often used to exploit them for work and sex. Girls are often bullied or pressured by teachers to have sex in exchange for a better grade. Even girls or women who escape situations of abuse including trafficking face formidable obstacles to a better life. A considerable number of Guatemalan and Central American women who are migrating through Mexico are trapped by trafficking networks and are forced again into a life of sexual exploitation. In addition, it has been estimated that eight out of ten migrant women from Central America traveling through Mexico suffer some kind of sexual abuse in Mexico. They start the journey aware that they may be raped once, twice, three times, or perhaps more.

11.3 Culturally Competent Strategies Recommended

Many healthcare professionals in the United States will come into contact with persons who have been sexually exploited in Guatemala or other Central America countries. "In fiscal 2016, the Border Patrol apprehended 58,819 unaccompanied children and 73,888 family units along the southwest border. Most were from El Salvador, Honduras, and Guatemala" (Sherman 2017). While some of these migrants are in immigration detention centers, others have been given immigration court dates and are living with relatives throughout the country. Some migrants who have applied for asylum are eligible for Medicaid and CHIP (Children's Health Insurance Program). There are also many free-standing clinics and urgent care centers that serve migrants in border regions and elsewhere. Many churches and nongovernmental agencies sponsor health clinics in the Central America countries, so it is possible that North American health professionals will be in contact with persons who have experienced sexual exploitation.

In view of the complexity involved in human trafficking in Guatemala, any response must be aimed at three priority areas: to eradicate trafficking for the purposes of sexual exploitation, to provide assistance to victims, and to impart justice to prevent offenses from remaining unpunished (CICIG and UNICEF p. 7). Such a massive undertaking involves the countries of the Northern Triangle (El Salvador, Honduras, and Guatemala), Mexico, and the United States. However, in this case study, we focus only on Guatemala.

11.3.1 Individual/Family-Level Interventions

- A victim of sexual trafficking suffers harm to their physical, psychological, social, and financial health. Conduct an in-depth assessment for sexually transmitted diseases, including HIV/AIDS, and injuries to the reproductive system such as syphilis, gonorrhea, and chlamydia that can cause serious long-term damage such as sterility, infertility, and pelvic inflammatory disease.

- Assess for drug and alcohol dependency as victims are forced from an early age to consume alcohol and drugs.
- Assess symptoms of emotional crises, low self-esteem, depression, and eating and sleeping disorders.
- Threats, beatings, and other forms of punishment take a tremendous toll on victims' psychological health and should be reported to local authorities.
- Refer to psychiatric care or counseling if available.

11.3.2 Organizational-Level Interventions

- Support activists in Guatemalan women's organizations who are speaking out and attempting to protect young women from exploitation.
- Collaborate with community organizations and churches to establish educational programs that explain trafficking and sexual exploitation to young persons as well as how to avoid being trafficked.
- Contact your congressional representatives to express your concern and urge them to support legislation that addresses poverty, education, and employment opportunities in Guatemala as opposed to focusing only on military solutions to gang violence and drug trafficking.

11.3.3 Community Societal-Level Interventions

- Criminal activities involve the participation of state authorities as well as police and municipal authorities. Trafficking and sexual exploitation in Guatemala must focus on criminal networks in Mexico and Central and Latin America and drug trafficking in the United States.
- Trafficking is a serious human rights violation, and the international magnitude of this offense has been recognized since the adoption of the Convention on the Abolition of Slavery that dates back to 1926 and ratified by the Guatemala State in 1983 (CICIG and UNICEF 2016, p. 15). Support anti-slavery or anti-trafficking organizations in your community.
- Publicize the US National Human Trafficking Research Center Hotline 1-888-373-7888.

Conclusion

Guatemala is a country of origin, transit, and destination of persons who are trafficked for purposes of sexual exploitation. Highly structured networks exist in Honduras and El Salvador that recruit and transfer victims to Guatemala where they are exploited. As a country of origin, thousands of families and children as well as unaccompanied minors have fled drug and gang violence in Guatemala and have made their way to the United States. Along the way through Mexico, sexual exploitation frequently occurs.

Maria Luisa was fortunate in many ways. While her home life was not ideal, her mother did rescue her from sexual exploitation. However, Geraldo continued to stalk and harass her, and there was little she could do legally to stop him.

A culture of patriarchy pervades Guatemala, influencing attitudes of ordinary Guatemalans, the police, and the judicial officials. Patriarchy condones the abuse and degradation of women. Maria Luisa knew that eventually Geraldo would find her and that there would be little she could do to resist sexual exploitation. She continually lived in fear of Geraldo who threatened and intimidated her; he actively participated, along with his mother, to lure Maria Luisa into a dangerous situation for purposes of trafficking her for sexual exploitation.

Maria finally fled to the United States to escape his harassment and unwanted attention. She applied for asylum in the United States but was terrified of the current political climate in the United States that denigrates migrants. While focusing on her needs secondary to her immigration status and fear of sexual exploitation, culturally competent care should promote her mental and physical health and a potential for participating as a productive citizen.

References

Comisión Internacional contra la Impunidad en Guatemala (CICIG), United Nations Children Educational Fund (UNICEF) (2016) Human trafficking for sexual exploitation purposes in Guatemala. Guatemala de la Asunción

Sherman C (2017) Mexico won't take 3rd-country deportees from US, official says. Associated Press, The Arizona Daily Star. Accessed 25 Feb 2017

United Nations Children Fund (UNICEF) (2014) Update: national diagnostic on the situation of unaccompanied boys, girls and adolescents in the migration process. Antigua, Guatemala, 2014

Case Study: A Young African American Woman with Lupus

12

Donna Shambley-Ebron

Nia Monroe is a 20-year-old African American woman who lives in a mid-sized city in the Midwestern United States. She, her mother, and her 3 younger siblings live in a large public housing community consisting of 700 individual units. Despite many obstacles, Nia graduated in the top of her class in high school and was a student athlete. She was awarded a full scholarship to the public university in her city where she planned to study nursing, as the first person in her family to attend college.

During her senior year in high school, Nia started experiencing joint and muscle pain, which she attributed to soreness or injury from her last athletic event. When symptoms did not subside and she began experiencing fever, she went to her neighborhood health center, where she was finally diagnosed with systemic lupus erythematosus (SLE). SLE, more commonly known as lupus, is an autoimmune disorder that disproportionately affects Black women. Lupus affects numerous organs, including the skin, brain, heart, and kidneys, and can lead to a significant lifelong disability. The disease may have periods of remissions and exacerbations, and Black women have an earlier onset and also greater severity of disease. Nia was given a pamphlet about lupus at the

health center and was referred to a rheumatologist, whom she has seen only once. The rheumatologist prescribed numerous medications that she is unable to afford.

Nia was able to begin her classes at the university; however, numerous lupus flares during her first year led her to withdraw from school, having fallen behind in all of her classes. Back at home with her family and being unemployed led to social isolation, frequent exacerbations, increasing debilitation, and major depression.

12.1 Cultural Issues

The Monroe family resides in a mid-sized Midwestern US city with a population of 300,000. It is estimated that about 44% of the city residents are African American. Nia and her family live in a public housing community for low-income residents operated by the Metropolitan Housing Authority. The public housing project in which Nia and her family reside is home to 3800 residents, 98% of whom are African American. Eighty-seven percent of the residents are women and their children under the age of 18. County residents have a median income of $50,000, which is similar to the state's median income; however within the city, the median income is $35,000. To qualify for public housing, residents must live below the federal poverty level, which for Nia's family of four is $24,600 (Office of the Federal Register 2017). Resources in

D. Shambley-Ebron, Ph.D., R.N., C.T.N.-A.
College of Nursing, University of Cincinnati, Cincinnati, OH, USA
e-mail: donna.shambley-ebron@uc.edu

© Springer International Publishing AG, part of Springer Nature 2018
M. Douglas et al. (eds.), *Global Applications of Culturally Competent Health Care: Guidelines for Practice*, https://doi.org/10.1007/978-3-319-69332-3_12

the community include a large recreation center with a swimming pool, two churches, a social service agency, a federally qualified healthcare center, and a K-8 elementary school. Crime is high in the community, often perpetrated by people who come in from outside of the community, with gun violence as a frequent occurrence.

Nia's mother works as a STNA (state-tested nurse aide) in a long-term care facility and takes evening classes to earn her LPN. Two of Nia's brothers attend the community school, and the oldest attends high school outside of the community. Nia's mother has an old, unreliable vehicle to drive to work, which leaves Nia at home without transportation.

Because Nia is over the age of 19, she is no longer eligible for Medicaid but cannot afford insurance under the Affordable Care Act and therefore remains uninsured. Nia and her family attend Sunday services at the community church in the neighborhood and rely on their spiritual family for emotional and social support. Also, Nia's aunts and cousins who live on the other side of town visit on weekends and provide some social support, although they do not understand her illness.

There is a small "corner store" in the neighborhood which is a "hangout" for young people in the community that sells snacks, soda, and beer; however, the closest full-service grocery store is 3 miles away, qualifying the community as a "food desert" or low-access community (USDA 2011).

Because Nia is uninsured, she has avoided going to see her rheumatologist. She is also unable to pay for the expensive medications and does not feel as if her provider genuinely cares about her condition. Even though she was able to secure a bus pass from the community social service agency for her first visit, to get to the rheumatologist required a long bus ride with several transfers that end up taking an entire day for a short visit.

12.2 Cultural Issues: Spirituality

For many African Americans, spirituality is a deeply held value that is manifested by the recognition of a spiritual world that has influence on one's everyday existence in the tangible world. Spirituality is often accompanied by a belief in the power of prayer to change adverse life circumstances, study of sacred scriptures, and often includes a spiritual community or family with whom believers congregate to worship, pray, and fellowship. Oftentimes, the spiritual leader provides counsel and advice to members. Spiritual beliefs often influence life decisions and choices, and the spiritual family serves as a source of support during illness, death, and other life difficulties.

According to the Pew Research Center on Religion and Public Life (2009), African Americans, when compared with other groups in the United States, are considered more religious, based on affiliation, attendance at church, frequency of prayer, and the importance of religion. The majority of African Americans practice Christianity; however, they are represented in other religious groups such as Islam, Buddhism, and Judaism. Others report no religious group affiliation (Pew Research Center 2009).

Although spirituality and religious beliefs can serve as a source of strength for African Americans, it may also lead to a failure to seek professional healthcare. This may be especially true for certain mental health conditions such as depression, which can be seen as evidence of spiritual weakness.

12.3 Mistrust of the Healthcare System

African Americans have had a long history of discrimination and maltreatment in the healthcare system (Washington 2006). Numerous historical offenses have been documented and also have been passed down by word of mouth, leading to mistrust of providers and the overall healthcare system by African Americans. This mistrust can lead African Americans to be reluctant in seeking healthcare and adhering to prescribed treatment plans.

12.3.1 Stigma

Among African Americans, stigma still exists as it relates to mental illness. Acknowledging mental illness, particularly depression, is often frowned upon and seen as a weakness. Treatment may not be sought or is discouraged by others, including family members. Moreover, African American women have had a history of being required to be "strong" in the face of adversity. This history of being strong has been passed down from generations since the time of their enslavement and has influenced African American women's responses to adverse life circumstances (Shambley-Ebron and Boyle 2006). This tradition of "being strong" is related to living and raising families independently, coping with illness, and caregiving for family members, among other situations. Although this perception may be useful for helping African American women to be resilient, it may also prevent them from seeking appropriate help and practicing needed self-care.

12.3.2 Extended Family Networks and Fictive Kin

African American families build networks of extended family for everyday subsistence. Often extended family members may share living arrangements and child-care responsibilities. In addition, non-blood-related relationships (fictive kin) are often considered family members and are called "auntie," "uncle," or "cousin" (Taylor et al. 2013).

12.4 Social Structural Factors

In spite of gains in education, 27% of all African American people live beneath the poverty line compared to only 11% of Whites (Black Demographics 2014). According to the report on race and inequality produced by The Century Foundation, African Americans are more likely to live in concentrated poverty, that is, segregated high-poverty neighborhoods and census tracts that place them in a type of "double jeopardy" from both individual and collective poverty (Jargowsky 2015). These high-poverty neighborhoods are often isolated and located a distance from resources needed to sustain health, such as affordable healthy foods, green space, safe walking spaces, and recreational areas. Living in such

neighborhoods, no doubt, is a contributor to poorer health and life expectancy, evidenced by the health inequities found between African Americans and White Americans in many areas, e.g., cardiovascular disease including hypertension, diabetes, SLE, high infant mortality rates, and many types of cancer. The chronic stress brought on by living in such conditions over an extended period of time leads to a diminished ability to resist illness and also a shortened lifespan (Williams et al. 2015). Moreover, even with the Affordable Care Act and Medicaid expansion, it is estimated that 12.2% of African Americans remain uninsured (Kaiser Family Foundation 2016).

SLE is one such illness that represents a substantial health disparity that negatively impacts the lives of African American women (Minority Women's Health 2010). Not only are African American women three times more likely to develop SLE than Caucasians, but they also have greater severity and earlier onset. Lupus can lead to significant disability and impairment, including neurologic, cardiovascular, and end-stage renal disease. In addition, women with lupus may have skin discoloration and hair loss, leading to low self-esteem and physical image issues (Beckerman et al. 2011). Although the reasons for this difference in incidence and severity of lupus among African American women are unknown, environment and stress, including discrimination, have been posited as risk factors in exacerbations and severity of the disease (Williams et al. 2015; Chae et al. 2015).

Another important societal factor that greatly influences African Americans and leads to chronic stress is the systemic racism and discrimination that daily impact their lives in the form of both micro and macro aggression and structural inequalities (Hollingsworth et al. 2017). Racism and discrimination have a direct impact on how healthcare is delivered and how it is accessed. Implicit bias has been studied among healthcare providers, particularly physicians. It has been found in studies of physicians' attitudes that many White physicians view their Caucasian patients more favorably and communicate with them differently than they do with their African American patients (Cooper et al. 2012). It has also been found that African Americans are less likely to receive aggressive treatments for many health conditions and under certain circumstances are less likely to receive needed pain medication (Oliver et al. 2014).

The neighborhood in which Nia and her family live is an example of an urban community of economic segregation and concentrated poverty in which the environmental stressors contribute to overall poor health and vulnerability. In spite of Nia's opportunity to leave her community, poor health has forced her back into the environment that has possibly contributed to her condition.

12.5 Culturally Competent Strategies Recommended

In order to address the complex health concerns faced by Nia, the following recommendations are made to provide culturally appropriate care on the individual, organizational, and societal levels.

12.5.1 Individual-/Family-Level Interventions

- Encourage monthly appointments with advanced practice nurse at the Federally Qualified Health Center (FQHC) for physical, mental health, and socioeconomic assessments.
- Educate patient about her condition and associated symptoms and comorbidities.
- Validate patient's feelings and emotions regarding her illness.
- Develop self-care plan using complementary therapies as needed.
- Refer to social services for assistance with needed resources regarding medication costs, assistance with applying for Medicaid under Medicaid expansion, and assistance with returning to school, part-time.
- Refer to free mental health services clinic for depression.
- Locate lupus support group and help enroll patient.
- Include family in education and planning with patient's permission.

- Investigate patient's comfort level with involving clergy in providing counsel.

12.5.2 Organizational Level

- Ensure all providers have adequate training in the promotion of culturally competent care. Provide ongoing and continuing education.
- Actively engage providers in community activities and organizations to enhance visibility and trust in the community.
- Develop a local media campaign about lupus to increase community awareness.
- Provide literature on lupus and other conditions that disproportionately impact African Americans in health centers and in the community.
- Identify community members with lupus and establish a support group that meets in the health center.

12.5.3 Community/Societal Level

- Establish community-empowerment groups for members to address concerns such as food access and safety in the community.
- Partner with local public safety to establish a plan to address neighborhood concerns such as high crime.
- Develop academic-community partnerships to address Lupus and other community health issues through community-based participatory research methods.
- Engage city policy makers and planners in a discussion around alleviating the burden of highly concentrated poverty neighborhoods.
- Collaborate with community churches and social service agencies to address the social and structural determinants of health in the community.

Conclusion

Systemic lupus erythematosus (SLE) is a chronic and sometimes acute autoimmune disease that destroys connective tissue and organs in the body. African American women carry a great burden of SLE, being impacted at three times the rate of Caucasian women. In addition, African American women have a much earlier onset and have a greater severity and higher mortality rate from the disease. The disease is characterized by remissions and exacerbations that can be brought on by numerous factors including stress.

Nia Monroe has developed the disease in young adulthood, and it has dampened her dreams of becoming the first college attendee in her family. Having had to drop out of school in her first year, she has returned to a low-resource community with concentrated poverty, a public housing project with her family. She is unable to adequately access the culturally competent healthcare and resources of which she is in need. She has become isolated and depressed because of her health status and living conditions. Nia's condition places her at increased vulnerability to frequent exacerbations, the development of comorbidities, and overall diminishing physical and mental health.

Interventions should focus on three levels of strategies that address not only the physical conditions that Nia is faced with but also the sociocultural and structural issues that influence her health and the health of her community. Only by addressing the root causes of poorer health in high-poverty communities can strides be made to reduce the health disparities that negatively impact African Americans and affect the health of our entire society.

References

Beckerman NL, Auerbach C, Blanco I (2011) Psychosocial dimensions of SLE: implications for the health care team. J Multidisc Healthcare 4:63–72. https://doi.org/10.2147/JMDH.A19303

Black Demographics.com (2014) Poverty in Black America. http://blackdemographics.com/households/poverty/. Accessed 3 July 2017

Chae DH, Drenkard CM, Lewis TT, Lim SS (2015) Discrimination and cumulative disease damage among African American women with SLE. Am J Public Health 105(10):2099–2107. https://doi.org/10.2105/AJPH

Cooper LA, Roter DL, Carson KA, Beach MC et al (2012) The associations of clinician's implicit attitudes about race with medical visit communication and patient ratings of interpersonal care. Am J Public Health 102(5):979–987. https://doi.org/10.2105/ajph.2011.300558

Federal Register. The Daily Journal of the United States Government (2017) Annual update of the HHS poverty guidelines. https://www.federalregister.gov/documents/2017/01/21/2017-02076/annual-update-of-the-hhs-poverty-guidelines. Accessed 3 July 2017

Hollingsworth DW, Cole AB, O'Keefe VM, Tucker RP et al (2017) Experiencing racial microaggressions influences suicide ideation through perceived burdensomeness in African Americans. J Couns Psychol 64(1):104–111. https://doi.org/10.1037/cou0000177

Jargowsky P (2015) Architecture of segregation: civil unrest, the concentration of poverty, and public policy. The Century Foundation. https://tcf.org/content/report/architecture-of-segregation/. Accessed 3 July 2017

Kaiser Family Foundation (2016) Key facts about the uninsured population. http://kff.org/uninsured/fact-sheet/key-facts-about-the-uninsured-population/. Accessed 3 July 2017

Minority Women's Health (2010) Lupus. https://www.womenshealth.gov/minority-health/african-americans/lupus.html. Accessed 3 July 2017

Oliver MN, Wells KM, Joy-Gaba JA, Hawkins CB et al (2014) Do physicians' implicit views of African Americans affect clinical decision-making? J Am Board Fam Med 27(2):177–188. https://doi.org/10.3122/jabfm.2014.02.120314

Pew Research Center: Religion and Public Life (2009) A religious portrait of African Americans. www.pewforum.ort/2009/01/30/a-religious-portrait-of-african-americans/. Accessed 3 July 2017

Shambley-Ebron D, Boyle JS (2006) In our grandmother's footsteps: perceptions of being strong in African American women. Adv Nurs Sci 29(3):195–206

Taylor RJ, Chatters LM, Woodward AT, Brown E (2013) Racial and ethnic differences in extended family, friendship, fictive kin, and congregational informal support networks. Fam Relat 62(4):609–624. https://doi.org/10.1111/fare.12030

United States Department of Agriculture, Food and Nutrition Locator (2011) https://www.fns.usda.gov/tags/food-desert-locator. Accessed 3 July 2017

Washington HA (2006) Medical apartheid: the dark history of medical experimentation on Black Americans from colonial times to the present. Doubleday, New York

Williams EM, Zhang J, Anderson J, Bruner L, Tumiel-Berhalter L (2015) Social support and self-reported stress levels in a predominantly African American sample of women with systemic lupus erythematosus. Autoimmune Dis 2015:401620. https://doi.org/10.1155/2015/4016

Case Study: Intimate Partner Violence in Peru

13

Roxanne Amerson

Sarah Moxley recently graduated from a baccalaureate nursing program in the United States. During nursing school, she participated in a 1-month immersion program in Guatemala to educate indigenous people about health issues. Recognizing her desire to continue working in a Latin American country, after graduation she accepted a volunteer position with a nongovernmental organization (NGO) to educate low-income women in a small community in the southeastern region of Peru. The mission of this organization is to empower women through education and to promote economic development for women and their children in the remote villages of the nearby Andes Mountains.

Sarah lives with a host family in a small town near the site of the NGO. Living and working in the small community allows Sarah to become friends with many of the local people within the town. The home where she lives shares adjacent walls with the neighbors' homes. The proximity of homes is representative of the collectivistic culture of Peru and allows for little privacy. It is quite common to hear the family activities of the neighbors.

Sarah has become a close friend of a young Quechua mother, Silvia Puma Quispe, who lives next door. Silvia is 18 years old, has two small children, and lives with an older man, Jorge, whom she plans to marry in the future. It is common for Peruvians to cohabit for several years before getting married. Silvia's family arranged her relationship with Jorge when she was 15 years old. While the legal age of marriage in Peru has increased to 18 years, the age of sexual consent remains at 14 years. Prior to this recent legislative change, the age of consent for marriage was 16 years. The common practice of early marriage is a major contributing factor to young girls dropping out of school early to assume the duties of wife and mother, rather than completing an education.

In the last week, Sarah has been hearing shouting and sounds of fighting coming from Silvia's house during the late hours of the night. This morning, Silvia arrived in the market with a swollen right cheek and a black eye. When Sarah asked Silvia, "What happened last night?," Silvia replied that Jorge sometimes has too much to drink and gets angry with her. If she argues with him, he will hit her or push her to the ground. Silvia starts to cry but tells Sarah it is her duty as Jorge's future wife to make her husband happy and not anger him. He is the father of her children, and it is important for her to stay with him. Because Silvia quit school early, she has a very limited education and no way to support her

R. Amerson, Ph.D., R.N., C.T.N.-A., C.N.E.
School of Nursing, Clemson University,
Greenville, SC, USA
e-mail: ROXANNA@clemson.edu

children financially. Silvia's mother and father are poor and have too many mouths to feed to take her back into their home.

Sarah is angry and frustrated by what she hears from Silvia. Sarah has been brought up in a culture where women are expected to be educated, have an equal voice in the marital relationship, and should not be hit by a man. She cannot understand why Silvia would choose to stay with a man who beats her. Nor does she understand why Silvia believes it is her duty to remain in a relationship for the sake of her children when she is being hurt and abused.

13.1 Cultural Issues

Intimate partner violence (IPV) represents a major public health problem in Peru. In 2009, over 45% of Peruvian women experienced physical, sexual, and emotional abuse (Cripe et al. 2015). Women who reside in rural areas of Peru experience even higher rates of IPV with estimates as high as 69% (Gelaye et al. 2010). Girls are taught the concept of *marianismo* (to model their behavior after the Virgin Mary) that encourages females to be submissive and to accept the burdens of life without complaint. Furthermore, boys are instilled with values of *machismo* (dominance and strength) which precipitates the power issues that often arise in a marriage or relationship. Men are expected to have control over the women in their lives.

Even the state of Peru has perpetuated violence against women in the past. Indigenous Quechua women underwent forced sterilization from 1996 to 2000 and were the frequent victims of sexual violence during the 20-year reign of the Sendero Luminoso (Shining Path), a communist terrorist group that operated in Peru starting in the 1970s. According to the World Health Organization Multi-Country Study on Domestic Violence Against Women, violence often begins early with one in five female children experiencing sexual abuse in urban Lima, Peru (Devries et al. 2011). While Peruvian legislation is now in place to reduce violence against women, the laws are poorly enforced.

Family values play an important role in the decision for women to remain in abusive relationships. The collectivistic nature of Peruvian culture supports the concept of *familismo* (the importance of putting the needs of the family before the needs of the individual) (Bernal and Rodriquez 2009). Women commonly will choose to remain in a relationship to ensure the needs of their children are met, even when the woman faces tremendous physical or emotional abuse. Only when her children's health or safety is at risk, then a woman may choose to leave the abusive relationship (Kelly 2009).

Economic status plays a major role in the decision to remain with an abusive partner. The illiteracy rate is approximately 20% with an average 6 years of school for women in rural communities (Pan American Health Organization 2012). Indigenous women of Quechua descent are more likely to be less educated and live in poverty in rural areas of Peru. A lack of education leads to fewer opportunities for work outside of the home. Poverty rates in rural areas exceed 50% with extreme poverty being present in more than 20% of the Quechua populations in Peru. Early marriage or cohabitation leads to greater risk of dropping out of school and fewer opportunity to engage in the workforce (Malé and Wodon 2016). Women with limited education and a lack of financial resources are much more likely to remain under the control of an abusive partner. Both low socioeconomic status and poverty are commonly linked with violence (Holtz 2017).

13.2 Cultural Competent Strategies Recommended

Nurses must engage in critical reflection to examine their own cultural beliefs and values and how these values influence the provision of culturally competent care (Douglas et al. 2014). Reflection is the process of "inner awareness of thoughts, feelings, beliefs, judgments, and perceptions" (Smith et al. 2015, p. 28). Critical reflection allows one to analyze personal perceptions to improve future care, especially in situations where the nurse's values conflict with the values of the patient or family.

Sarah engages in critical reflection when she asks herself the following questions:

1. How do my own cultural values of relationships between men and women affect my response to Silvia's experience with IPV?
2. How do my values of individualism influence my expectation that Silvia will leave her abusive partner?
3. If I were Silvia and based on her worldview in rural Peru, what options would I see available to me to leave an abusive situation?
4. How can I provide culturally competent recommendations for IPV to Silvia based on the resources available in her situation?

13.2.1 Individual- or Family-Level Interventions

- Examine one's own personal values, beliefs, perceptions, and biases related to IPV.
- Encourage Silvia to discuss her previous experiences with violence, including any history of sexual violence.
- Help Silvia to recognize that abuse is not acceptable (Cripe et al. 2015).
- Assess Silvia for signs of depression, suicidal behaviors, anxiety, or alcohol dependency, which are common in women who have experienced IPV (Gelaye et al. 2010).
- Determine if Silvia engages in violent self-defense behaviors with Jorge during periods of conflict. Women who are severely abused are more likely to respond in a violent manner to defend themselves, therefore, increasing the amount of violence witnessed by children in the home (Gelaye et al. 2010).
- Encourage Silvia to participate in a secondary IPV prevention program available through the local NGO to learn about help-seeking behaviors, rather than remaining a victim.
- Assist Silvia to enroll in a microcredit (small loan to promote self-employment) program available through the local NGO if available.

- Provide information in a nonjudgmental manner about the childhood effects of witnessing violence in the home (Amerson et al. 2014).
- Respect Silvia's autonomy to decide whether to stay or leave (Cripe et al. 2015).

13.2.2 Organizational-Level Interventions

- Encourage the NGO where Sarah volunteers to start a primary IPV prevention program to help break the cycle of violence (Gelaye et al. 2010).
- Design an intervention program to teach self-help behaviors for abused women (Gelaye et al. 2010).
- Maintain a database of available microcredit programs or other financial program to help women become more self-sufficient.

13.2.3 Community- or Societal-Level Interventions

- Begin gender equality education in primary school to break the cycle of violence.
- Recognize "gate-keepers" such as forensic doctors, police, and nurses who can affect the outcome of IPV cases that go to trial; therefore, training for service providers is crucial to prevent further victimizing of women who come forward to report IPV (Cripe et al. 2015).
- Start a support group for women who are victims of IPV where they can find and maintain supportive relationships (Cripe et al. 2015).
- Work with community and government leaders to establish professional counseling services and legal services to assist battered women (Cripe et al. 2015), while recognizing that resources will be minimal in more rural, isolated areas.

Conclusion

Sarah now realizes that her initial reaction to Silvia's situation and the expectation that Silvia should leave her partner are based on

Sarah's own cultural values; therefore this may not be the best solution for Silvia and her children. The combination of economic, cultural, and educational factors has a crucial impact on a woman's decision to leave an abusive situation. Simply telling a woman to leave may actually create new problems when a community does not have resources in place to protect or provide shelter to a woman and her children. Few rural communities in rural Peru will have battered women shelters, and many members of the community will simply see IPV as a "burden the woman must bear."

Teaching self-help behaviors, providing psychological counseling, and establishing support groups may be the best choice for helping women cope with abusive relationships when there is simply no place to go in the short term. Helping the woman to become more financially independent may be a good long-term solution to helping escape the abuse. Each woman has a unique situation where one size does not fit all. Finding the right solution involves weighing the risks and benefits to have an optimal outcome while maintaining a safe environment for the woman and her children.

References

Amerson R, Whittington R, Duggan L (2014) Intimate partner violence affecting Latina women and their children. J Emerg Nurs 40(6):531–536

Bernal G, Rodriguez M (2009) Advances in Latino family research: cultural adaptations of evidence-based interventions. Fam Process 48(2):169–178

Cripe SM, Espinoza D, Rondon MB, Jimenez ML et al (2015) Preferences for intervention among Peruvian women in intimate partner violence relationships. Hisp Health Care Int 13(1):27–37

Devries K, Watts C, Yoshihama M, Kiss L et al (2011) Violence against women is strongly associated with suicide attempts: evidence from the WHO multi-country study on women's health and domestic violence against women. Soc Sci Med 73(1):79–86

Douglas M, Rosenkoetter M, Pacquiao D, Callister L et al (2014) Guidelines for implementing cultural competent nursing care. J Transcult Nurs 25(2):109–121

Gelaye B, Lam N, Cripe S, Sanchez S et al (2010) Correlates of violent response among Peruvian women abused by an intimate partner. J Interpers Violence 25(1):136–151

Holtz C (2017) Global health care: issues and politics, 3rd edn. Jones & Bartlett Learning, Burlington

Kelly U (2009) I'm a mother first: the influence of mothering in the decision-making process of battered immigrant Latino women. Res Nurs Health 32:286–297

Malé C, Wodon Q (2016) Basic profile of child marriage in Peru. Knowledge brief: health, nutrition and population global practice. World Bank Group. http://documents. worldbank.org/curated/en/765701467991927389/ pdf/106417-BRI-ADD-SERIES-PUBLIC-HNP-Brief-Peru-Profile-CM.pdf. Accessed 3 July 2017

Pan American Health Organization (2012) Health in the Americas, 2012 edition: country volume. http://www.paho.org/salud-en-las-americas-2012/ index.php?option=com_docman&task=doc_ view&gid=143&Itemid=. Accessed 3 July 2017

Smith M, Carpenter R, Fitzpatrick J (2015) Encyclopedia of nursing education. Springer, New York

Useful Websites

Summary Report: Violence Against Women in Latin America and the Caribbean: a comparative analysis of population-based data from 12 countries (2013) PAHO, Washington. http://www.endvawnow.org/ uploads/browser/files/paho-vaw-exec-summ-eng.pdf. Accessed 3 July 2017

Understanding and addressing violence against women (2012) World Health Organization. http://www.end-vawnow.org/uploads/browser/files/paho-vaw-exec-summ-eng.pdf. Accessed 3 July 2017

Country Reports: Peru Facts and Culture (2017) http:// www.countryreports.org/country/Peru.htm. Accessed 3 July 2017

Part IV

Guideline: Cross Cultural Communication

Cross Cultural Communication: Verbal and Non-Verbal Communication, Interpretation and Translation

14

Larry Purnell

Guideline: *Nurses shall use culturally competent verbal and nonverbal communication skills to identify clients' values, beliefs, practices, perceptions, and unique healthcare needs.*

Douglas et al. (2014: 112)

14.1 Introduction

Despite decades of attention and awareness, healthcare disparities persist across the United States and other countries throughout the world. Racial and ethnic minorities, people with limited English proficiency (LEP) and low health literacy, sexual and gender minorities, and people with disabilities experience worse health outcomes, decreased access to healthcare services, and lower-quality care than the general population (Building an Organizational Response to Health Disparities 2016). Vast demographic changes are occurring around the world; inherent in these demographics are cross-cultural communication issues between patients and healthcare providers. Communication is culture bound: what works in one culture may not work in another culture. Thus, the onus on effective cultural communication is on healthcare providers. Cross-cultural communication combines anthropology, cultural studies, psychology, and communication theory. The goal of cross-cultural communication is to understand how people from different cultures communicate among insiders such as family and friends and with outsiders. Healthcare providers are considered outsiders.

Effective cross-cultural communication can be challenging because it provides people with ways of thinking and interpreting the world. Cross-cultural communication includes verbal and nonverbal components as well as the health literacy of patients.

14.2 Verbal Communication

The components of verbal communication consist of a number of elements: a dominant language and its dialects; contextual use of the language; paralanguage variations, such as voice volume, tone, and intonations; the willingness to share thoughts and feelings; degree of formality; and name format (Galanti 1991; Papadopoulos 2006; Purnell 2013). In addition, the healthcare provider needs to pay attention to the nonverbal communication such as a grimace or lack of eye contact during verbal communication. Dialects, regional variations of a language, can be troublesome

L. Purnell, Ph.D., R.N., FAAN
School of Nursing, University of Delaware, Newark, DE, USA

Florida International University, Miami, FL, USA

Excelsior College, Albany, NY, USA
e-mail: lpurnell@udel.edu

© Springer International Publishing AG, part of Springer Nature 2018
M. Douglas et al. (eds.), *Global Applications of Culturally Competent Health Care: Guidelines for Practice*, https://doi.org/10.1007/978-3-319-69332-3_14

because specific words may have a different meaning or the provider has difficulty understanding an accent as is the case in some parts of Appalachia in the United States where Elizabethan English is still spoken. In addition, sometimes the word does not exist in another language. In Mexico, while Spanish is the most widely spoken language, the government also recognizes 68 Mexican indigenous languages as official national languages (Mexican Languages 2017). India has 18 major languages and over 1600 regional dialects. Even though Hindi is the official language, many people in India do not speak it at all. Hindi is spoken by about half the population, mostly in North India (How many Languages do Indian People Speak? 2017). The current estimate of languages spoken in Nigeria is 521 with English being the official language, although only 75% of the people speak it. Yoruba, Hausa, Igbo, Fulfulde, Kanuri, and Ibibio are also popular (Languages of Nigeria n.d.). When a patient speaks a dialect for which there is no interpreter, use an interpreter using the language of popular radio stations because most people will understand this language.

The same words can mean different things to people from different cultures, even when they speak the same language. The use of idioms, slang, colloquialisms, and technical jargon should be avoided because they may not be understood by everyone, even by those who have good language proficiency. In addition, they do not translate well into other languages. Even though a patient might be somewhat bilingual, it can be difficult to fully understand the nuances of a language, especially with words that sound alike but spelled differently (homonyms) and must be viewed in context. For example, a "case" can be something that contains papers or other paraphernalia, a "case" as in a lawsuit, or as an adjective as in a "case" study. Another example is "glass," something to hold liquid for drinking, or "glass" as in a window. "Iron" could be an element or something used to iron clothing.

Slang and colloquial expressions can be particularly difficult and cause communication concerns. Some slang expression are the buck (versus as male deer) stops here and sweet to describe a person (versus the sweet taste in a drink). Colloquialisms, using informal words or phrases, can be troublesome, especially for whom the host language is not the patient's primary language. Some examples of colloquialisms are "go bananas" for going insane or angry, "feel blue" for feeling sad, and "y'all" (yawl) for you all. Health providers must make a concerted effort and avoid slang and colloquialisms. When the patient uses colloquialisms or slang, ask the patient to explain the terms.

In some cultures, people disclose very personal information about themselves, such as information about sex, recreational drug use, sexual orientation, and family problems to friends (and even casual acquaintances) and healthcare providers. However, in other cultures, it is taboo to disclose this information to others, even among healthcare providers. Even though some cultures willingly share their thoughts and feelings among family members and close friends, they may not easily share them with "outsiders" until they get to know them. Outsiders may include healthcare providers. By engaging in small talk and inquiring about family before addressing the patient's health concerns, healthcare providers can help establish trust and, in turn, encourage more open communication and sharing important health information (see Chap. 2 for more on collectivistic and individualistic cultures).

In some cultures, having well-developed verbal skills is seen as important, whereas in other cultures, such as among some Appalachians, the person who has very highly developed verbal skills is seen as having suspicious intentions (Huttlinger 2013). In addition, health literacy and limited language proficiency can compromise cross-cultural communication and lead to incomplete or inaccurate diagnoses. Such miscommunication can affect the ability to follow healthcare recommendations and prescriptions, even when the patient is in agreement with them (Andrews and Boyle 2016; Helman 2000; Purnell 2011; Sagar 2014).

Paralanguage is an area that combines verbal and nonverbal communication using nuances such voice volume, tone, and posturing as means of expressing thoughts and feelings. People normally use paralanguage multiple times per day and are sometimes not even aware they are doing so; this can include healthcare providers during assessments and at other times communicating with patients. The ability to interpret this kind of human communication correctly is considered an important competency in both personal and professional settings. Good communicators also have the ability to gauge how their own paralanguage affects others and to alter it so as to gain patients' trust and to project confidence.

In collectivistic cultures, such as Amish, Chinese, Filipino, Indigenous Indian, Vietnamese, Korean, and Panamanian cultures to name a few, implicit indirect communication is common. People are more likely to tell the healthcare providers what they think they want to hear (Bui and Turnbull 2003).

In collectivistic cultures a formal greeting is usually required by using the surname of the patient or family member with a title. This can be a first step in gaining trust. Names are important to people, and name formats differ among cultures. The most common Western system is to have a first or given name, a middle name, and then the family surname. The person would usually write the name in that order. In formal situations, the person would be addressed with a title of Mr., Mrs., Ms., or Miss and the last name. Friends and acquaintances would call the person by the first name or perhaps a nickname. Married women may take their husband's last name, keep their maiden name, or use both their maiden and married names. However, in some cultures, such as many in Asia, the family or surname name comes first, followed by the given name and then the middle name. The person would usually write and introduce himself or herself in that order. Married women usually, but not always, keep their maiden name. Diversity in naming formats can create a challenge for healthcare workers keeping a medical record; it is important to ask for the family name and then for their given names. The healthcare provider should always ask what is the legal name for medical record keeping and by which name the patient wishes to be addressed.

In some cultures, the concept of "saving face" is highly valued and is reflected in communication patterns (Baron 2003). Sharing intimate life details of self or family is discouraged because it could stigmatize the person and the family. "Yes" may mean I hear you or I understand. "Yes" does not necessarily mean agreement with what is being asked or being explained but rather I hear you. Therefore healthcare providers need to exercise caution in framing questions and interpreting responses to Yes/No questions. Instead of asking a patient if he/she took a medicine today, ask what time did you take your medicine today?

For the healthcare provider, deciding to whom to direct the conversation can also be complicated. In some cultures, decision-making is a responsibility of the male or most respected family member. And in some cases, the male may be the spokesperson for the family, even though he may not be the decision-maker.

In individualistic cultures, such as those of Western Europe, European American, and Canadian to name a few, explicit, direct, straight forward communication is the expected norm (Rothstein-Fisch et al. 2001). More informal greetings using the given name early in an encounter are common, especially among the younger generation. Healthcare providers should introduce themselves by the name they preferred to be addressed. Again, asking the individual by what name they wish to be addressed is the better plan of action.

In individualistic cultures individuals will usually respond to the healthcare provider with straightforward answers or evade the question completely if they do not want to answer it. Questions requiring "yes" or "no" are answered frankly. Sharing intimate life details is encouraged, even with non-intimates, and does not carry a stigma for patients or their families. Egalitarian decision-making is the norm, that is, patients/clients are empowered to make health-related decisions for themselves, although there are variations. When in doubt, ask who the primary decision-maker is for health-related concerns.

14.3 Nonverbal Communication

Nonverbal communication includes touch; eye contact; facial expressions; body language; temporality in terms of past, present, and future orientation; clock versus social time; and dress and adornment. Touch has substantial variations in meaning among cultures. For the most part, individualistic cultures (see Chap. 2 for individualistic and collectivistic cultural values) are low-touch cultures, which have been reinforced by sexual harassment guidelines and policies in the United States and many other countries. For many, even casual touching may be seen as a sexual overture or taboo and should be avoided whenever possible as is the case with traditional Muslims and Orthodox Jews as examples. In many cultures, people of the same sex (especially men) or opposite sex do not generally touch each other unless they are close friends (Purnell 2013; Purnell and Finkl 2018). However, among most collectivist cultures, two people of the same sex can touch each other without it having a sexual connotation, although modesty remains important (Black-Lattanzi and Purnell 2006; Hall 1990a). Being aware of individual practices regarding touch is essential for effective health assessments. Always explain the necessity and ask permission before touching a patient.

Under Islamic law, it is *haram* (forbidden) for a man to expose himself to any woman other than his wife. Likewise, for a woman to expose herself to a man who is not her husband is also forbidden. Therefore, except for an emergency, a full physical examination generally must be carried out by a healthcare professional of the same sex as the patient unless it is an emergency situation (Kulwicki and Ballout 2014), and even then the patient may be reluctant or refuse touching. When a same-sex healthcare professional is not available, some patients may give permission to touch using gloves, having the healthcare provider's hand over the patient's hand for palpation or through a layer of clothing. When examining women, especially young unmarried girls, a female chaperone must be present. The chaperone could be a member of the family, allowing the patient to feel more at ease. Married women may wish their husbands to be present. Moreover, the patient should also be examined in an area where the sudden intrusion of other people is not possible.

In general, the physical health assessment progresses from head to toe, touching less intimidate areas of the body first such as the head, arms, and hands. However, traditional Vietnamese never touch another's head because it is deemed disrespectful, especially that of a child, and is something that only an elder may do (Mattson 2013).

Personal space needs to be respected when working with multicultural patients and staff. Among more individualistic cultures, conversants tend to place at least 18 in. of space between themselves and the person with whom they are talking. Most collectivist cultures require less personal space when talking with each other (Hall 1990a). They are quite comfortable standing closer to each other than are people from individualistic cultures; in fact, they interpret physical proximity as a valued sign of emotional closeness (Hall 1990a). However, patients who stand very close and stare during a conversation may offend some healthcare providers. Thus, an understanding of personal space and distancing characteristics can enhance the quality of communication among individuals (Gardenswartz and Rowe 1998; Hall 1990b; Ritter and Hoffman 2010).

Regardless of the class or social standing of the conversants, people from individualistic cultures are expected to maintain direct eye contact without staring. A person who does not maintain eye contact may be perceived as not listening, not being trustworthy, not caring, or being less than truthful (Hall 1990b). Among some traditional or collectivist cultures, sustained eye contact can be seen as offensive. Furthermore, a person of lower social class or status is expected to avoid eye contact with superiors or those with a higher educational status (Purnell 2010). Thus, eye contact must be interpreted within its cultural context to optimize relationships and improve health assessments and recommendations.

Although many people in individualistic cultures consider it impolite or offensive to point with one's finger, many do so and do not see it as impolite. In other cultures, beckoning is done by waving the fingers with the palm down, whereas extending the thumb, like thumbs-up, is considered a vulgar sign. Among some cultures, signaling for someone to come by using an upturned finger is a provocation, usually done to a dog (Purnell 2013).

Temporal relationships—people's worldview in terms of past, present, and future orientation—vary among individuals and among cultural groups. Highly individualistic cultures are primarily future-oriented, and people are encouraged to sacrifice for today and work to save and invest in the future. The future is important in that people can influence it (Gudykunst and Matsumoto 1996).

In terms of healthcare, more future-oriented cultures are more likely to have at least yearly preventive health checkups and prenatal visits, adhere to immunizations, take advantage of flu vaccines, engage in healthy physical activities, and strive to consume a healthy diet. Present-oriented patients may have difficulty incorporating the future into long-term plans. For example, present-oriented patients might not take their antihypertensive medications if they are asymptomatic, although this occurs among some from individualistic cultures as well. Patients with diabetes might be reluctant to perform glucose monitoring unless they are symptomatic. Stress, poverty, and other social issues may exacerbate present-oriented beliefs on healthcare.

In past-oriented cultures, laying a proper foundation by providing historical background information can enhance communication. Past-oriented societies are concerned with traditional values and ways of doing things. They tend to be conservative in healthcare management and slow to change those things that are tied to the past. Past-oriented patients strive to maintain harmony with nature and look to the land to provide treatment for disease and illness. Herbal remedies are important and patients usually prefer traditional approaches to healing rather than accepting each new procedure, treatment, or medication that comes out. However, for people in many societies, temporality is balanced among past, present, and future in the sense of respecting the past, valuing and enjoying the present, and saving for the future (Hall 1990a, c).

Most people from individualistic cultures see time as a highly valued resource and do not like to be delayed because it "wastes time" (Hall 1990d). When visiting friends or meeting for strictly social engagements, punctuality is less important, but one is still expected to appear within a "reasonable" time frame. In the healthcare setting, if an appointment is made for 1300 hour (1:00 *PM*), the person is expected to be there 15 min early to be ready for the appointment and not delay the healthcare provider. For collectivistic cultures, the concept of time may be more fluid. Expectations for punctuality can cause conflicts between healthcare providers and patients, even if one is cognizant of these differences. These details must be carefully explained to individuals when such situations occur. Being late for appointments should not be misconstrued as a sign of irresponsibility or not valuing one's health (Hall 1990d; Purnell and Pontious 2014).

14.4 Sign Language

Sign language is a combination of verbal and nonverbal communication. Although signing is primarily nonverbal, it also includes multiple facial expressions and may have guttural sounds to accompany the signed words. It is important to note that signing is not a direct word-for-word interpretation, but rather the interpreter must extract the meaning from a message and then convey that meaning. No one form of sign language is universal. Different sign languages are used in different countries or regions. For example, British Sign Language (BSL) is a different from American Sign Language (ASL), and Americans who know ASL may not understand BSL (Lingua translations 2016). Belgium and India have more than one sign language. More diversity in sign languages can be found with Japanese Sign Language (or Nihon Shuwa, JSL), Spanish Sign Language (Lengua de signos o señas española, or LSE), and Turkish Sign Language (or Türk İşaret Dili, TID) (World Federation of the Deaf 2016). In addition, there are numerous country-/language-specific sign languages such as Filipino and Hebrew (Abdel-Fattah 2004).

Only recently has sign language in the Arab world been recognized and documented. Many efforts have been made to establish the sign languages used in individual countries, including Jordan, Egypt, Libya, and the Gulf States by trying to standardize the language. Such efforts produced many sign languages, almost as many as Arabic-speaking countries. Levantine Arabic Sign Language, also known as Syro-Palestinian Sign Language, is the deaf sign language of Jordan, Palestine, Syria, and Lebanon (Abdel-

Fattah 2004). Some hospitals in the United States and Great Britain have used Skype to connect with Arab countries in order to communicate with deaf and hearing impaired patients.

14.5   Communicating with Communities

Communicating with community populations can be critical for culturally competent care to better understand issues that affect the lives of the vulnerable and to assist them to make informed decisions for themselves and their community (Public Health Assessment Guidance Manual (2005: Update) 2011). At all times, the message should be in the language(s)/dialect(s) of the populations served.

Strategies to communicate with the community include announcements on public radio and television stations, local newspapers and media outlets, partnering with community organizations and associations, newsletters, neighborhood grocery stores, local libraries, town hall meetings, focus group discussions, and distributing brochures at public venues such as the Post Office, utility companies, restaurants, houses of worship, barber shops and beauty salons, and on public transportation systems if available. Even partnering with local gangs and cults can help gather and disseminate information.

14.6   Health Literacy

Health literacy is the degree to which individuals have the capacity to obtain, process, and understand basic health information and healthcare services required to make health decisions and follow treatment recommendations (Egbert and Nanna 2009). Studies have shown that people from all ages, races, income, and educational levels are challenged by this problem. Individuals with limited health literacy incur medical expenses that are up to four times greater than

patients with adequate literacy skills, resulting in higher costs to the healthcare system, unnecessary visits to healthcare providers, and increased hospital stays (National Academy on an Aging Society 1999). Seeking medical care, taking medications correctly, and following prescribed treatments require that people understand how to access and apply health information (US Department of Health and Human Services 2015). People with limited literacy are less likely to (a) ask questions during the medical encounter, (b) seek health information from print resources, and (c) understand medical terminology and jargon (National Association of the Deaf (n.d.), US Department of Health and Human Services 2015).

Many health-related documents are written at a college level and contain a large amount of text in small print and complex terminology (Neilsen-Bohlman et al. 2004). However, the recommendation is that patient education materials should be written at the sixth grade reading level, although this level varies somewhat by the language (Cotunga et al. 2005). Those with limited language proficiency have difficulty understanding written information, including medication dosage instructions and warning labels, discharge instructions, consent forms for treatment, participation in research studies, and basic health information about diseases, nutrition, prevention, and health services. The inability to read and comprehend such materials also impacts patients' ability to understand medical advice, engage in self-care behaviors, and make informed decisions about their healthcare (US Department of Health and Human Services 2015).

One of the recommendations found in the literature for patients taking medicines is to instruct them to take the "green," "blue," "yellow," etc. pill. This practice **is not recommended** for a number of reasons. Some patients may not be able to distinguish colors, or the color of a pill may change given the numerous generic medications. Moreover, the word for green and blue are the same in some languages (World Heritage Encyclopedia 2017).

14.7 Interpretation Versus Translation

The key difference between interpretation and translation is the choice of communication channels. Translation deals with written communication, while interpretation deals with the spoken word (Bureau of Labor Statistics, Department of Labor; Occupational Outlook Handbook 2006; Lionbridge 2012). Both channels require linguistic and cultural knowledge of the working languages. While translators usually provide word-for-word translation, interpreters must know both the original speech and the target language and transpose one language into another in real-time situations. They also act as facilitators between the speakers and listeners (Translation Central n.d.). Although, in the past, interpretation occurred in real time and only face-to-face, the advent of technology has changed this dramatically. Systems can accommodate (a) headphones used by the patient, healthcare provider, and interpreter, (b) Skyping, (c) television/video service, and (d) other distance methodologies 24 hours a day. Interpreters must capture the tone, inflection, voice quality, and other intangible elements of the spoken word and convey the meaning of the words. Interpretation, unlike translation, is not word-for-word but a paraphrasing of the words (American Translators Association 2015; Federation of Interpreters and Translators 2015; National Council on Healthcare Interpreting n.d.).

14.8 Recommendations for Using Medical Interpreters

1. Use certified interpreters whenever possible. Certified interpreters are trained to be ethical and nonjudgmental. Noncertified interpreters might not report information that he/she perceives as superstitious or not important. Certified interpreters take an oath of confidentiality.
2. Normally, children should never be used as interpreters for their family members. Not only does it have a negative bearing on family dynamics, but sensitive information may not be transmitted. However, the healthcare provider must also be aware that in some cultures, family or other people in the community might be preferred as an interpreter because they are more trusted then outsiders.
3. Avoid the use of relatives if possible because they may distort information or not be objective.
4. If possible, give the interpreter and patient time alone to get acquainted.
5. Use dialect-specific interpreters whenever possible.
6. Use a same-sex interpreter as the patient if desired.
7. Maintain eye contact with both the patient and the interpreter.
8. Direct your question to the patient, not the interpreter.
9. Some patients may want an interpreter who is older. Ask the patients if they have an age preference of the interpreter and accommodate this preference if possible.
10. Social class differences between the interpreter and the patient may affect interpretation.
11. Some patients may desire an interpreter of the same religion.

14.9 Recommendations

Recommendations for clinical practice, administration, education, and research follow.

14.9.1 Recommendations for Clinical Practice

Ascertain the possibility that cultural differences may cause communication problems; pay attention to nonverbal as well as verbal communication. Clinical staff must consider factors that govern diversity within a culture that can affect cross-cultural communication such as age, generation, nationality, race, color, sex, gender roles, religion, military status, political beliefs, educational status, occupation, socioeconomic status, sexual orientation, urban versus rural residence, limited language proficiency, health literacy, physical characteristics of patients and providers, and reasons for immigration/migration including documentation status. Refugees and asylees may have considerable difficulty trusting healthcare providers based on discrimination in their home country (Purnell and Finkl 2018).

Effective communication is a key to providing culturally competent and congruent care in clinical practice. Therefore, healthcare providers need to understand their own cultural communication practices as well as being knowledgeable of the communication practices of their patients. Concerted efforts must be made for translating educational materials according to the patient's health literacy level and language proficiency. Every attempt should be made to obtain certified interpreters when needed. Recognize that it is not always possible to have an interpreter for every language and dialect. Family members and significant others should only be used as a last resort and for nonconfidential information such as dietary and medication instructions. Moreover, if possible, it is best to refrain from using interpreters known to the patient or family.

Because it is not always possible to know the cultural characteristics and attributes of all diverse patients, using a collectivistic and individualistic communication framework and guide can be helpful when you are not familiar with the culture of the patient (see Chap. 2). The caregiver should always address the patient formally until told to do otherwise and ask how he/she wishes to be identified, along with their legal name for medical record keeping. Likewise, the care providers should introduce themselves by their titles and positions. Patients have a right to know who is providing care to them.

For the hearing impaired, determine whether the patient uses American Sign Language, Signed English, or other specific sign languages. A writing system for communication when a signer is not available should be provided.

Develop pain scales in the patient's preferred language as well as "Faces of Pain" specific to ethnicities. Recognize that some people might

not show their amount of pain in facial expressions. Using numerical pain scales might be more helpful.

When providing instructions for medications, the provider should explain them in the correct sequence and one step at a time. For example, (a) at 9:00 every morning, get the medicine bottle, (b) take two tablets out of the bottle, (c) get your hot water, and (d) swallow the pills with the water. Do not use complex and compound sentences or use contractions when giving instructions. Many languages do not use contractions, and they can cause confusion for some patients. The patient should always demonstrate procedures and how medications are prescribed; simply repeating the instructions does not demonstrate understanding. Upon discharge, educational materials should be in the patient's preferred language and at a level that meets the needs of patients with low health literacy and limited language proficiency (Purnell 2008; Purnell and Finkl 2018).

14.9.2 Recommendations for Administration

Administration has a prime responsibility for obtaining resources to ensure that culturally competent clinical practice can occur. Resources include finances as well as recruiting adequate staff from the population the organization serves. In addition, financial resources are needed for interpretation and translation services which are a federal requirement in the United States and highly recommended in many other countries.

Symbols and pictograms should be included in hospitals, clinics, and other healthcare organizations whenever possible. These symbols and pictograms need to be validated with members of the specific ethnic community to assure that they are accurate and not culturally offensive. Intranet websites should be developed and in different languages for diverse patient populations. General health information on illnesses, infections, diseases, and injury protection in languages of the patient population can be developed and distributed in areas where patients, families, and significant others shop, congregate, and use public transportation. Patients and families should be informed about their existence upon admission. Disease-oriented practice guidelines for culturally diverse populations served in the organization can be developed and shared with all staff. When feasible, consider short video clips in languages spoken by the patient population.

Administration has the responsibility of keeping abreast of assistive technology used with the hearing and visually impaired and perhaps collaborating with communities to develop training for interpreters if certified interpreters are not feasible. In addition, satisfaction surveys should be translated into the languages of the populations served; otherwise only part of the information is gathered. Direct care providers and others who work with patients, families, and significant others from diverse cultures should be surveyed on their most pressing issues. Develop disease-oriented practice guidelines for culturally diverse populations served in the organization.

14.9.2.1 Recommendations for Education and Training

Culturally competent clinical practice begins with formal classes in educational programs of all healthcare professionals. Individual healthcare professionals must continue their education on cultural values, beliefs, and skills because cultures change over time. In addition, culturally congruent care should be included in orientation programs for all staff. Cultural assessment tools need to be included on admission forms. Classes with common foreign phrases could be included, specific to areas of clinical practice for when interpreters are not available.

Ongoing continuing education classes and seminars on the cultures and religions of the patient population served should be conducted on a yearly and on an as-needed basis. Train-the-trainer programs can help assure staff have access to information on a 24/7 basis. Evidence-based printed and electronic resources specific to the diversity of patients and staff in the organization could be in the organization's Intranet so staff can access it on a 24/7 basis. Intranet with articles, book chapters, and books could be included with the organizations' library as well as having them in printed format for staff to take home.

14.9.2.2 Recommendations for Research

Research needs to continue on population-specific health beliefs and values to assure culturally competent clinical practice. Resource-poor organizations may not have the human and material resources to conduct research, but with newer technologies and the Internet, partnering with educational organizations is a viable alternative. At a minimum, staff, educators, and administrators and managers can identify gaps in the literature of patients cared for in the organization, conduct research on those topics, and conduct quality improvement projects. A culture of nursing research can be accomplished by initiating a journal club devoted to evidence-based practice and research studies. Advanced practice nurses with a background in research and evidence-based practice can help staff obtain literature and assist them with quality improvement projects.

Conclusion

The importance of effective verbal and non-verbal cross-cultural communication cannot be overemphasized as it is the basis of establishing trust and obtaining accurate health assessments and providing instructions. Both interpretation and translation have some inherent troublesome concerns. Due to the complexity of languages and multiple dialects of a language, specific words may not exist in the host language and require an explanation of the word or phrase; the exact meaning may still be lost (Van Ness et al. 2010). For example, having knowledge of the cultures to whom care is provided, the variant cultural characteristics, and the complexities of interpretation and translation is a requisite for decreasing/eliminating health and healthcare disparities (International Medical Interpreters Association 2017). A healthcare provider cannot possibly know all worldwide cultures; however, an understanding of the differences between collectivistic and individualistic cultures is a starting point and can be used as a framework for assessing cross-cultural communication styles and improving health assessments (Keeskes 2016). Intercultural pragmatics, dealing with things sensibly and realistically, can bring some new insight into theories.

Appendix 1: Communication Exercise

Effective communication is essential in the delivery of culturally congruent health and nursing care. For cultural communication to be effective, the healthcare providers need to understand their own communication practices. The following exercise will assist providers to understand their own communication practices.

Instructions
1. Identify your own cultural identity and personal communication practices and how they differ with family, friends, and strangers, including patients.
2. Investigate the scholarly literature on your culture after you have completed the exercises.
3. Identify how your communication patterns differ from what was in the scholarly literature.
4. Posit why these personal practices differ.

Note: Variant characteristics within a culture can be used as a guide to addressing the statements below. These variant cultural characteristics include:

Nationality	Age	Skin color
Race	SES	Physical characteristics
Ethnicity	Occupation	Parental status
Gender	Marital status	Political beliefs
Sexual orientation	Educational status	Religious affiliation
Gender issues	Health literacy	Military experience
Enclave identity	Urban vs. rural residence	

Length of time away from country of origin
Reason for migration: sojourner, immigrant, undocumented status

Once this exercise is completed, it should be shared with others for a discussion. This exercise can be used in academic classes, continuing education classes, and in-services.

- Identify your cultural ancestry. If you have more than one cultural ancestry, choose one for the sake of this exercise.
- Explore the willingness of individuals in your culture to share thoughts, feelings, and ideas. Can you identify any area of discussion that would be considered taboo?
- Explore the practice and meaning of touch in your culture. Include information regarding touch between family members, friends, members of the opposite sex, and healthcare providers.
- Identify personal spatial and distancing strategies used when communicating with others in your culture. Discuss differences between friends and families versus strangers.
- Discuss your culture's use of eye contact. Include information regarding practices between family members, friends, strangers, and persons of different age groups.
- Explore the meaning of gestures and facial expressions in your culture. Do specific gestures or facial expressions have special meanings? How are emotions displayed?
- Are there acceptable ways of standing and greeting people in your culture?
- Discuss the prevailing temporal relation of your culture. Is the culture's worldview past, present, or future oriented?
- Discuss the impact of your culture on your nursing and/or healthcare. Be specific, that is, not something that is very general.

Appendix 2: Reflective Exercises

The following reflective exercises can be used in formal courses at any level and discipline or interdisciplinary. They can also be used in staff development.

1. What changes in ethnic and cultural diversity have you seen in your community over the

last 5 years? Over the last 10 years? Have you had the opportunity to interact with newer groups?

2. What health disparities have you observed in your community? To what do you attribute these disparities? What can you do as a professional to help decrease these disparities?

3. Who in your family had the most influence in teaching you cultural values and practices? Mother, father, or grandparent?

4. How do you want to be addressed? First name or last name with a title?

5. How do you address older people in your culture? First name or last name with a title?

6. What activities have you done to increase your cultural competence?

7. Given that everyone is ethnocentric to some degree, what do you do to become less ethnocentric?

8. How do you distinguish a stereotype from a generalization?

9. How have your variant characteristics of culture changed over time?

10. What ethnic and racial groups do you encounter on a regular basis? Do you see any racism or discrimination among these groups?

11. What does your organization do to increase diversity and cultural competence?

12. What barriers do you see to culturally competent care in your organization? School, work, etc.

13. How many languages are spoken in your community?

14. Do different languages pose barriers to healthcare, including health literacy? What affordability concerns for healthcare do you see in your community?

15. What complementary/alternative healthcare practices do you use?

16. What complementary/alternative healthcare practices are available in your community?

17. Is public transportation readily available to healthcare services in your community? What might be done to improve them?

18. What do **you** do when you cannot understand the language of your patient?

19. In what languages are healthcare instructions provided in your organization?

20. Does your organization offer both interpreter and translation services?

21. Given the heritage and diversity of the population in your community, what cultural, social, and material issues do you consider important?

References

Abdel-Fattah MA (2004) Arabic sign language: a perspective. J Deaf Stud Deaf Educ 10(2):212–221

American Translators Association (ATA) (2015) www.atanet.org. Accessed 29 July 2017

Andrews MM, Boyle JS (eds) (2016) Transcultural concepts in nursing care, 7th edn. Wolters Kluwer, Philadelphia

Baron, M (2003) Beyond intractability. http://www.beyondintractability.org/essay/cross-cultural-communication. Accessed 29 July 2017

Black-Lattanzi J, Purnell L (eds) (2006) Exploring communication in a cultural context. In: Developing cultural competence in physical therapy practice. F.A. Davis Co., Philadelphia

Bui YN, Turnbull A (2003) East meets west: analysis of person-centered planning in the context of Asian American values. Educ Train Ment Retard Dev Disabil 38(1):18–31

Building an Organizational Response to Health Disparities (2016) A practical guide to a practical guide to implementing the national CLAS standards: for racial, ethnic and linguistic minorities, people with disabilities, and sexual and gender minorities. https://www.cms.gov/About-CMS/Agency-Information/OMH/Downloads/CLAS-Toolkit-12-7-16.pdf. Accessed 15 Oct 2017

Bureau of Labor Statistics: Department of Labor, Occupational Outlook Handbook (2006) Interpreters and translators. http://www.bls.gov/oco/ocos175.htm. Accessed 29 July 2017

Cotunga N, Vickery CE, Carpenter-Haefele KM (2005) Evaluation of literacy level of patient education pages in health-related journals. J Community Health 30(3):213–219

Douglas M, Rosenketter M, Pacquiao D, Callister C et al (2014) Guidelines for implementing culturally competent nursing care. J Transcult Nurs 25(2):109–221

Egbert N, Nanna K (2009). Health literacy: challenges and strategies. Online J Issues Nurs 14, 3, Manuscript 1. http://www.nursingworld.org/MainMenuCategories/ANAMarketplace/ANAPeriodicals/OJIN/TableofContents/Vol142009/No3Sept09/Health-Literacy-Challenges.html. Accessed 29 July 2017

Federation of Interpreters and Translators. (2015) www.ift-fit.org. Accessed 29 July 2017

Galanti G (ed) (1991) Communication and time orientation. In: Caring for patients from different cultures: case studies from American hospitals. University Pennsylvania Press, Philadelphia

Gardenswartz L, Rowe A (eds) (1998) Communication in diverse environments. In: Managing diversity in health care. Jossey-Bass, San Francisco

Gudykunst WB, Matsumoto Y (1996) Cross-cultural variability of communication in personal relationships. In: Gudykunst WB, Ting-Toomey S, Nishida T (eds) Communication in personal relationships across cultures. Sage Publishing, Thousand Oakes

Hall E (1990a) The silent language. Doubleday, New York

Hall E (1990b) The hidden dimension. Doubleday, New York

Hall E (1990c) Beyond culture. Doubleday, New York

Hall E (1990d) The dance of life. Doubleday, New York

Helman C (ed) (2000) Culture, health, and illness, 4th edn. Butterworth Heinemann, Oxford

How Many Languages do Indian People Speak?. http://www.answers.com/Q/How_many_languages_do_indian_people_speak. Accessed 14 Sept 2017

Huttlinger KW (2013) People of Appalachian heritage. In: Purnell L (ed) Transcultural health care: a culturally competent approach, 4th edn. F.A. Davis Co, Philadelphia

International Medical Interpreters Association (2017) www.imiaweb.org. Accessed 29 July 2017

Keeskes I (2016) Can intercultural pragmatics bring some new insight into pragmatic theories? In: Capone A, Mey JL (eds) Interdisciplinary studies in pragmatics, culture and society. Springer, New York

Kulwicki A, Ballout S (2014) People of Arab heritage. In: Purnell L (ed) Transcultural health care: a culturally competent approach, 4th edn. F.A. Davis Co., Philadelphia

Languages of Nigeria (n.d.) http://language.nigerianunion.org/. Accessed 14 Sept 2017

Lingua Translations (2016) http://www.lingua-translations.com/blog/asl-bsl/. Accessed 21 Sept 2017

Lionbridge: Professional Translation and Localization Services (2012) http://www.lionbridge.com/. Accessed 29 July 2017

Mattson S (2013) People of Vietnamese heritage. In: Purnell L (ed) Transcultural health care: a culturally competent approach, 4th edn. F.A. Davis Co., Philadelphia

Mexican Languages (2017) http://www.donquijote.org/culture/mexico/languages/index.asp. Accessed 14 Sept 2017

National Academy on an Aging Society (1999) Fact sheets. www.agingsociety.org/agingsociety/publications/fact/fact_low.html. Accessed 29 July 2017

National Association of the Deaf (n.d.) Interpreting American Sign Language. http://nad.org/issues/american-sign-language/interpreting-american-sign-language. Accessed 29 July 2017

National Council on Healthcare Interpreting (NCIHC) (n.d.) www.ncihc.org. Accessed 29 July 2017

Neilsen-Bohlman L, Panzer AM, Kindig DA (2004) Health literacy: a prescription to end confusion. National Academies Press, Washington, DC

Papadopoulos, I. (ed.). (2006). The Papadopoulos, Tilki, and Taylor model for developing cultural competence. Transcultural health and social care. London: Churchill Livingston.

Public Health Assessment Guidance Manual (2005 Update) (2011) Involving and communicating with the community. https://www.atsdr.cdc.gov/hac/phamanual/ch4.html#4.8. Accessed 29 July 2017

Purnell L (2008) The Purnell model for cultural competence. In: Purnell L, Paulanka B (eds) Transcultural health care. A culturally competent approach. F.A. Davis Co., Philadelphia

Purnell L (2010) Cultural rituals in health and nursing care. In Esterhuizen P, Kuckert A (eds) Diversiteit in de verpleeg-kunde [Diversity in Nursing]. Bohn Stafleu van Loghum, Amsterdam

Purnell L (2011) Application of transcultural theory to mental health-substance use in an international context. In: Cooper D (ed) Intervention in mental health-substance use. Radcliffe Publishing, London

Purnell L (ed) (2013) The Purnell model for cultural competence. In: Transcultural health care. A culturally competent approach. F.A. Davis Co., Philadelphia

Purnell L, Finkl E (2018) Guide to culturally competent health care. F.A. Davis Co., Philadelphia

Purnell L, Pontious S (2014) Cultural competence. In: Gurung RAR (ed) Multicultural approaches to health and wellness in America: Volume 1. Praeger, Santa Barbara

Ritter LA, Hoffman NA (2010) Cross cultural concepts of health and illness. Multicultural health. Jones & Bartlett Publishing, Boston

Rothstein-Fisch C, Greenfield PM, Quiroz B (2001) Continuum of "individualistic" and "collectivistic" values. National Center on Secondary Education. http://www.ncset.org/publications/essentialtools/diversity/partIII.asp. Accessed 29 July 2017

Sagar P (2014) Transcultural concepts in adult health courses. In: Sagar P (ed) Transcultural nursing education strategies. Springer, Philadelphia

Translation Central (n.d.) Translation versus interpretation. http://www.translationcentral.com/. Accessed 29 July 2017

U.S. Department of Health and Human Services (2015) National Institute of Deafness and other Communication Disorders. http://www.nidcd.nih.gov/health/hearing/pages/asl.aspx. Accessed: 29 July 2017

Van Ness F, Abma T, Jonsson J (2010) Language differences in qualitative research: is meaning lost in translation. Eur J Aging 7:313–316

World Federation of the Deaf (2016) https://wfdeaf.org/. Accessed 29 July 2017

World Heritage Encyclopedia (2017) Distinguishing "blue" from "green" in different languages. http://self.gutenberg.org/articles/Distinguishing_%22blue%22_from_%22green%22_in_language. Accessed 29 July 2017

Case Study: Korean Woman with Mastectomy Pain

15

Sangmi Kim and Eun-Ok Im

Jina, a 57-year-old Korean immigrant woman with a high school education, has been a housewife since getting married to her husband who ran a small business until they immigrated to the United States (USA). Jina and her husband immigrated to the USA in 2000 with their two daughters after her husband's company faced extreme financial difficulties in the middle of the economic crisis that hit South Korea in the late 1990s. There were no families, relatives, or friends living in the USA, but they settled in a suburban neighborhood within a Korean community on the East coast. They have run a dry cleaning business since their arrival in the USA. Their adult daughters currently work in other states after completing their college education. They regularly visit their parents during holidays and for special occasions.

Although Jina has lived in the USA for an extended period of time, she still finds it challenging to communicate with others in English. She predominantly speaks Korean and socializes only with Korean friends who she met at her Korean church. Mostly, she cooks Korean cuisine at home, watches Korean TV shows, and listens to Korean songs.

S. Kim, Ph.D., R.N. (✉)
E.-O. Im, Ph.D., R.N., FAAN (✉)
School of Nursing, Duke University,
Durham, NC, USA
e-mail: sangmi.kim@duke.edu; eun-ok.im@duke.edu

Three years ago, she was diagnosed with a Grade III infiltrating ductal carcinoma in her right breast with an enlarged lymph node in the axilla. She underwent chemotherapy followed by a mastectomy and postoperative radiation therapy. Since then, she has experienced chronic pain in her chest and underarm as if a wire was wrapping around these body parts. The pain becomes worse at night. After the surgery, she tried over-the-counter and prescribed painkillers and physical therapy, but none of them helped relieve the pain. She once talked about her constant pain to her physician, but was told, "Some pain will go away with time, but it does not get too much better. You just need to learn to live with it."

After the conversation with her physician, she did not bring up her pain-related issues again during her physician's visits because it was difficult to verbally describe the characteristics/patterns of pain and her pain experiences in English. She was also hesitant to ask the physician because she did not want to challenge him by questioning his attitudes toward her pain as well as the care plans and their effectiveness to relieve it.

Jina tries not to tell her family that she is in pain since she does not want them to worry about her condition. She thinks that her family already shoulders the financial burden caused by her surgery and cancer treatment, and she does not want to add even an emotional burden on her husband and daughters. The couple has experienced financial strain to some degree since her diagnosis with breast cancer. Even though the health insurance covers her cancer treatment, she is responsible for paying some of the medical bills with out-of-pocket money. The limited range of motion of her right arm and pain discouraged her from continuing to work in the dry cleaner. Instead, she stays at home and takes care of household chores, while her husband works longer hours on weekdays and often during weekends to keep their business running. She tries to act normal by handling all the household chores because she wants to be a strong mother to her daughters. Nevertheless, she is often frustrated and stressed by a lack of instrumental and emotional support from her family and friends. She feels like no one understands what she is going through.

Jina does not depend on pain medications because they are ineffective and because they are costly. She is worried about becoming addicted to them. Instead, she manages her pain with an intermittent use of acupuncture and yoga. As a religious Christian, she goes to church every morning and prays to God to help her overcome this physical and emotional suffering. After the prayer, she feels stronger and less fearful. She thinks that she can stand her pain if her suffering is part of God's plan for her, although she cannot understand it right now.

15.1 Cultural Issues

Korean women tend to minimize pain due to their cultural beliefs toward pain. Korean culture is under the influence of Confucianism and Taoism that highly value stoicism. Specifically, Confucianism teaches people to live in harmonious social relations and subsequently deters people from expressing potentially disruptive and unpleasant emotions, including pain (Im et al. 2008, 2009). Moreover, Korean women have a tendency to consider pain as a natural human experience. If the pain is unavoidable, people should be brave and strong to face and embrace it so that they can be role models for others in the same situation. A cultural belief among Koreans is that pain helps to build one's strong character;

complaining about pain merely signals weakness (Im et al. 2008). Thus, opting out of aggressive treatment through Western medicine, Korean women try to maintain normal lives and use natural modalities for pain management such as massage, meditation, and Qigong (Im et al. 2009).

Other reasons that Korean women with cancer pain reduce the magnitude of the problem are due to the negative meanings attached to breast cancer and cancer in general as well as the patriarchal Korean culture. Specifically, a victim-blaming tendency is observed among Korean women with cancer (Im et al. 2002). They believe that pain is a consequence of bad karma or punishment of sins committed in the past (Im et al. 2009). In addition, traditional Korean medicine posits that one's misconduct or negative attitudes bring about cancer such that cancer patients need to change their reactions to or perspectives toward situations rather than modifying the situations themselves. Some feel that one should not think too much about cancer because that would ultimately make the person sick (Tam Ashing et al. 2003). Thus, positive thinking and strong mentality are values to deal with cancer pain.

A belief that the mind has control over the physical body seems to contribute to passive pain management among Korean women cancer survivors by relying not only on mental therapies such as yoga, deep breathing, and reading other cancer patients' stories but also a religion (Im et al. 2008). Indeed, spirituality plays an essential role in a journey of recovery from cancer among Korean women. Reportedly, Korean Americans are prone to perceive less control over illness and treatment than some other groups (Tam Ashing et al. 2003). They believe that God wills a diagnosis of breast cancer or the outcome of the disease is in God's hands (Tam Ashing et al. 2003). Through religious activities (e.g., prayer), Korean women find comfort and strength to undergo their life crisis, such as cancer (Im et al. 2008).

The Korean patriarchal culture emphasizes family as an essential social unit with women's low status in traditional family systems. The culture expects women to sacrifice themselves for their families (Im et al. 2002). Even, the family expects women to function the same as before the breast cancer surgery, providing little or no help with household tasks (Im et al. 2002; Tam Ashing et al. 2003). Women place their family as a priority ahead of their personal needs such as health, resulting in delaying treatment and medical services (Tam Ashing et al. 2003). Women's health problems tend to be regarded as trivial even by women themselves and by their family members (Im et al. 2000). This applies especially to those of lower socioeconomic status (SES) and those who are uninsured; they are more concerned with supporting their families than seeking early care (Tam Ashing et al. 2003). As a result, Korean women tolerate cancer pain so as not to become a financial or emotional burden on the family and make them worry (Im et al. 2008; Tam Ashing et al. 2003). Also, the most common concern as barriers to pain control among Korean cancer survivors pertains to analgesic use, such as developing tolerance to pain medication; taking pain medication on an around-the-clock versus as on a needed basis; and developing addiction (Edrington et al. 2009).

Cancer pain experience is gendered. Relative to men, women may be disadvantaged in cancer pain management. For example, people may take men's cancer pain more seriously and pay more attention to their pain experience than women's (Im et al. 2009). Women are also more likely to tolerate pain than men not only due to biological differences but also normative gender roles in the household. Specifically, women experience pain throughout their lives caused by menstruation and childbirth (Im et al. 2009). Household tasks and child rearing have been considered as women's responsibilities. Women think that they should be stronger to endure pain from cancer treatment and survive for their children who depend on them (Im et al. 2009).

Furthermore, many Korean cancer survivors lack information about their diagnosis, treatments, and cancer-related terminology. This may be attributed to healthcare providers' failure to adequately educate them, language barriers, and survivors' belief that they should leave most of the treatment decisions to their physicians (Im et al. 2002; Tam Ashing et al. 2003). Lack of fluency and discomfort in speaking English and

unfamiliarity with healthcare systems contribute to the lack of active pain management among Korean women, especially among those who are less acculturated and newly immigrated (Tam Ashing et al. 2003). Even those with higher education and those who are bilingual may find it difficult to navigate healthcare systems and feel uncomfortable with asking questions about their health conditions (Tam Ashing et al. 2003). Korean women often do not seek second opinions and tend not to ask their physicians' advice. This is derived from their cultural respect for medical physician's status as an authority figure and their cultural belief that physicians know what they are doing and will provide the best care (Im et al. 2002; Tam Ashing et al. 2003). Korean women desire to be perceived as good patients by their healthcare providers (Im et al. 2008).

15.2 Social Structural Factors

Racial/ethnic minorities and socioeconomically disadvantaged groups disproportionately face system-level barriers to pain management that include inequalities in high costs of pain medication, insufficient/lack of health insurance reimbursement for pain services and medications, and the availability of analgesics in pharmacies (Stein et al. 2016; Sun et al. 2007). For example, they are more likely than their non-minority or privileged counterparts to be underinsured/uninsured and have fewer resources for out-of-pocket expenses (Anderson et al. 2009; Stein et al. 2016). The inadequate health insurance coverage among racial/ethnic minorities limits the availability and affordability of analgesic medications for pain relief (Anderson et al. 2009; Stein et al. 2016).

When minority patients receive a prescription for pain medication, they may face limited availability of opioids in their hospital or neighborhood pharmacy (Anderson et al. 2009; Stein et al. 2016). Morrison et al. (2000) documented that only 25% of New York City pharmacies in predominantly non-White neighborhoods (i.e., those in which less than 40% of residents were White) had adequate opioids, while 72% of pharmacies in predominantly White neighborhoods stocked sufficient opioids. More specifically, in predominantly Korean neighborhoods, the proportion of pharmacies with sufficient opioid stocks was 25% as compared with 54% in predominantly non-Korean neighborhoods.

15.3 Social Stratification

Negative attitudes toward racial/ethnic minorities or prejudicial racial stereotyping by healthcare providers can also contribute to ineffective pain care among racial/ethnic minorities (Lasch 2000; Mossey 2011; Stein et al. 2016). For example, some healthcare providers are inclined to underestimate pain severity among racial/ethnic minorities and prescribe less effective analgesics to them (Anderson et al. 2009; Mossey 2011). NSAIDs rather than opioid analgesics or opioids at lower doses are more likely to be prescribed to Blacks, Hispanics, and Asians than to Whites, even though pain severity is comparable among the groups (Mossey 2011).

15.4 Culturally Competent Strategies Recommended

15.4.1 Individual-/Family-Level Interventions

- Assess Jina's linguistic preferences, SES, cultural beliefs about and attitudes toward her pain, coping strategies, and perceived barriers to pain control.
- Examine healthcare providers' cultural beliefs and implicit negative stereotypical perceptions toward Korean women.
- Appreciate the importance to Jina of her beliefs about pain, even though they may not be scientifically grounded or conflict with the healthcare provider's beliefs.
- Dispel misconceptions about opioid analgesics.
- Be open, authentic, sensitive, and caring when communicating with Jina and her husband.
- Coach Jina on how to report her pain and empower her to do it accurately.

- Provide Jina and her husband with information about her pain and pain management options and resources.
- Prescribe long- vs. short-acting opioid analgesics and an aggressive bowel regimen to prevent opioid-related constipation.

15.4.2 Organizational-Level Interventions

- Train healthcare providers in communication skills, use of interpreters, and cultural competence.
- Educate healthcare providers on the central concepts relevant to pain care (e.g., addiction and tolerance), pain assessment, and management techniques.
- Develop or implement recommended pain treatment guidelines and protocols based on research evaluating the efficacy of the pain treatments for minority patients with cancer, and regularly monitor if the healthcare providers execute the guidelines and protocols during the care.
- Provide certified interpreters for better communication between healthcare providers and patients with limited language fluency.
- Implement educational campaigns in Korean communities for improved pain control among cancer survivors in concert with local Korean churches and organizations.
- Establish a referral system to supportive care/social services that can address socioeconomic concerns of cancer patients and families.

15.4.3 Community Societal-Level Interventions

- Build community-based partnerships and initiatives to increase the availability of opioids medications in minority neighborhood pharmacies.
- Evaluate regulations that may act as disincentives for pharmacists to stock controlled substances.

Conclusion

Inaccurate assessment and undertreatment of Jina's cancer pain is a manifestation of the deeply rooted social and racial/ethnic disparities in opportunities and resources to maintain an optimal health/functional status. Jina's cancer pain is less appreciated because she is a woman and racial/ethnic minority; her healthcare providers are ignorant about her cultural beliefs and attitudes toward pain, and her English is not fluent enough to communicate her pain experience with healthcare providers. Jina receives an insufficient treatment due to healthcare providers' racial bias toward pain of minority patients and her limited affordability and availability of opioid pain medications. High cost of opioid pain medications is financially burdensome for Jina and her husband considering their financial instability resulting from her cancer treatment and limited health insurance coverage. Even though she can afford the medication, having access to them is another hurdle when pharmacies in the segregated neighborhood do not have sufficient opioid stock.

Concerted efforts at multiple levels (i.e., individual, organization, and community) are called for to address undertreatment of cancer pain that many Korean breast cancer survivors like Jina experience. Such individual-level efforts as cultivating healthcare providers' cultural sensitivity and empowering Korean breast cancer survivors and their families to engage in their pain management plans may not sustain without organizational support through increasing awareness of the issue and providing resources, monitoring, and regulating. Upstream risk factors for pain care for Korean breast cancer survivors (e.g., not affordable or available pain medications) can be addressed by community involvement through partnerships with social service organizations and local pharmacies. Finally, healthcare providers and Korean breast cancer survivors can form a united front to advocate the unequal pain care as a significant public health issue. Persuade or negotiate with policymakers to change laws or health policies that affect cancer patients' pain care options.

References

Anderson KO, Green CR, Payne R (2009) Racial and ethnic disparities in pain: causes and consequences of unequal care. J Pain 10(12):1187–1204. https://doi.org/10.1016/j.jpain.2009.10.002

Edrington J, Sun A, Wong C, Dodd M, Padill G, Paul S, Miaskowski C (2009) Barriers to pain management in a community sample of Chinese American patients with cancer. J Pain Symptom Manag 37(4):665–675. https://doi.org/10.1016/j.jpainsymman.2008.04.014

Im EO, Hautman MA, Keddy B (2000) A feminist critique of breast cancer research among Korean women. West J Nurs Res 22(5):551–570. https://doi-org.proxy.lib.duke.edu/10.1177/01939450022044593

Im EO, Lee EO, Park YS (2002) Korean women's breast cancer experience. West J Nurs Res 24(7):751–765. https://doi.org/10.1177/019394502762476960

Im EO, Liu Y, Kim YH, Chee W (2008) Asian American cancer patients' pain experience. Cancer Nurs 31(3):E17–E23. https://doi.org/10.1097/01.ncc.0000305730.95839.83

Im EO, Lee SH, Liu Y, Lim HJ, Guevara E, Chee W (2009) A national online forum on ethnic differences in cancer pain experience. Nurs Res 58(2):86–94

Lasch KE (2000) Culture, pain, and culturally sensitive pain care. Pain Manag Nurs 1(3, Supplement 1):16–22. https://doi.org/10.1053/jpmn.2000.9761. Accessed 4 July 2017

Morrison RS, Wallenstein S, Natale DK, Senzel RS, Huang LL (2000) "We don't carry that"—failure of pharmacies in predominantly nonwhite neighborhoods to stock opioid analgesics. N Engl J Med 342(14):1023–1026. https://doi.org/10.1056/nejm200004063421406

Mossey JM (2011) Defining racial and ethnic disparities in pain management. Clin Orthop Relat Res 469(7):1859–1870. https://doi.org/10.1007/s11999-011-1770-9

Stein KD, Alcaraz KI, Kamson C, Fallon EA, Smith TG (2016) Sociodemographic inequalities in barriers to cancer pain management: a report from the American Cancer Society's study of cancer survivors-II (SCS-II). Psychooncology 25(10):1212–1221. https://doi.org/10.1002/pon.4218

Sun V, Borneman T, Ferrell B, Piper B, Koczywas M, Choi K (2007) Overcoming barriers to cancer pain management: an institutional change model. J Pain Symptom Manag 34(4):359–369. https://doi.org/10.1016/j.jpainsymman.2006.12.011

Tam Ashing K, Padilla G, Tejero J, Kagawa-Singer M (2003) Understanding the breast cancer experience of Asian American women. Psychooncology 12(1):38–58. https://doi.org/10.1002/pon.632

Case Study: An 85-Year-Old Saudi Muslim Woman with Multiple Health Problems

16

Sandra Lovering

In a hospital in Saudi Arabia, an 85-year-old Saudi woman, Umm Khalid, was admitted with end-stage heart failure, diabetes mellitus, and infected diabetic foot ulcers. She is a widow with one son, two daughters, and many grandchildren. She lives with her eldest son, Khalid, and his family in a remote rural community. Her older daughter and eldest granddaughter take turns staying with her as a "sitter" throughout the day and night while in the hospital.

The primary consultant reviewed her results and advised the family that due to her age and general condition the plan was for palliative care. The adult children discussed the care of their mother, and the son requested the nurses and physicians not to tell their mother her diagnosis as they felt she would lose hope.

A few days later, the daughter told the nurse that they had called for a sheik, a religious healer, to visit the patient because a relative suggested that heart failure was caused by the evil eye. The daughter said the sheik would read from the Qu'ran, say ruqyah, special verses, and encourage her to drink water from a special well called Zamzam in Mecca. After the visit of the sheik, the family appeared more accepting of their mother's condition.

During the admission assessment, the daughter shared that Umm Khalid took Shamar, *Foeniculum vulgare* (fennel) and *Trigonella foenum-graecum* L (fenugreek), in a hot drink for her "sugar" (diabetes) and treated the diabetic ulcer with honey and myrrh. Cupping marks (Hejama) were noted on her back during the skin assessment.

During visiting hours, the room was overcrowded with visitors including children. Concerned at the overcrowding, the nurses requested visitors to leave, which was refused, so the nurses called security to handle the situation. The son was angry that the hospital security made visitors leave and made the decision to take his mother home against medical advice so she could spend her final days with the family.

16.1 Cultural Issues

Arab is a cultural and linguistic term referring to those who speak Arabic as a first language and are united by culture and history. Twenty-two Arab countries stretching across the Middle East and North Africa have a rich diversity of ethnic, linguistic, and religious communities including Christians and Jews. Most Arabs are Muslims, but most Muslims are not Arabs.

Large social inequalities and health inequities exist among Arab countries related to social and economic factors such as access to drinking water, sanitation, and healthcare as well as

S. Lovering, R.N., B.S.N., M.B.S., D.H.Sc.
King Faisal Specialist Hospital and Research Center, Jeddah, Saudi Arabia
e-mail: slovering@kfshrc.edu.sae

© Springer International Publishing AG, part of Springer Nature 2018
M. Douglas et al. (eds.), *Global Applications of Culturally Competent Health Care: Guidelines for Practice*, https://doi.org/10.1007/978-3-319-69332-3_16

degree of urbanization. Twenty percent (20%) of Arab countries with low economic development such as Yemen and Sudan have high maternal and child mortality and the burden of communicable diseases. In contrast, the top 3% of Arab countries such as Qatar, Bahrain, and the United Arab Emirates with high urbanization have high life expectancy, good access to education and healthcare, and low levels of maternal and infant mortality. However, these are offset by the burden of noncommunicable diseases such as obesity, diabetes mellitus, and injuries from road traffic accidents. The remaining 77% of the Arab countries such as Saudi Arabia, Oman, and Jordan have shifted from a desert nomad to a modern, urbanized society within the past two generations. Significant economic and social progress has led to improved life expectancy, reduced maternal and infant mortality, and a shift from communicable diseases to high rates of obesity, diabetes mellitus, heart disease, and mortality due to road traffic accidents (Boutayeb and Serghini 2006).

Saudi Arabia's population is 31.5 million, of which 19.9 million (63.21 %) are Saudi citizens, while 11.5 million (36.78%) are foreign residents. The population profile is similar to other countries in the Eastern Mediterranean region with over 29.12% of the population under the age of 15. The population is expected to double by 2030. Only 2.93% of the population is over the age of 65 with total life expectancy of 74.3 years (Ministry of Health KSA Statistics 2015). Chronic diseases such as diabetes mellitus, hypertension, heart diseases, cancer, genetic blood disorders, and childhood obesity have emerged with the change from communicable to noncommunicable disease patterns in the past generation (Almalki et al. 2011). Free and available health services are provided by the government; however, Saudis tend to seek healthcare after developing disease symptoms or reaching an advanced stage of illness despite organized screening programs and protocols (El Bcheraoui et al. 2015).

The Arab Muslim worldview is derived from the religion of Islam. Islam means total submission and obedience to the will of Allah and is a complete way of life. The teachings and laws of Islam are derived from the Holy Qur'an and the Sunnah (a path of virtue). Muslims believe in divine predestination and in life after death when Allah judges people on the Day of Judgment for how they have lived their life on earth. A practicing Muslim lives in a way that reflects unity of mind and body with Allah with no separation of physical and spiritual health (Al-Shahri and Al-Khenaizan 2005; Lovering 2012).

Health is defined as complete physical, psychological, social, and spiritual well-being with spiritual health an essential component of the Muslim health belief model. God is the source of health, illness, and treatment. Health is a gift or reward from God, while illness, suffering, and dying are part of life and a test of faith or atonement for sins. While accepting medical treatment, spiritual healing practices are widely used including curing disease caused by the evil eye or jinn (spirits). Spiritual healing practices, also called prophetic medicine, include reading from the Holy Qur'an, use of prayer, religious supplications, eating honey, black cumin seeds (nigella), myrrh, and drinking Zamzam water, holy water from Makkah (Al-Shahri and Al-Khenaizan 2005). Traditional medicine and folk remedies such as the use of wet cupping, cautery, and herbal medications are used alongside Western medicine and spiritual healing, particularly by the elderly and rural populations (Alrowais and Alyousefi 2017).

16.2 Family and Decision-Making

Family is the core institution in Arab Muslim populations and includes husband, wife, children, and parents and close relatives and relations across all generations. The family is the basis of an individual's identity. Marriage is the only institution that connects family members; sex outside of marriage is not permitted.

The roles within the family are based on Islamic tradition and Arab culture. The father is usually the leader, breadwinner, provider, protector, and spokesperson of the family. The mother is the homemaker and main nurturer of the children. Grandparents have significant level of decision-making authority on family matters; parents are regarded with high respect and children encouraged to obey parents (Al Mutair et al. 2014). Loyalty to family and respect for the elderly are the most important social obligations (Ezenkwele and Roodsari 2013).

Traditionally, the elderly live with the oldest son. The son or daughter will accompany the parent during the hospital stay and mediate the communication between their parent and the health professional. Care giving is a responsibility shared by all family members (Al Mutair et al. 2014). It is culturally unacceptable and shameful for elderly family members to be institutionalized, such as in a nursing home, because caring for parents is a cultural and religious obligation. For this reason, nursing homes are not available in most Middle East countries; however, some chronic care facilities are developing for patient requiring chronic medical care.

It is the role of the family to protect and care for the patient and to relieve the patient of the burden of significant treatment decisions while ill. A cultural expectation is that the family decision-maker, usually the older male, will take responsibility for decisions concerning the patient after consultation with other family members. This consultation may or may not include the patient, depending on the patient's wishes and the cultural norms. It is important for the health professional to work through the family in providing care and building trust. In this dynamic pattern, the health professional treats the patient and family as the unit after confirming with the patient who is their delegated decision-maker.

Visiting is a religious and cultural requirement on family members (Al Mutair et al. 2014), and it is considered shameful not to visit ill relatives. Support for the extended visitation is important to the well-being of the patient and to the family, with the family "in charge" of the visiting process. The family may need support from the nurse to ensure a balance of psychological support through visiting and the need for rest. Dismissal of visitors by healthcare providers is culturally unacceptable (Al-Shahri 2002).

16.3 Modesty

Modesty is an important religious and cultural value. The need to protect modesty and dignity in the healthcare encounter is from the religious value to promote chastity and purity. The wearing of hijab (head scarf and/or face veil) is to protect the modesty of females, including during the healthcare encounter. Unnecessary touch, including shaking hands between unrelated adults of the opposite sex, is not acceptable within traditional Islam.

A woman must cover all the parts of her body except the hands and face, while a male will wish to cover parts of the body from the navel to the knee. Modesty is maintained by covering during procedures and examinations and avoidance of skin to skin contact between the sexes. Depending on the degree of conservatism, some patients may request sex concordant caring such as in maternity or gynecology settings (Al-Shahri and Al-Khenaizan 2005; Lovering 2012).

16.4 Communication

Arabs value interpersonal relationships. Indirect communication with meaning embedded in sociocultural context and nonverbal messages and avoidance of direct conflict are important. Establishing a trusting relationship with the patient and family is important through the use of formal greetings, such as Asalaam alaikum (peace be upon you), and nonverbal communication conveying a calm and respectful approach. Use of Arabic words, such as saying Bism'allah (in the name of God) before doing a procedure and Insh'allah (if God wills) when discussing the future, is a meaningful way to connect and establish trust with the patient and family, even when used by a non-Arab non-Muslim person (Lovering 2012).

Cultural rules need to be understood when interpreting eye contact and use of body language in the healthcare encounter. To show respect, touch and direct eye contact between male health workers and female Arab Muslim patients should be avoided unless necessary. Listening skills are important with interpretation of other body language signals, particularly when a female is wearing a face veil, which may be challenging for non-Muslims. When communicating with the elderly, it is disrespectful to call an older person by their own name (Al Mutair et al. 2014). For example, in Saudi Arabia the elderly will be called father (Baba) or mother (Mama), or by the name of the eldest son, Abu Khalid, meaning father of Khalid or Umm Khalid, meaning mother of Khalid.

16.5 Culturally Competent Strategies Recommended

Culturally competent strategies for Umm Khalid, mother of Khalid, need to address cultural and spiritual caring needs, communication strategies, and working within the sociocultural context of patient- and family-centered care within the Arab Muslim context.

16.5.1 Individual/Family Interventions

- Assess the role of the patient within the family and family support systems.
- Determine the structure of the family (multi-generational), main family decision-maker, family roles related to the care of the patient, and the impact of illness and hospitalization on the patient's role within the family.
- Assess the patient's relationships with other family members and family support systems for the patient.
- Elicit family members in assessing and interpreting the patient's psychosocial needs, level of anxiety and stress, as well as coping mechanisms.
- Assess the family's need for emotional support because they may bear the burden of coping with bad news rather than the patient.

16.5.2 Assessment of Health Beliefs and Use of Traditional Healing Methods

- Assess the use of traditional healing methods such as herbs, traditional medicines, oil, and honey because some traditional methods may be harmful to the patient condition, such as

diabetes mellitus, or be substituted by the patient and family for allopathic medicine.
- Conduct skin assessment to identify the use of cupping or cautery healing practices for skin integrity issues and need for wound care.
- Use "medical honey" dressings to replace use of raw honey for wound care.
- Accommodate family requests for a religious healer for treating the evil eye, jinn, or for reading special religious supplications.

16.5.3 Support for Religious Caring Practices

- Support use of prayer by providing prayer mats and support for patient doing ablutions, (washing ritual prior to performing prayers), providing a basin with water, and turning the bed to face Makkah (Mecca) for prayers if requested by patient or family.
- Modify the care routine to accommodate prayer prior to procedures.
- Do not interrupt the patient or family members during the prayer ritual.
- Accommodate listening to/reading of the Holy Qur'an as a religious healing practice.
- Accommodate requests for using Zamzam water, holy water, to wash the patient, for taking Zamzam water with medications, and for flushing a nasogastric tube.
- Do not place objects on the Holy Qur'an as it is a holy book and ask permission to touch or move the holy book if the provider is a non-Muslim.

16.5.4 Decisions About Care

- Ask the patient or the family the preferred way of addressing the patient, i.e., what "name" to use.
- Use Arabic words such as Asalaam alaikum (peace be upon you) as a greeting and Bism'allah before performing a procedure as part of establishing a trusting relationship with patient and family.
- Seek permission before touching the patient, in particular if male/female touching is required for a procedure.

- If a female patient wears a hijab (head and/or face cover), ensure that the hijab, or similar such as an operating room cap or a towel, remains in place under all circumstances when a male is present.
- Use an interpreter for communication with patients as family members may not fully disclose information due to the need to protect the patient from distress.
- Ask the family decision-maker to be responsible for the control of visitors in respect for their family member and in respect for the hospital rules.

16.5.5 Organizational-Level Interventions

- Provide support to the family to care for the patient and for the family members to stay within the patient room at all times.
- Adjust ward routines for supporting prayer by providing prayer mats.
- Support extended visiting hours, in particular if end-of-life care is instituted.
- Support the use of religious healers/sheiks.
- Encourage the use of family conferences by the healthcare team for decision-making about the care of Arab Muslim patients.
- Modify organization policies to accommodate a process for patients to elect a family member as decision-maker on behalf of a competent patient.
- Teach non-Arab Muslim staff about cultural values and beliefs of Arab Muslim patients.

16.5.6 Societal Level

- Develop home health services to support families in caring for loved ones at end-of-life care, consistent with the need for family caring practices.
- Collect data on the use of complimentary alternative medicine (traditional and folk) within the community.
- Target health education strategies on harmful practices within the community. Engage with religious community leaders on teaching

about harmful traditional practices such as cautery.
- Engage with the religious community to promote healthy living as a religious obligation to prevent obesity and diabetes mellitus.

Conclusion

Working within the Arab Muslim sociocultural context is the key to caring for Umm Khalid. Umm Khalid is an elderly woman who has seen a massive transformation from her early life as a desert nomad to experiencing modern medicine. Her family is her world, who she expects to completely protect her and care for her to the end of her life. She believes that her health and illness are from Allah and that she must bear suffering as a test of her faith while depending on prophetic medicine and spiritual healing. The modern healthcare team must place the Western medicine model alongside the traditional practices while working with the family to prevent harm.

The family is the key to planning the care of Umm Khalid with the son as the family decision-maker and the daughters most knowledgeable of the patient's spiritual and cultural needs. Healthcare organizations in Arab Muslim societies need to refocus care models on the patient-family unit as the center of care to be consistent with the sociocultural beliefs. At a community level, the religious community support for health promotion strategies is the key to tackling the "new" diseases of obesity, diabetes mellitus, and cardiovascular disease.

References

Al Mutair Abbas S, Plummer V, O'Brien A, Clerehan R (2014) Providing culturally congruent care for Saudi patients and their families. Contemp Nurse 46(2):254–258

Almalki M, Fitzgerald G, Clark M (2011) Health care system in Saudi Arabia: an overview. East Mediterr Health J 17:784–793

Alrowais N, Alyousefi N (2017) The prevalence extent of complementary and alternative medicine (CAM) use among Saudis. Saudi Pharm J 25:306–318

Al-Shahri M (2002) Culturally sensitive caring for Saudi patients. J Transcult Nurs 13(2):133–138

Al-Shahri M, Al-Khenaizan A (2005) Palliative care for Muslim patients. J Support Oncol 3:432–436

Boutayeb A, Serghini M (2006) Health Indicators and human development in the Arab region. J Health Geogr 5:61. https://ij-healthgeographics.biomedcentral.com/articles/10.1186/1476-072X-5-61. Accessed 4 July 2017

El Bcheraoui C, Marwa T, Farah D, Kravitz H, Almazroa M, Al Saeedi M, Memish Z, Basulaiman M, Al Rabeeah A, Mokdad A (2015) Access and barriers to healthcare in the Kingdom of Saudi Arabia: findings from a national multistage survey. BMJ Open 5:e007801. https://doi.org/10.1136/bmjopen-2015-007801

Ezenkwele U, Roodsari G (2013) Cultural competencies in emergency medicine: caring for Muslim-American patients from the Middle East. J Emerg Med 45(2):168–174

Lovering S (2012) The crescent of care: a nursing model to guide the care of Arab Muslim patients. Divers Equality Health Care 9:171–178

Ministry of Health KSA Statistics (2015) http://www.moh.gov.sa/en/Ministry/Statistics/book/Documents/StatisticalBook-1436.pdf. Accessed 25 May 2017

Case Study: Communication, Language, and Care with a Person of Mexican Heritage with Type 2 Diabetes

17

Rick Zoucha

Mr. Jose Garcia is a 57-year-old man who identifies culturally as Mexican American or a person of Mexican heritage. He recently presented at the behest of his wife to his primary care physician (PCP) with symptoms of type 2 diabetes such as frequent urination, increased thirst, blurry vision, and tingling in his hands (American Diabetes Association 2017). His blood glucose was 210 and his A1C was 9.5. Mr. Garcia was diagnosed with type 2 diabetes and was provided with educational information in English and a prescription for metformin 500 mg two times per day. Mr. Garcia went to his PCP appointment alone since his wife was not able to get off work. After leaving the office, Mr. Garcia felt confused and not sure how to proceed with his prescription and suggestions for managing his new diagnosis of type 2 diabetes. He did not understand much of the discussion and instructions with the nurse and physician regarding his diagnosis. The interactions were in English, and Mr. Garcia did not feel confident in both comprehension and speaking English. Mr. Garcia has certain beliefs about diabetes and was not sure if those beliefs were consistent with what he heard and understood during his visit with the nurse and physician.

Mr. Garcia was born and raised in a State in central Mexico, in the capital city of that State in central Mexico. The city is located in the center of the country in a mountainous region. The climate is dry with warm days and cool evenings. There is no need for in-house heating and air-conditioning. The population of the city is estimated to be around 70,800 but varies historically (Consejo Nacional de Población, México 2015). For Mr. Garcia's family, life was difficult with few jobs, crowded housing, and little opportunity economically, socially, and personally. Mr. Garcia's uncle and his family immigrated to the USA in search of a better life. They found a better life in the USA and shared that news frequently with family members and friends still living in Mexico. In the late 1970s and early 1980s, there was an increase in foreign-born immigration (14.1 million) to the USA including people from Mexico. The numbers of immigrants continued to grow and by 2009 Mexican-born immigrants accounted for over 29% of the foreign-born residents of the USA (Batalova and Terrazas 2010).

Mr. Garcia, his parents, grandparents, and siblings spoke frequently about leaving Mexico for the USA. It was a difficult discussion because the family would leave a large extended family for an unknown country. In addition, no one in the family spoke English, which was of concern to the family. However, Mr. Garcia's uncle assured the family that he did not speak much English and

R. Zoucha, PhD, PMHCNS-BC, FAAN
Professor and Joseph A. Lauritis Chair for Teaching and Technology, School of Nursing, Duquesne University, Pittsburgh, PA, USA
e-mail: zoucha@duq.edu

that he was doing well and supporting his family.

Mr. Garcia immigrated to the southwest region of the USA from Mexico with his parents, his five siblings (four brothers and one sister), and his maternal set of grandparents when he was 17 years old. He completed the equivalency of high school in Mexico prior to coming to the USA. In Mexico, the educational system children complete school until ninth grade. While in ninth grade, students and families make the decision to stop their education and go directly into the workforce or study for the entrance exams for preparatoria (preparatory) or commonly called prepa. Successful entrance exams allow students to be admitted to a 3-year college preparatory program. This program prepares student to then be able to apply to a college or university in Mexico. Unlike many of his friends and family, Senior Garcia decided to stop and graduate from the ninth grade and work. This was a joint decision between him and his parents due to the financial needs of the family.

Since Mr. Garcia immigrated with his family, he has lived in a multigenerational household: first with his siblings, parents, and grandparents and now with his wife and his parents, one daughter, son-in-law, and one grandchild. Mr. Garcia has one son in addition to his daughter who lives in the same city near the Garcia family. His son is married with three children. In total Mr. Garcia has four grandchildren living either with him or near his family. Spanish is the primary language spoken in the home and work. Both of Mr. Garcia's adult children and all the grandchildren speak both Spanish and English. However, the entire family speaks mainly Spanish with Mr. Garcia. Mr. Garcia lives in a large metropolitan city in the southwestern part of the country in a predominately Mexican American neighborhood. Spanish is the primary language spoken in the neighborhood including the stores, restaurants, and businesses.

Mr. Garcia, along with his father, cousin, son, and grandson, runs a small roofing business in the city. There are four generations working together to provide for the family and extended family. Mr. Garcia's father continues to join the roofers to work sites and offers suggestions and advice but no longer performs roofing. Each male member of the four generation provides different skills to keep the small business profitable. While at work, the primary language spoken is Spanish.

17.1 Cultural Issues

There are several cultural issues to consider when caring for Mexican Americans through prevention and/or treatment of type 2 diabetes. These issues include prevalence and beliefs about diabetes, family roles, and communication and will be discussed.

Mexican Americans experience an 87% higher risk for diabetes relative to non-Hispanic Whites (CDC 2011). This significant fact is important to consider when working with Mexican Americans regarding diabetes care. In addition, considering Mexican Americans perceptions and beliefs about diabetes is imperative in promoting culturally congruent care. According to Coronado et al. (2004), Mexican Americans believe that diabetes is caused by eating a high-fat or high-sugar diet, family history of diabetes, and little to no exercise. Included in this belief is a precipitating event that is thought to cause diabetes called sustos. This precipitating event is viewed and experienced as strong emotions and described as fright or soul loss. Some Mexican Americans believe that diabetes is in the body through heredity and sustos activates the disease. It is believed that some life events have caused the person to be frightened such as witnessing an accident or a traumatic event of a child and essentially the soul is frightened out of the body (Caballero 2011). Many believe that sustos is the eventual cause of diabetes (Lemley and Spies 2015). It is important for nurses and healthcare professionals to understand the cultural belief and perception to focus care in a culturally congruent manner.

It is critical to understand the role of family when promoting culturally congruent care in Mexican Americans. There is a saying in the culture that God is first, family is second, and the individual is third. During times of health and illness, understanding the role of family is imperative. Illness affects not only the individual but the entire family. The idea of presence and attending to family members in which care is either directed or self-directed is important to understand (Zoucha 1998). In some traditional Mexican American families, the female members (wife, daughter, mother, grandmother, aunt) of the family may assume the role of caregiver and health promoter (Caballero 2011; Hatcher and Whittemore 2007). It would be prudent to include women in the care of male members of the family if indicated. This practice may be changing over time but should be considered with some families.

There are specific communication patterns that are present in many people of Mexican heritage. It is estimated that over 41 million people speak Spanish in the USA (U.S. Census Bureau 2015a, b). Many people living in the USA speak both Spanish and English in and outside of the home. Some, depending on their age, may feel less confident speaking English outside of the home and with healthcare professionals. Whether the individual prefers speaking Spanish or English or both, it is important to approach communication with a sense of *personalismo* and respect (Zoucha and Zamarripa 2013). The first meeting may be more formal and respectful when introduced; however, the remaining interactions may be less formal. *Personalismo* is the process or interaction in which the person (healthcare professional) behaves like a friend and is less formal when communicating. It is common to engage in conversations that may include questions and conversations on both sides related to family or friends. When using *personalismo* it can build *confianza*, confidence, in the relationship between the healthcare provider and people of Mexican heritage (Zoucha 2017).

17.2 Social Structure Factors

The total Hispanic population in the USA is 56.6 million, and Mexican Americans represent approximately 63.4% of the Hispanic pop-

ulation (U.S. Census Bureau 2015a, b, 2016). The median income of Hispanic households is $45,150, and the poverty rate among Hispanics is 21.4% in the USA. The percentage of Hispanics who lacked health insurance was 16.2%, and the 66% of Hispanics age 25 and older hold at least a high school education.

The census data do not report specifically on Mexican American voting trends, but it is important to note that in the Hispanic community there have been increases in voting within this community. In 1996, 4.7% of all voters were Hispanic with an increase in 2012 to 8.4% for presidential elections. In 2014, 7.3% of voters were Hispanic for congressional election. This upward trend may suggest increased influence on policy and politics in the USA.

The changing political climate in the USA has produced much anxiety regarding immigration and residency issues for Mexican Americans and non-Mexican Americans alike. Recent presidential executive order related to the DACA (Deferred Action for Childhood Arrivals) is promoting perceived uncertainty regarding healthcare and healthcare issues for many in the Mexican American community. Regardless of actual immigration, residency, and US citizenship, people of Mexican heritage have common concerns about the perceptions of the government and some citizens regarding their place in US society (C. Zamarripa, personal communication, August 17, 2017). This most certainly will and can impact heath, health status, and healthcare access for people of Mexican heritage in the USA.

17.3 Culturally Competent Strategies

Past and current social structures have affected Mr. Garcia's health, illness, and well-being experiences and reality. The following presents ideas and suggestions about individual-, organizational-, and societal-level strategies to promote care that is competent and congruent with Mr. Garcia's cultural context.

17.3.1 Individual-/Family-Level Interventions

- Since Mr. Garcia has some difficulty with the English language, the individual provider and those in the office can provide interpreters through a variety of services on site or mobile/phone or computer-assisted services.
- If Mr. Garcia comes to his appointments alone, healthcare providers can make aftercare calls to his wife and/or other family members to assure that Mr. Garcia has understood any medical or nursing interventions.
- If Mr. Garcia comes to his appointment with any family members, it is imperative that they are included in the discussion about the reason and intervention for the visit.
- Healthcare providers should provide educational and instructional materials in Spanish for Mr. Garcia and his family.

17.3.2 Organizational-Level Interventions

- Healthcare systems that include hospitals, PCP offices, clinics, and community centers should adopt policies that are consistent throughout the health system.
- Consistent policy and implementation of procedures regarding family inclusion, interpreters, and educational materials in Spanish will promote best practices and potentially positive health outcomes.
- Large and small healthcare institutions should partner with businesses, institutions, and leaders in the community to plan and provide care that is consistent with people in the community in their cultural context.
- Professional schools such as nursing, health sciences, pharmacy, social work, and medicine can form a multidisciplinary effort to promote communication and interventions that are consistent with the cultural care needs of people of Mexican heritage.
- Professional schools such as nursing, health sciences, social work, pharmacy, and medicine can utilize a common approach to education that includes concepts important to understanding the cultural care needs of the people they serve, including people of Mexican heritage.

17.3.3 Societal-Level Interventions

- Encourage people of Mexican heritage to vote for candidates that promote healthcare access for all people and more specifically to include people of Mexican heritage.
- Healthcare professionals can influence policy through their professional organizations and elected officials.
- Encourage health policy that includes social justice application for people of Mexican heritage for universal access to healthcare.
- Influence and promote policy that is culturally congruent with provisions for not only cultural care needs but in language of choice (verbal and written materials) for people of Mexican heritage.

Conclusion

The USA demographically will continue to evolve and change well into the future. It is predicted that the Hispanic population will grow to 119 million or 28.6% of the total population in the USA by 2060 (US Census Bureau 2014). With the continued growth and prediction by the US Census Bureau of the increases in the Hispanic population and more specifically the Mexican American population, the quest to promote culturally congruent care will continue. Nurses and other healthcare professionals must continue to be vigilant as advocates for people of Mexican heritage as suggested in the levels of interventions outlined earlier. In order to promote health outcomes for people of Mexican heritage, it remains imperative that nurses and healthcare professionals always consider their unique cultural care needs.

References

American Diabetes Association (2017) www.diabetes.org. Accessed 10 Aug 2017

Batalova J, Terrazas A (2010) Frequently requested statistics on immigration and immigration in the United States. Migration Policy Institute. http://www.migrationpolicy.org/article/frequently-requested-statistics-immigrants-and-immigration-united-states-1. Accessed 20 May 2017

Caballero AE (2011) Understanding the Hispanic/Latino patient. Am J Med 124(10 Suppl 5):511–515

Centers for Disease Control and Prevention (CDC) (2011) National diabetes fact sheet: national estimates and general information on diabetes and prediabetes in the United States, 2011. U.S. Department of Health and Human Services, Center for Disease Control and Prevention, Atlanta

Consejo Nacional de Población, [National Population Council] México (2015) https://www.citypopulation.de/Mexico-Guanajuato.html. Accessed 20 May 2017

Coronado GD, Thompson B, Tejeda S, Godina R (2004) Attitudes and beliefs among Mexican Americans about type 2 diabetes. J Health Care Poor Underserved 15(4):576–588

Hatcher E, Whittemore R (2007) Hispanic adults' beliefs about type 2 diabetes: clinical implications. J Am Acad Nurse Pract 19:536–545

Lemley M, Spies LA (2015) Traditional beliefs and practices among Mexican American immigrants with type II diabetes: a case study. J Am Assoc Nurs Pract 27:185–189

U.S. Census Bureau (2015a) American community survey 1-year estimates, selected social characteristics in the United States. https://factfinder.census.gov/faces/tableservices/jsf/pages/productview.xhtml?src=bkmk. Accessed 11 Sept 2017

U.S. Census Bureau (2015b) American community survey 1-year estimates, Hispanic or Latino origin by specific origin. https://factfinder.census.gov/faces/tableservices/jsf/pages/productview.xhtml?src=bkmk. Accessed 11 Sept 2017

U.S. Census Bureau Population Division (2016) Annual estimates of the resident population by sex, age, race, and Hispanic origin for the United States and States: April 1, 2010 to July 1, 2015. Source: U.S. Census Bureau, Population Division. https://factfinder.census.gov/faces/tableservices/jsf/pages/productview.xhtml?src=bkmk. Accessed 11 Sept 2017

U.S. Census Bureau Population Projections (2014) 2014 National population projections datasets. https://www.census.gov/data/datasets/2014/demo/popproj/2014-popproj.html. Accessed 11 Sept 2017

Zoucha RD (1998) The experiences of Mexican Americans receiving professional nursing care. J Transcult Nurs 9(2):34–44

Zoucha R (2017) Understanding the meaning of Confianza (confidence) in the context of health for Mexicans in an urban community: a focused ethnography. Unpublished raw data.

Zoucha R, Zamarripa C (2013) People of Mexican heritage. In: Purnell LD (ed) Transcultural health care: a culturally competent approach, 4th edn. F. A. Davis, Philadelphia, pp 374–390

Case Study: Stigmatization of a HIV+ Haitian Male

18

Larry Purnell, Dula Pacquiao, and Marilyn "Marty" Douglas

Ronald is a 27-year-old homosexual man with a high school education who recently emigrated from Haiti to a large urban area in the United States. His parents and two siblings emigrated 8 years earlier because of the country's political unrest. At that time, Ronald remained with relatives because he did not want to leave his friends. While working in Haiti, Ronald was hospitalized for pneumonia, at which time he was diagnosed with HIV. He did not reveal his HIV status for fear of discrimination. Even though homosexuality in Haiti is legal, it remains a taboo. Ronald joined the local voodoo community because of its acceptance of homosexuals. Ronald joined his parents in the United States to receive better healthcare for his HIV+ condition than was possible in Haiti. He was concerned, however, about his poor English language proficiency. His parents successfully applied for Ronald to immigrate under the Cuban Haitian Entrant Program (US Citizenship and Immigration Services 2015).

Currently Ronald and his family live in a predominantly Haitian community in southeastern United States that has a median household income of $38,525, which is below the state median household income of >$47,000 (US Census Bureau 2015). His father works as a bank clerk despite being an accountant back in Haiti. His mother, trained as a teacher in Haiti, now works as a teacher's aide in the United States. The neighborhood lacks adequate bus service and is a long distance from the nearest hospital. Occasionally a mobile health clinic will be available, but the visits are unpredictable. The high crime rate in the neighborhood has driven out large-scale grocery stores that would provide healthy, fresh food, leading to a "food desert" environment. The crime rate also is a personal safety issue, preventing walking to maintain a healthy lifestyle.

His family is well-respected in the community for their strong Catholic faith and display of positive moral values. Ronald is reluctant to attend church because he perceives a lack of acceptance due to both the community's and the Church's view of homosexuality. For similar reasons,

L. Purnell, Ph.D., R.N., FAAN (✉)
School of Nursing, University of Delaware, Newark, DE, USA

Florida International University, Miami, FL, USA

Excelsior College, Albany, NY, USA
e-mail: lpurnell@udel.edu

D. Pacquiao, Ed.D., R.N., C.T.N.-A.
Center for Multicultural Education, Research and Practice, School of Nursing, Rutgers University, Newark, NJ, USA

School of Nursing, University of Hawaii, Hilo, Hilo, HI, USA
e-mail: dulafp@yhaoo.com

M. Douglas, Ph.D., R.N., FAAN
School of Nursing, University of California, San Francisco, San Francisco, CA, USA
e-mail: martydoug@comcast net;
marilyn.douglas@nursing.ucsf.edu

© Springer International Publishing AG, part of Springer Nature 2018
M. Douglas et al. (eds.), *Global Applications of Culturally Competent Health Care: Guidelines for Practice*, https://doi.org/10.1007/978-3-319-69332-3_18

Ronald has not disclosed either his sexual orientation or HIV status to his parents. He tried unsuccessfully to find a voodoo community. Three months after his arrival in the United States, Ronald was hospitalized for pneumonia and is diagnosed with AIDS. He disclosed his sexual orientation to the doctor but still feels he cannot tell his parents for fear of bringing shame to the family. He was offered the services of an interpreter because of his lack of language proficiency, but he refused for fear that the interpreter would discuss his condition with members in the community and word would ultimately reach his parents (Colin and Paperwalla 2013).

Since Ronald is unemployed, he does not have health insurance and feels that he cannot ask his family for financial assistance to purchase the expensive drugs. In addition, he has difficulty understanding the directions and information about his medication prescriptions. Ronald agreed to a visit from a social worker, who informed him of the Haitian Community Coalition, which provides health education, English language classes, and certified interpreters. They have taken an oath of confidentiality and could help him understand his medications.

In addition, the social worker assisted Ronald in contacting the Ryan White AIDS Drug Assistance Program, a program that provides HIV drugs to low-income people (US Department of Health and Human Services n.d.). Ronald was also referred to an organization named Dignity, a community of homosexual Catholics, their families, and their friends who could help him disclose to his parents about his HIV/AIDS status (Dignity USA 2015).

18.1 Cultural Issues

In the Haitian culture, any action taken by one family member has repercussions for the entire family; consequently, all members share prestige and shame. The prestige of a family is very important and is based on attributes such as honesty, pride, trust, social class, and history. Homosexuality is taboo in the Haitian culture, so gay and lesbian individuals usually remain closeted because of this stigma and the fear of discrimination. If a family member discloses that he or she is gay, everyone is silent; there is total denial. Within the Catholic Haitian community, there is a strong stigma associated with both being gay and being infected with HIV (Colin and Paperwalla 2013).

The literature cites some cases in which Haitians' communication patterns include loud, animated speech and touching in the form of handshakes and taps on the shoulder to define or reconfirm social and emotional relationships, including with healthcare providers. Haitians with lower levels of education generally hide their lack of knowledge to non-Haitians by keeping to themselves, avoiding conflict, and, sometimes, projecting a timid air or attitude. They may smile frequently and may respond in this manner when they do not understand what is being said. Traditional Haitians generally do not maintain eye contact because it is considered rude and insolent, especially when speaking to persons of authority. Due to the stigma associated with certain sensitive cases, such as HIV/AIDS, some Haitians may prefer to use professional interpreters who they will likely never see again (Colin and Paperwalla 2013).

Even though most Haitians are deeply religious, spiritual beliefs of many are combined with voodoo (voodooism), a complex religion with its roots in Africa (Religious Tolerance: Religions of the World 2010). Voodoo involves communication by trance between the believer and ancestors, saints, or animistic deities. Voodoo believers may attribute some of their ailments or medical problems to the actions of evil spirits and therefore not readily seek Western medical care for these problems. For many Haitian patients, the belief in the power of the supernatural can have a great influence on the psychological and medical concerns of the patients (Colin and Paperwalla 2013).

18.2 Social Structural Factors

Haiti is habitually ranked as the poorest country in the Western Hemisphere (Slatten and Egset 2004). In 2012, 58.5% of the Haitian population was at or below the poverty level (World Bank 2016). As an indicator of their poor health and healthcare system, Haitians have a life expectancy of only 57 years, as compared to an average of 69 years for all Latin Americans. Only about 25% of children are vaccinated, and safe water is accessible to only a quarter of the population (World Bank 2016). Coming from a lifetime of these conditions places a huge allostatic load on Ronald and his family, as well as the Haitian community in the United States. The chronic stress affects the autoimmune system, among others, and makes recipients less resilient in the face of illnesses and disease threat (Global Health Policy 2015).

In Haiti, HIV/AIDS is a significant health problem, with approximately 141,300 Haitians living with the infection (US Central Intelligence Agency 2015). As in the case of Ronald, migrants bring their health problems with them to their new country. In the United States, the HIV/AIDS prevalence rate among Haitian-born residents is 1.3% or 12,789 (Marc et al. 2010).

Haitian immigration to the United States has continued for many years, with most living in seven states along the eastern coast (Fact Sheet on Haitian Immigrants in the United States 2010). A majority of those who emigrated before 1920 were members of the upper class. In 1920, the United States occupied Haiti, and the first wave of poverty-stricken Haitian migration to North America soon followed (Colin and Paperwalla 2013). Today, many Haitians are in low-paying jobs that do not provide health insurance, and they cannot afford to purchase it themselves. Thus, economics acts as a barrier to health promotion. In addition, for those who do not speak English well, it is difficult for them to access the healthcare system, fully explain their needs, or understand prescriptions and treatments.

The Haitian neighborhood in which Ronald and his family live exemplifies the environmental and socioeconomic issues that contribute to the vulnerability of this population. The lack of health services, unhealthy food choices, high crime rate, and personal safety issues influence how the inhabitants are able to address their health problems. With so many social structural

factors impinging on their lives, they face huge challenges to maintain health for themselves and their families without the assistance and support of the broader society.

18.3   Culturally Competent Strategies Recommended

Haitian refugees are one of the most at-risk populations living in the United States. Besides those actions already employed to assist Ronald, the following are recommendations to enable the development of strategies that are culturally appropriate, adequate, and effective (Colin and Paperwalla 2013).

18.3.1 Individual-/Family-Level Interventions

- On admission, conduct an in-depth assessment of the person's cultural self-identity, linguistic preferences, and environmental, occupational, socioeconomic, and educational status.
- Be aware of the stigma that HIV+ has with the patient's family and the community.
- Respect patient's privacy regarding his reluctant to share his diagnosis of HIV/AIDS.
- Provide a thorough explanation of the role and confidentiality of certified interpreters and resources available.
- Ascertain upon admission if the patient wishes a visit from pastoral care. A referral to chaplaincy services might help Ronald with discussions of his family situation and HIV/AIDs status.
- Secure a psychiatric liaison professional to assist Ronald with his fear of discrimination and assistance with informing his family about his lifestyle.
- Secure a referral to social services early in Ronald's admission to help him apply for health insurance and other social programs for which he would qualify, such as English classes, job training, and housing, food, and transportation support.

- Provide education on sexually transmitted infections and HIV prior to discharge and in the preferred language of the patient. These documents are available in Haitian Creole from the Centers for Disease Control and Prevention (CDC).

18.3.2 Organizational-Level Interventions

- Establish organization-wide committees to address the promotion of culturally competent care delivery to all patients.
- Allocate financial resources to fund certified interpreters in the major languages of the populations served.
- Provide a certified interpreter when the patient has limited language proficiency in the language that is different from the healthcare providers.
- Provide signage and printed materials on multiple conditions in the major languages of the population served.
- Partner with local Haitian community centers and coalitions, churches, and businesses including bars, nightclubs, and radio and television stations to provide information on HIV and sexually transmitted infections in English, French, and Haitian Creole.

18.3.3 Community Societal-Level Interventions

- Collect demographic, socioeconomic, and health data, including morbidity and mortality, of the Haitian community.
- Establish a partnership with the Haitian Community Coalition to assist with health education.
- Collaborate with the Haitian community to organize health fairs to address HIV and other infections common among their population.
- Collaborate with the Haitian community in working toward an environment that fosters healthy lifestyles.

Conclusion

Several social structural factors have enormous impact on Ronald's health and illness experience. Ronald has high school education and limited English proficiency that limit his ability to seek better-paying jobs. He is currently unemployed, and his capacity for employment will be further compromised by his HIV condition. The stigma associated with homosexuality and HIV compounded by the fact that he is Haitian descent can potentially isolate Ronald from his family which is his main financial support, as well as the Haitian community. This stigma will ultimately shape the quality of his interaction with others including healthcare providers. All these factors create cumulative risks and vulnerability as well as Ronald's dependence on others.

In order to promote his health, strategies should not be limited to the disease alone but rather on the multiple problems that impact the outcomes of his condition. Therefore, culturally competent strategies should focus not only on him and his family in managing his disease but to seek organizational and societal resources to promote his integration in the community and potential participation as a citizen in society. While focusing on his needs secondary to the disease, culturally competent care should promote the socioeconomic, cultural, and environmental supports that can make a difference in the way he lives and enhance his potential for an autonomous and productive life.

References

Colin J, Paperwalla G (2013) People of Haitian heritage. In: Purnell L (ed) Transcultural health care: a culturally competent approach, 4th edn. F. A. Davis Co., Philadelphia, pp 269–287

Dignity USA (2015) https://www.dignityusa.org/. Accessed 14 Sept 2017

Fact Sheet on Haitian Immigrants in the United States (2010) http://www.cis.org/HaitianImmigrantFactSheet. Accessed 14 Sept 2017

Global Health Policy (2015) The global HIV/AIDs epidemic. http://kff.org/global-health-policy/fact-sheet/the-global-hivaids-epidemic/. Accessed 14 Sept 2017

Marc LG, Patel-Larson A, Hall HI, Hughes D, Alegria M, Jeanty G, Eveilland YS, Jean-Louis E (2010) HIV among Haitian-born persons in the United States, 1985–2007. AIDS 24(13):2089–2097

Religious Tolerance: Religions of the World (2010) Vodun, Voodoo, Vodoun, Vodou. http://www.religioustolerance.org/voodoo.htm. Accessed 14 Sept 2017

Slatten P, Egset W (2004) Poverty in Haiti. Fafo

U.S. Census Bureau (2015) New York Quick Facts. http://quickfacts.census.gov/qfd/states/36000.html. Accessed 14 Sept 2017

U.S. Central Intelligence Agency (2015) The World Fact book, 2015. https://www.cia.gov/library/publications/ the-world-factbook/geos/ha.html. Accessed 15 Sept 2017

U.S. Citizenship and Immigration Services (2015) Cuban Haitian Entrant Program. http://www.uscis.gov/ humanitarian/humanitarian-parole/cuban-haitian-entrant-program-chep. Accessed 14 Sept 2017

U.S. Department of Health and Human Services (n.d.) Health Resources and Services Administration: Ryan White HIV/AIDS Program Guarantee. http://www. hrsa.gov/opa/eligibilityandregistration/ryanwhite/ index.html. Accessed 14 Sept 2017

World Bank (2016) World development indicators. http:// data.worldbank.org/country/haiti#cp_wdi. Accessed 14 Sept 2017

Part V

Guideline: Culturally Congruent Practice

Integrating Culturally Competent Strategies into Health Care Practice

19

Marilyn "Marty" Douglas

Guideline: *Nurses shall use cross cultural knowledge and culturally sensitive skills in implementing culturally congruent nursing care.*

Douglas et al. (2014)

19.1 Introduction

Integrating the principles of cultural competence into our health-care practice is the ultimate definition of individualized patient care. Providing such care requires an understanding first of how the individual and family define health and illness and then the measures they take to cure illnesses and maintain wellness. These beliefs about health are constructed by cultural groups within a society. The foundation of these beliefs is laid down in infancy but is later modified by education and life experiences. In order for health-care providers to deliver quality care that is meaningful to the individual, that care must be integrated within the health belief framework of the individual. If not, then there is a risk that the expected outcomes will not be realized because the prescription of the provider cannot be incorporated into the individual's belief system. This asynchrony between the values of the mainstream health-care providers and individuals of socio-cultural and economically diverse populations may be one reason for the disparity in health outcomes. Therefore, it is incumbent upon the health-care provider to partner with the individual to explore ways in which care can be blended and adapted to be mutually acceptable and meaningful so that the desired outcomes are achieved by both.

19.2 Cultural Definitions of Health and Illness

In the preamble to its constitution, the World Health Organization (WHO) defines health as "…a state of complete physical, mental and social well-being and not merely the absence of disease or infirmity" (WHO 1946). This definition remains today, although it is controversial because it is too broad, unmeasurable, and difficult to operationalize in policies and health strategies. One reason for these difficulties is because health is culturally defined and practiced. "In all human societies, beliefs and practices related to ill health are a central feature of the culture" (Helman 2007). These beliefs about the causes of illness and how to cure and prevent them are linked to how they view the world around them and the social structure in which they live.

In some societies, ill health can be blamed on the intervention by a supernatural being (a deity), an evil spirit, a witch, or another person wishing harm, such as in the "evil eye" (Anderson 2010). Others, notably some persons in Latin America, the Middle East, and Asia, may also ascribe to a naturalistic framework that originated in China and India and was elaborated upon by

M. Douglas, Ph.D., R.N., FAAN
School of Nursing, University of California, San Francisco, San Francisco, CA, USA
e mail: martydoug@comcast.net; marilyn.douglas@nursing.ucsf.edu

© Springer International Publishing AG, part of Springer Nature 2018
M. Douglas et al. (eds.), *Global Applications of Culturally Competent Health Care: Guidelines for Practice*, https://doi.org/10.1007/978-3-319-69332-3_19

Hippocrates. Named the humoral theory, the cause of illness is an imbalance of the four body humors. In this system, the four humors are characterized as follows: (1) blood (hot and moist), (2) phlegm (cold and moist), (3) black bile (cold and dry), and (4) yellow bile (hot and dry). More recently, this system has been distilled into the "hot" and "cold" theory whereby foods and therapies are ascribed "hot" or "cold" attributes, unrelated to their actual temperature. Achieving a healthy state then requires the individual to maintain an equilibrium of the body humors by treating "hot" illnesses with "cold" therapies and vice versa (Helman 2007).

Both the Indian Ayurvedic system and traditional Chinese medicine, for example, equate health with balance. Within these Eastern worldview systems are the cosmic concepts of yin and yang. Yin is defined as negative, cold, moist, dark, soft, and female, whereas yang is positive, hot, dry, light, hard, and male (Macdonald 1984). The individual is expected to maintain a balance or harmony of these positive and negative forces in all aspects of life. Balancing these opposing forces is necessary in order to achieve optimal health.

A religious and spiritual worldview rooted in a strong belief in God can also have a health dimension. Adherents may believe that faith in God and prayer will assure health. Their faith in God helps them deal with illness and disabilities, and they may believe that God allows diseases in order to test their faith. Health-care practitioners need to be aware that this strong belief in God's will may explain some of a person's resistance to some forms of prolonged intensive treatments.

19.3   Culturally Based Health Beliefs and Practices

It is particularly important to begin this discussion with a cautionary note. Certain health-care practices and beliefs may be common among specific cultural groups. However, health-care professionals should be aware that these are just a framework, a baseline from which to begin a discussion with a patient regarding the patient's

health concerns and an optimal treatment program. Obviously not all persons within a cultural group believe the same, act the same, or use the same therapies for specific conditions. But if the health-care professional is equipped with the knowledge of cultural beliefs and practices that are different from those of the dominant culture, then questions can be framed in such a way as to validate which beliefs and practices the individual patient adheres to. To avoid stereotyping, it is absolutely essential to evaluate each patient independently as to which health-care beliefs and practices they ascribe. The following discussion presents some examples of these alternative belief systems.

19.3.1 Maternity Care

Cultural variations in the beliefs and practices surrounding childbirth have been studied extensively in the past decades (Fishman et al. 1988; Jordan 1980; Rice and Manderson 1996; Morse 1989; Manderson 1981). Traditional practices for pregnancy and childbirth center on food choices, herbal prescriptions, massage, rest and exercise restrictions, bathing, and postpartum confinement periods (Small et al. 1999), many of which are based on the humoral medical theory of "hot" and "cold." However, there is great variation within countries and even regions within countries. Many cultures adhering to the humoral theory consider pregnancy a "hot" condition or one that depletes the body of heat and causes the woman to be vulnerable to cold. But some consider the mother and fetus to be "cold" during some portion of the pregnancy (Manderson 1981). Similarly, cultural prescriptions vary widely for the herbs used during pregnancy and during the postpartum period and the prescriptions for foods, bathing, and exercise during the postpartum confinement period.

These differences are illustrated in reports of studies investigating maternity care of cultural groups around the world. Shewamene et al. (2017) performed a systematic review of 20 studies conducted in 12 African counties representing 11,858 women, which found that the use of various complementary and alternative medicines (CAM) or traditional medicine was as high as 80%. Boerleider et al. (2014) describe the maternity care experiences of non-Western immigrants in the Netherlands, whereas Shahawy et al. (2015) describe the health care practices of Muslim mothers. Wandel et al. (2016) performed in-depth qualitative interviews with Somali mothers living in Norway, while Chen et al. (2013) explored the differences between maternal behaviors and infant care of South Asian immigrants and Taiwanese women in Taiwan. Naser et al. (2012) compared the birthing practices of Chinese, Malay, and Indian women in Singapore. And finally, Hadwiger and Hadwiger (2012) described some of the health beliefs Filipina mothers have about health. But in all these studies, there remained a wide range of adherents to specific beliefs and practices. Therefore, it is problematic to classify the treatment of pregnancy and childbirth according to one's culture. For that reason, it is imperative that the health-care practitioner ask the mother broad questions about the general areas of cultural diversity in maternal care, such as:

- What types of foods do you prefer during pregnancy or after childbirth?
- Do you use any particular herbs or spices, such as ginger, during pregnancy/after birth?
- What types of drinks do you prefer during this period (hot or cold)?
- Do you have any restrictions on bathing after childbirth?
- Do you have any restrictions on exercise before and after childbirth?
- Do you observe a period of "confinement" after childbirth? If so, for how long?

Discussion of the mother's practices not only provides the health-care provider with ways in which care can be adjusted to the benefit of the new mother but also identifies potential risks, such as thrombophlebitis due to prolonged inactivity both before and after childbirth.

One area of maternity care that requires a great deal of cultural sensitivity is that of female genital circumcision (FGC), or sometimes known as female genital cutting or female genital mutilation (FGM), which is a term used in the medical literature but not preferred by the women themselves. The World Health Organization (2017) reports that at least 200 million girls and women currently alive have undergone some form of FGC. Although this procedure is performed mainly in Africa, it is also practiced in some parts of the Middle East and Asia. With migration from these countries currently increasing, health-care practitioners in Western countries are increasingly caring for these women who have had FGC.

Female genital circumcision has been a tradition dating back thousands of years. Hearst and Molnar (2013) provide illustrations of the geographical distribution of its prevalence as well as detailed photos of the four major types of FGC, which range from partial to full excision of the clitoris to infibulation or the stitching or narrowing of the vaginal opening. These illustrations can be seen at http://www.mayoclinicproceedings.org/article/S0025-6196(13)00264-4/fulltext#appsec1. The proponents cite a number of traditional, cultural, and religious reasons for this procedure. They believe that this procedure will promote cleanliness, preserve femininity, and ensure marriage. They also believe that this will prevent stillbirths in primigravidae, increase fertility, prevent promiscuity, and enhance male sexual performance because of the smaller vaginal opening (El-Shawarby and Rymer 2008).

Health-care professional may see young girls or women who have been circumcised for a number of both early and late complications. Early complications include bleeding that may have occurred due to laceration of the pudendal or clitoral artery. Local infection due to unsterile instruments can be severe enough to lead to tetanus or sepsis. Urinary retention is also seen in some cases due to injury to the urinary meatus, vagina, perineum, or bladder. Higher rates of these early immediate complications are seen with those types of FGC that involve more tissue excision and more extensive infibulation (Hearst and Molnar 2013). Common long-term complications of this procedure are most frequently urinary in nature. These include urinary strictures and stenosis, frequent urinary tract infections due to retention, urinary crystal formation in stagnant urine in the vestibule created by closed labia, poor urinary flow below the infibulated scar, and occasionally urinary incontinence. Scarring as a result of this procedure can cause fibroids, keloid fusion of the labia, and clitoral neuromas, all of which cause severe pain and may require surgical intervention. Other types of pain commonly encountered in women with FGC are painful intercourse, lower abdominal pain, and dysmenorrhea (Momoh et al. 2001). Complications related to infections include an increased incidence of yeast infections, bacterial vaginosis, and herpes simplex virus. It is yet to be determined whether there is a clear association between FGC and sexually transmitted diseases and HIV (Olaniran 2013). Psychological disorders are also sequelae of FGC, such as anxiety, depression, and sexual dysfunction.

Providing care for a woman with FGC requires a culturally sensitive approach that is kind, empathetic, and nonjudgmental. Using the term "circumcision" is more readily understood by the patients and their interpreters than *female genital mutilation*, since they don't view this procedure as mutilation. Women who have undergone FGC should not be treated as "specimens" wherein the presence of this condition is more interesting to the health-care providers than the woman's present condition. A level of trust must be established before the woman will be forthcoming and share the information that is critical to her care. Some broad questions follow that a health-care professional can use to begin the discussion with a woman who has undergone FGC who is seeking care.

- Can you share/tell me about your experience with being circumcised? At what age were you circumcised? By whom? Where was it done?
- What do you think is good about being circumcised?
- Does your religion recommend circumcision?
- Does your culture recommend it?
- Do you have any pain/discomfort/problems because of your circumcision?
- Other problems?

- What help would you like for any of these problems?

The health-care provider cannot be expected to know everything about every culture. However, every person who seeks health care is entitled to respect and the willingness on the part of the health-care practitioner to listen to their concerns. In a study of 318 Vietnamese, Turkish, and Filipino immigrants seeking maternity care in Australia, Small et al. (1999) found that the women were less concerned that the health-care providers were knowledgeable about their cultural beliefs. On the other hand, they were more concerned that these Western caregivers were unkind, rushed, and unsupportive. Although language difference could explain some of this interpretation, there still remains a considerable portion of these feelings that can be attributed to the attitude of the caregiver.

19.3.2 Pain Assessment: Does Culture Play a Role?

Pain is a symptom reported by patients to their health-care professionals in all specialties and all settings. The experience of pain is a synthesis of physiological, psychological, and sociocultural factors, only one of which is ethnicity. But as a subjective experience, pain can have very wide interindividual and group variability in expression. Complicating the picture is that ethnicity and pain are both fluid and multidimensional in nature. Yet, for more than half a century, numerous investigators have been trying to determine the exact relationship between the two.

Leininger (1979) states that how one reacts to illness—pain, for example—is linked to cultural values and experiences. Culture defines not only health beliefs and practices but also what is expected and how to behave, including how to react to painful stimuli. Embedded within the cultural context are the perception, expression, and management of pain. In a landmark and classic study that stimulated subsequent studies on the relationship between pain and culture, Zborowski (1952) studied four cultural groups in the United States: "Old Americans" (Anglo-Saxon), Irish, Italian, and Jewish hospitalized patients. He concluded that pain behaviors are influenced by culture and social conditioning and that these patterns of attitudes toward pain may have different functions in various cultures. He described the Anglo-American response as stoic, restrained, avoiding any outward expressions of pain and withdrawing in the event of severe pain. Unfortunately, the hospital staff were inclined to use the Anglo-American response as the "acceptable" model and to judge all others as either complaining, overacting, or emotional.

Numerous subsequent studies attempted to further explore this relationship between culture and the response to pain. These investigations can be categorized into either a study of experimental pain or clinical pain. Although studies of experimental pain are greatly limited by solely measuring pain tolerance and pain threshold in essentially healthy participants, they can act as proxies for clinical pain when trying to evaluate the basic mechanism of pain, and they can control for ethnicity through subject selection.

In one large-scale review of 26 studies of ethnic differences in experimental pain, Rahim-Williams et al. (2012) examined the effect of cold stimuli, ischemic stimuli, mechanical or pressure stimuli, and electrical stimuli via acupuncture on the report of pain tolerance (the highest intensity of painful stimulation an individual is able to tolerate) and pain threshold (the lowest level of stimulation at which a stimulus can be perceived as painful). The majority of the studies compared non-Hispanic Whites (NHW) with African-Americans (AA), but other comparison groups studied included Hispanics, South and East Asians, British, Danish and Belgian Whites, Eskimos, and Nepalese, among others. Many of these studies did report ethnic differences in the response to these painful stimuli, but their explanations of these differences varied. Of the 26 studies reviewed, 15 compared AA with NHW; analysis revealed that there were moderate to large effect sizes for pain tolerance, with AA demonstrating lower pain tolerance than NHW. In those investigations comparing NHW with other ethnic groups, there was a wide range of effect sizes for both pain tolerance and pain threshold.

In a more recent systematic review performed by Kim et al. (2017), 41 studies investigated the use of the same types of experimental stimulation, i.e., cold, pressure, electrical, ischemic, and thermal, with populations of AA, Hispanics, Asians, and NHW. Meta-analysis showed that AA, Asians, and Hispanics had higher pain ratings and lower pain tolerance as compared with NHW, but no differences in pain threshold. The type of painful stimuli and demographic variables did not contribute to these variations.

Faculty members of schools of dentistry also studied cultural differences in pain sensitivity, using only mechanical and electrical stimulation. Al-Harthy et al. (2016) used a case control method to study 122 women from three cultures, Italians, Swedes, and Saudis, all living in their country of origin. The Italian females reported statistically significant scores that were lower in both pain threshold and tolerance than the Swedes and Saudis. The Swedes reported the highest levels of pain tolerance.

These experimental pain studies only address a fraction of the pain experience. In the clinical setting, there is also the psychological aspect of fear and anxiety if pain signals a worsening condition, fear of disability, interference in life activities, impact on employment, potential burden on family, and anticipation for treatment or nontreatment. Therefore, clinical pain studies are needed to provide the human perspective to this experience.

Lavin and Park (2014) performed a systematic review of 27 articles addressing pain in racially and ethnically diverse older adults. Race and ethnicity was a statistically significant factor in 17 of these 27 studies. As compared with NHW, minority older adults reported a greater prevalence of pain, higher pain intensity ratings, were less likely to receive prescription pharmacologic agents and surgery and were more likely to use complementary and alternative medicines to treat their pain. Almost 15 years ago, Green et al. (2003) unveiled racial and ethnic disparities in pain treatment of minorities in a large-scale review of 118 clinical pain research studies investigating pain treatment across a range of clinical conditions: acute postoperative pain, cancer pain, occupational orthopedic injuries, sickle cell disease, pain treatment in emergency departments, and in geriatric patients both hospitalized and in hospice care.

In addition to the undertreatment of pain, racial and ethnic minorities carried a larger burden of the pain, particularly with more disability and depression. The mechanisms for this disparity remain unclear and therefore mandate for further research in this area if culturally competent care is to be provided to these populations. More information is needed about the influence of the social context on the painful condition. In the meantime, culturally competent health-care professionals need to be aware of not only the intercultural differences in perception and verbal expression of pain but also the disparities of care that exist.

When caring for diverse populations, more focused attention needs to be paid to pain assessment, especially pain severity and the meaning and impact of the painful condition on the life situation and social context of the person. A nonjudgmental communication style that engenders patience and trust can encourage the individual to more willingly share their experiences and ways of treating their pain, even though they may be different from those of the health-care professional. When there is a lack of racial and language concordance between patient and health-care provider, more effort and time is required to accomplish these goals of culturally competent health care. With an increase in refugee populations migrating throughout the world, health-care professionals in all parts of the globe will be caring for racially and ethnically diverse populations and thus require culturally competent skills (Schiltenwolf and Pogatzki-Zahn 2015).

19.3.3 Traditional and Complementary Medicine

Complementary and alternative medicine (CAM) has many synonyms, namely, traditional medicine (TM), folk medicine, ethnomedicine, and native healing, among others. The earliest humans used the plant, animal, and mineral substances in their immediate environment to keep healthy and deal with diseases that threatened their survival. As people spread across the globe and into new environments, each culture found new sources to help them survive in their current environment. Hence, traditional medicine is as wide-ranging and diverse as the regions and cultures of the world. As such, traditional medicine is the oldest form of health-care system and one that persists in the present day and is increasing in demand. In almost every culture, from those in developing nations to the most industrialized, some form of complementary therapy is used to maintain health, whether it be massages, hot mineral baths, sweat lodges, acupuncture, Indian Ayurveda, herbal teas, Arabic unani medicine, or many others. The challenge for the health-care practitioner is to be aware that almost every patient uses some form of these therapies and to provide a therapeutic milieu in which the patient feels safe in sharing what other therapies he or she is using.

The World Health Organization (2013) defines traditional medicine as "…sum total of the knowledge, skill, and practices based on the theories, beliefs, and experiences indigenous to different cultures, whether explicable or not, used in the maintenance of health as well as in the prevention, diagnosis, improvement or treatment of physical and mental illness" (WHO 2013, p. 15). WHO acknowledges that in some countries, the terms traditional medicine and complementary medicine are used synonymously but adds that CAM also refers to health-care practices that are not fully integrated into the dominant health-care system. In *Traditional Medicine Strategy 2014–2023* (WHO 2013), the global health organization outlines its aims to develop a TM knowledge base, evaluate the safety and efficacy of TM/CAM therapies, design policies and regulations for their use, and promote the integration of therapies into national health-care systems. The result of this work will hopefully be a valuable tool of health-care practitioners and planners around the world as they implement TM and

CAM into their systems to the ultimate benefit of those who seek their care.

To provide culturally competent care, the health-care practitioner must be knowledgeable about those TM and CAM therapies most commonly seen within their specialty areas of practice and used by populations they serve. Abdullahi (2011) provides a review of 12 herbs and spices that are commonly used in 15 African countries, as well as the barriers and challenges to integrating TM in Africa. Kumar et al. (2017) summarize the key principles of Ayurvedic medicine and the indications, side effects, and rationale for many common herbs and plants used in Indian traditional medicine. Their reference list will be valuable to clinicians in many specialties who care for Indian populations. Investigations in a number of cultures have documented the extensive prevalence of the use of CAM in a wide variety of conditions: in racial and ethnic groups in the United States (Upchurch and Rainisch 2012), Iran (Ghaedi et al. 2017; Mahjoub et al. 2017; Shokoohi et al. 2017), and Caribbean immigrants in Canada (Braithwaite and Lemonde 2017).

One area of significant importance to clinicians is the pharmacokinetic drug interaction between TM herbal extracts and the synthetic medicines used in many Western and dominant health-care systems. Co-administration of herbal drugs with conventional drugs can modulate the uptake and elimination pathways when they are metabolized. One example is *Ginkgo biloba*, a popular herbal extract used mainly in Asian countries but also in Europe and the United States for conditions as varied as cognitive impairment, diabetes, vertigo, hypertension, rheumatism, peripheral vascular disease, and GERD. In an extensive investigation of *Ginkgo biloba*, Unger (2013) reviewed more than 150 studies conducted both in vitro and in vivo. He found evidence that the extracts of *Ginkgo* can be both inhibitors and inducers of drug-metabolizing enzymes, but usually the effects were weak in each direction. He concluded that the risk for drug interactions is minimal but only if the recommended low dose of 120–240 mg/day is ingested and other comorbidities are controlled. However, much more research is needed because of the lack of quality control and standardization of the product on the open market and small sample sizes of some of the research studies.

Another source for information on drug interactions with herbal medicines is provided by Meng and Liu (2014). These authors outline the pharmacokinetic interactions of seven widely used herbal remedies: *Ginkgo biloba*, ginseng, garlic, black cohosh, *Echinacea*, milk thistle, and St. John's wort. And in the area of oncology, Haefeli and Carls (2014) estimate that 30–70% of cancer patients use CAM, with herbal remedies particularly frequent. They reviewed the pharmacokinetic drug reactions of those herbs most commonly used by patients with cancer: garlic, *Ginkgo*, ginseng, *Echinacea*, and St. John's wort. Of this group of herbs studied, two have the most notable clinical relevance. Because of ginseng's effect on the clearance of vitamin K antagonists, close monitoring is warranted when co-administered with warfarin. St. John's wort had the greatest impact on drug metabolism, with the potential for decreasing the efficacy of some drugs by as much as 70%. Finally, using a systematic review of the literature, Kooti et al. (2017) compiled brief descriptions of actions and effectiveness of 36 Iranian plants used in cancer treatment in Iran. The studies cited above should provide the health-care practitioner with a beginning knowledge of herbal-drug interactions.

CAM, particularly herbal supplements, are most commonly used for chronic illnesses. With the rising incidence of chronic illnesses around the world, the demand for and use of herbal remedies is also increasing. Some of the barriers to communication with the health-care practitioner about TM and CAM were a lack of trust and a perception of superiority (van der Watt et al. 2017). Culturally competent health-care practitioners need to project cultural humility and a sense of respect for the persons seeking care who use TM and CAM in order for those persons to divulge the therapies they use. Only then can the culturally competent practitioner begin to jointly develop a plan of care that safely integrates both the person's cultural meaning of their illness and their ways of treating it with the treatment plan of the dominant health-care system provider. With the safety and efficacy of many CAM therapies still unknown and with the lack of quality control of these agents, this integration remains a challenge.

19.4 Cultural Competence Skills

19.4.1 Cultural Assessment

A thorough health assessment is a composite of physical, psychological, social, and cultural factors that contribute to the person's current state of wellness or illness. Particularly in the case of a mismatch between the cultures of the caregiver and the recipient of that care, a thorough cultural assessment is needed to reveal the cultural beliefs, the context of the illness, and the social structure in which the person exists. Information gained from a cultural assessment is crucial in formulating a diagnosis, preparing a culturally appropriate plan of care, and possibly adapting the intervention to one that is mutually acceptable to both the provider and recipient. With such adjustments, there is a greater likelihood that the plan will be implemented and the expected health outcomes achieved, thus contributing to decreasing the health disparities seen in culturally diverse populations.

A cultural assessment can be conducted with varying degrees of detail depending on a number of factors: the needs of the individual seeking care, the familiarity and clinical experience of the health-care practitioner with the culture of the population involved, and the availability of resources, such as interpreter services and the time the health-care practitioner can devote to the assessment. The process begins with a face-to-face interview in which the health-care practitioner uses active listening skills to establish rapport, build trust, and demonstrate respect, which is essential if individuals are to share beliefs and practices they may perceive as different from the practitioner. The next step is to frame open-ended questions and then delineate the issues to be addressed so that interventions and rehabilitation plans can be tailored to the beliefs of the individual. An example of an open-ended question is:

- Are there any traditional practices or cultural aspects of your care that we need to be aware of?

There are a number of cultural assessment tools available that health-care practitioners can use to select the questions and discussion points appropriate to the clinical situation and cultural populations being served. One that can be used in many different situations is the Purnell Cultural Assessment Tool (Purnell 2014) provided below in the Appendix. The practitioner can use questions from this tool to design a tool specific to the desired clinical situation and population. In addition, Andrews and Boyle (2016) provide detailed cultural assessment guides that can be used with specific types of clients: (1) Andrews/Boyle Transcultural Nursing Assessment Guide for Individuals and Families, (2) Andrews/Boyle Transcultural Nursing Assessment Guide for Groups and Communities, and (3) Boyle/Baird Transcultural Nursing Assessment Guide for Refugees.

Cultural assessment also involves integrating biological variations into all relevant clinical skills checklists. For example, skin color is one of the most significant biological variations when providing culturally competent care. The assessment of the skin for rashes, sclera for jaundice, presence of cyanosis, or capillary refill can all be more challenging in persons with darker pigmentation. In such cases, a careful baseline examination best performed in bright daylight is recommended during the initial evaluation. If the clinician is unaware of normal variations, not only inaccurate assessment but also detrimental effects can result. For example, the presence of Mongolian spots, common in a number of ethnic groups, may be interpreted erroneously as signs of child abuse and the parents subsequently reported to the authorities. Giger and Davidhizar (2008) provide detailed descriptions on the biological differences, enzymatic and drug metabolism variations, and disease susceptibilities among people in 23 racial or ethnic groups. This book serves as a useful resource for clinicians of all specialty areas.

If the health-care practitioner serves a significant number of a particular racial or ethnic population, then it would be useful to design a cultural assessment tool specifically designed for that population. Balaratnasingam et al. (2015) describe the process of developing, implementing, and evaluating two cultural assessment tools to assess the mental health and social and emotional well-being of Aboriginal and Torres Strait Islanders. In their practice, they found that current tools used for the dominant culture lacked normative data on their population, relied heavily on written responses in English, and lacked cultural relevance. Early evaluations of their new tools suggest they were effective and easy to use. The authors acknowledged the lack of generalizability of their tool because it was tested only in the clinical service where it was developed. However, the description of their process of designing a culture-specific assessment tool may be beneficial to other clinicians.

19.4.2 Negotiation or Shared Decision-Making

The purpose of the cultural assessment is to gain an accurate and comprehensive picture of the context of the individual, family, and community so that the care decisions made are specific, meaningful, and beneficial to them. The information collected from the cultural assessment is the baseline from which negotiating a plan of care begins. The practitioner also needs a knowledge of the culture and culturally competent communication skills in order to initiate the decision-making process. Access to expert cultural consultants or peers with the appropriate cultural knowledge and skills can also be useful to assist in this process (Marion et al. 2016; Owiti et al. 2014).

The culturally competent practitioner, prepared with the assessment data and cultural knowledge and skills, begins discussion with a summary of the practitioner's interpretation of the data and clinical situation. Then the clients, as in the case of the individual, family, and community members, are offered the opportunity to identify and correct any misinterpretations of the practitioner's interpretation. Next, all parties partake in identifying the nature, meaning, and significance of the problem so that the full context is

appreciated. Finally, all potential solutions are discussed and a plan of care developed, with the clients suggesting their preferences for care.

When there are incongruences between cultural beliefs and practices and institutional standards of practices, usual procedures, and policies, creativity and flexibility are required. With patient safety being nonnegotiable, options can be explored as to how to adapt usual policies and procedures to accommodate the patient's beliefs. The classic example is the use of intraoperative normovolemic hemodilution or "bloodless" cardiopulmonary bypass (CPB) for persons of Jehovah's Witnesses faith whose beliefs forbid the use of blood during surgery (Marinakis et al. 2016; McCartney et al. 2014). This change of procedure not only avoided harmful adverse effects of the use of blood products for persons of Jehovah's Witnesses faith but also led to the use of "bloodless" CPB as a routine procedure in many other eligible patients. Another example is adapting hospital visiting hours rules to accommodate cultural and family customs that require a larger number of visitors and longer hours than hospital policy dictates. Family support is an important ingredient of the healing process, so flexibility in visiting hours whenever possible is warranted for the benefit of the patient rather than solely for staff routines. However, some issues may be more complex to negotiate. Placing a lighted candle in a dying patient's oxygen-filled room may require extra flexibility and creativity to explore a compromise in which an at least some portion of the request is granted. In this case, one suggestion might be to allow the lighted candle immediately upon the patient's death and once the oxygen has been discontinued (Marion et al. 2016).

The aim of mutual decision-making is to design a plan of care that is beneficial to the health of the client and is feasible within the environmental, social, and cultural context of the client. If the client is a partner in designing the plan, there is greater likelihood that the client will be motivated to implement the plan. Designing and implementing a culturally competent plan of care has the potential of reducing racial and ethnic disparities in health outcomes.

19.5 Recommendations for Culturally Competent Practice

19.5.1 Direct Care Providers

Direct care providers, whether they are a physician, clinical nurse, physical or occupational therapist, or other direct caregiver, are the first point of an encounter that a person from an ethnically diverse population has with the health-care system. Therefore, it is the initial greeting, which can be culturally defined, that begins the process of establishing a trusting relationship in which the person can feel safe to share disparate viewpoints and practices. The culturally competent practitioner is knowledgeable and respectful of the person's cultural beliefs and practices and possesses the cultural humility to admit unfamiliarity and seek expert opinions when needed. Direct care providers have the responsibility to participate in educational opportunities about the cultural knowledge that they lack about the populations they serve. Continuing education courses and service learning experiences in the communities are some ways to improve their knowledge base.

An essential element of care of all direct care providers is assessment. By conducting a cultural assessment, the culturally competent health-care provider can determine the person's language preference and the need for interpreters, identify the designated decision-maker within the family, and ascertain the person's perceptions of the cause of the current health problem and any culturally prescribed treatment modalities. This information is crucial in formatting a plan of care and negotiating any adaptations in the event of cultural conflicts.

19.5.2 Health-Care System Administrators

An important function of administrators within a health-care organization is to provide the staff with the resources it needs to deliver culturally competent care. To accomplish this, accountability for culturally competent practice should be made at the executive level of the organization, starting with writing it into its mission statement. If a substantial portion of population served is racially and ethnically diverse, the organization should establish a baseline of health data on those within its catchment area so that health programs can be designed to address those with the greatest morbidity and mortality outcomes.

Organizational policies and procedures should reflect a respect for the cultural beliefs and practices of the community it serves and a willingness to partake in shared mutual decision-making in the event of conflicting cultural beliefs. Recruitment of community members from racially and ethnically diverse populations to become permanent members on such organization-wide committees as the ethics committee, patient education committee, or nursing practice committee would be helpful in incorporating cultural relevance, content, and sensitivity into the policies and procedures.

Budget allocations are necessary for interpreters to work with patients and translators to develop patient education materials and important standard forms, for example, the informed consent form (Marrone 2016) for procedures or discharge instructions. Funds are also needed for signage in various languages around the organization to guide those who are unfamiliar with the dominant language.

Administrators are also responsible for providing the funds and opportunity for staff to attend education and training in culturally competent practice, for example, during orientation and continuing education classes. Following these classes, the administrators are responsible for supervising the staff and evaluating whether effective cross-cultural practice is being delivered.

19.5.3 Educators

At the academic level, students should be exposed to general cultural content at their earliest opportunity, in their basic prerequisites for professional schools. Then, in each specialty, cultural-specific beliefs in their area of practice should be integrated into the coursework and practical experiences. Incorporating cultural case studies in simulation labs allows students to explore the cultural components of care in a safe environment. In addition, student clinical practice should include service learning experiences with racial and ethnic groups that have high incidences of negative health outcomes. These experiences can be both within their own communities or abroad, where students have the opportunity to observe health-care delivery models that are adapted to the needs of a different cultural group.

Educators in both academic and clinical settings are increasingly using simulation modules in labs to teach clinical skills, but where resources are limited, role-playing and mannequins also serve. Cultural competence skills can also be taught through simulations, in which the students are presented with cross-cultural situations and feel "safe" to negotiate cultural conflicts before going into the practice setting (Roberts et al. 2014; Gallagher and Polanin 2015). Simulation content can begin with a preliminary cultural self-assessment ("What is your cultural heritage"?) and a module on the cultural knowledge of some of the populations the students will be caring for later in the clinical setting. A module on performing a cultural assessment can also be part of the preparation. After this preparation, the student is exposed to simulated experiences that portray realistic clinical scenarios. Biological, cultural, social, and physical characteristics as well as cultural conflicts are integrated. The students are asked to perform a cultural assessment using culturally sensitive interview techniques and negotiate any cultural conflicts that present themselves. To conclude the session, debriefing and self-reflection is a final important stage in the process of learning cultural competence.

For educators teaching within a health-care organization, the primary responsibility is to develop and coordinate in-service and continuing education programs to prepare staff to provide culturally competent care. In addition, these educators can participate on practice committees, patient education committees, and policy and procedure committees, among others, to integrate elements of culturally competent care into their respective contents. The educators can also assist supervisors to develop mechanisms and performance evaluation tools to evaluate whether the staff is performing culturally competent practice.

19.5.4 Researchers

Much of the cross-cultural research done to date has been describing the cultural beliefs, norms, and practices of specific cultural groups. Although this descriptive research is necessary, it is yet insufficient upon which to base practice. Much more research is needed to design and test interventions to determine whether the intervention is capable of sufficient improvement to affect the racial and ethnic disparities in health outcomes. Furthermore, scores of educators have tested whether their students have greater "cultural sensitivity" and cultural knowledge after their educational offerings, but we don't know whether this translates into improved outcomes for the patients they care for. In both these areas of intervention testing and education, research on culturally competent practice is still in its infancy.

Another critical need in the area of culturally competent practice is to determine whether certain traditional medicine practices are safe. If the practitioner is to be able to negotiate with a person who wishes to use a complementary/alternative or traditional medicine practice, the practitioner must be aware of its safety or adverse effects. Combining some herbal medicines with conventional pharmacologic agents can have serious consequences. In recent years, the World Health Organization and the National Institutes of Health, among others, have begun to compile a database on these folk medicines. Much more research is needed on their interactions with an ever-increasing number of drugs put on the market by pharmaceutical companies.

Conclusion

Health and illness are culturally defined. Providing culturally competent practice involves using knowledge of the cultures of the populations served in combination with the skills of cross-cultural communication, cultural assessment, and negotiation for mutual care decisions. Health-care providers are responsible for learning about the cultures of the diverse populations they care for in order to provide culturally competent practice. However, while knowledge is necessary, it is insufficient. The health-care practitioner uses that knowledge to develop cross-cultural communication skills (Chap. 14) as the first step in adapting knowledge to practice. Conducting a baseline cultural assessment requires this knowledge and these skills in order to establish an atmosphere of openness and respect that allows the individual to share beliefs and practices that may be unfamiliar to the health-care providers. The ultimate goal is to integrate the cultural knowledge with the communication skills and cultural assessment data to negotiate a mutually agreed upon plan of care that is feasible within the sociocultural context of the person. An understanding of the social determinant of health, particularly for minority populations who have limited financial and community resources, is also necessary when negotiating a plan of care that the person is able to accomplish. If the cultural beliefs and practices and the sociocultural context of the person are incorporated into the treatment plan, and if the person is motivated to adhere to a feasible plan, then the potential for achieving the desired health outcome is more probable. It is only with improved health outcomes for racially and ethnically diverse populations that the disparities will decrease and the health of their communities improve. Culturally competent practice shares these goals.

Appendix: Purnell Cultural Assessment Tool(version 2.1)

An extensive cultural assessment is rarely completed in the clinical setting because of time and other circumstances. A seasoned clinical practitioner will know when further assessment is required. Thus, this tool should be used as a guide. *Shaded items in italics are part of any standard assessment. Other items may also be part of a standard assessment, depending on the organization, setting, and clinical area.*

Cultural assessment question	Comments
Overview, inhabited localities, and topography	
Where do you currently live?	
What is your ancestry?	
Where were you born?	
How many years have you lived in this country?	
Were your parents born in this country?	
What brought you (your parents/ancestors) to this country?	
Describe the land or countryside where you live. Is it mountainous, swampy, etc.?	
Have you lived in other places in the United States/world?	
What was the land or countryside like when you lived there?	
What is your income level?	
Does your income allow you to afford the essentials of life?	
Do you have health insurance?	
Are you able to afford health insurance on your salary?	
What is your educational level (formal/informal/self-taught)?	
What is your current occupation? If retired, ask about previous occupations	
Have you worked in other occupations? What were they?	
Are there (were there) any health hazards associated with your job(s)?	
Have you been in the military? If so, in what foreign countries were you stationed?	

Cultural assessment question	Comments
Communications	
What is your full name?	
What is your legal name?	
By what name do you wish to be called?	
What is your primary language?	
Do you speak a specific dialect?	
What other languages do you speak?	
Do you find it difficult to share your thoughts, feelings, and ideas with family? Friends? Health-care providers?	
Do you mind being touched by friends? Strangers? Health-care workers?	
How do wish to be greeted? Handshake? Nod of the head, verbal greeting only, etc.?	
Are you usually on time for appointments?	
Are you usually on time for social engagements?	
Observe the patient's speech pattern. Is the speech pattern high- or low-context? Note: patients from highly contexted cultures place greater value on silence	
Observe the patient when physical contact is made. Does he/she withdraw from the touch or become tense?	
How close does the patient stand when talking with family members? With health-care providers?	
Does the patient maintain eye contact when talking with the nurse/physician, etc.?	
Family roles and organization	
What is your marital/partner status?	
How many children do you have?	
Who makes most of the decisions in your family?	
What types of decisions do(es) the female(s) in your family make?	
What types of decisions do(es) the male(s) in your family make?	
What are the duties of the women in the family?	
What are the duties of the men in the family?	
What should children do to make a good impression for themselves and for the family?	

Cultural assessment question	Comments
What should children not do to make a good impression for themselves and for the family?	
What are children forbidden to do?	
What should adolescents do to make a good impression for themselves and for the family?	
What should adolescents not do to make a good impression for themselves and for the family?	
What are adolescents forbidden to do?	
What are the priorities for your family?	
What are the roles of the older people in your family? Are they sought for their advice?	
Are there extended family members in your household? Who else lives in your household?	
What are the roles of extended family members in this household? What gives you and your family status?	
Is it acceptable to you for people to have children out of wedlock?	
Is it acceptable to you for people to live together and not be married?	
Is it acceptable to you for people to admit being gay or lesbian?	
What is your sexual preference/ orientation? (ask only if appropriate and later in the assessment after a modicum of trust has been established)	
Workforce issues	
Do you usually report to work on time?	
Do you usually report to meetings on time?	
What concerns do you have about working with someone of the opposite gender?	
Do you consider yourself a "loyal" employee? How long do you expect to remain in your position?	
What do you do when you do not know how to do something related to your job?	
Do you consider yourself to be assertive in your job?	
What difficulty does English (or another language) give you in the workforce?	
What difficulties do you have working with people older (younger) than you?	

Cultural assessment question	Comments
What difficulty do you have in taking directions from someone younger/older than you?	
What difficulty do you have working with people whose religions are different from yours?	
What difficulty do you have working with people whose sexual orientation is different from yours?	
What difficulty do you have working with someone whose race or ethnicity is different from yours?	
Do you consider yourself to be an independent decision-maker?	
Biocultural ecology	
Are you allergic to any medications?	
What problems did you have when you took over-the-counter medications?	
What problems did you have when you took prescription medications?	
What are the major illnesses and diseases in your family?	
Are you aware of any genetic diseases in your family?	
What are the major health problems in the country from which you come (if appropriate)?	
With what race(s) do you identify?	
With what ethnic group(s) do you identify?	
Observe and document skin coloration and physical characteristics	
Observe for and document physical handicaps and disabilities.	
High-risk health behaviors	
How many cigarettes a day do you smoke?	
Do you smoke a pipe (or cigars)?	
Do you chew tobacco?	
For how many years have you smoked/chewed tobacco?	
How much alcohol do you drink each day? Ask about wine, beer, spirits	
How many energy drinks do you consume each day?	
What recreational drugs do you use?	
How often do you use recreational drugs?	
What type of exercise do you do each day?	
Do you use seat belts?	
What precautions do you take to prevent getting sexually transmitted infections or HIV/AIDS?	

Cultural assessment question	Comments
Nutrition	
Are you on a special diet?	
Are you satisfied with your weight?	
Which foods do you eat to maintain your health?	
Do you avoid certain foods to maintain your health?	
Why do you avoid these foods?	
Which foods do you eat when you are ill?	
Which foods do you avoid when you are ill?	
Why do you avoid these foods (if appropriate)?	
For what illnesses do you eat certain foods?	
Which foods do you eat to balance your diet?	
Which foods do you eat every day?	
Which foods do you eat every week?	
Which foods do you eat that are part of your cultural heritage?	
Which foods are high-status foods in your family/culture?	
Which foods are eaten only by men? Women? Children? Teenagers? Elderly?	
How many meals do you eat each day?	
What time do you eat each meal?	
Do you snack between meals?	
What foods do you eat when you snack?	
What holidays do you celebrate?	
Which foods do you eat on particular holidays?	
Who is present at each meal? Is the entire family present?	
Do you primarily eat the same foods as the rest of your family?	
Where do you usually buy your food?	
Who usually buys the food in your household?	
Who does the cooking in your household?	
How frequently do you eat at a restaurant?	
When you eat at a restaurant, in what type of restaurant do you eat?	
Do you eat foods left from previous meals?	
Where do you keep your food?	
Do you have a refrigerator?	
How do you cook your food?	

Cultural assessment question	Comments
How do you prepare meat?	
How do you prepare vegetables?	
What type of spices do you use?	
What do you drink with your meals?	
Do you drink special teas?	
Do you have any food allergies?	
Are there certain foods that cause you problems when you eat them?	
How does your diet change with each season?	
Are your food habits different on days you work versus when you are not working?	
Pregnancy and childbearing practices	
How many children do you have?	
What do you use for birth control?	
What does it mean to you and your family when you are pregnant?	
What special foods do you eat when you are pregnant?	
What foods do you avoid when you are pregnant?	
What activities do you avoid when you are pregnant?	
Do you do anything special when you are pregnant?	
Do you eat nonfood substances when you are pregnant?	
Who do you want with you when you deliver your baby?	
In what position do you want to be when you deliver your baby?	
What special foods do you eat after delivery?	
What foods do you avoid after delivery?	
What activities do you avoid after you deliver?	
Do you do anything special after delivery?	
Who will help you with the baby after delivery?	
What bathing restrictions do you have after you deliver?	
Do you want to keep the placenta?	
What do you do to care for the baby's umbilical cord?	
Death rituals	
What special activities need to be performed to prepare for death?	
What special activities need to be performed after death?	
Would you want to know about your impending death?	

Cultural assessment question	Comments
What is your preferred burial practice? Interment, cremation?	
How soon after death does burial occur?	
How do men grieve?	
How do women grieve?	
What does death mean to you?	
Do you believe in an afterlife?	
Are children included in death rituals?	
Spirituality	
What is your religion?	
Do you consider yourself deeply religious?	
How many times a day do you pray?	
What do you need in order to say your prayers?	
Do you practice meditation, such as TM, mindfulness meditation, etc.?	
What gives strength and meaning to your life?	
In what spiritual practices do you engage for your physical and emotional health?	
Health-care practices	
In what prevention activities do you engage to maintain your health?	
Who in your family takes responsibility for your health?	
Who takes care of family members when they are sick?	
What over-the-counter medicines do you use?	
What herbal teas and folk medicines do you use?	
For what conditions do you use herbal medicines?	
What do you usually do when you are in pain?	
How do you express your pain?	
How are people in your culture viewed or treated when they have a mental illness?	
How are people with physical disabilities treated in your culture?	
What do you do when you are sick? Stay in bed, continue your normal activities, etc.?	
What are your beliefs about rehabilitation?	
How are people with chronic illnesses viewed or treated in your culture?	
Are you averse to blood transfusions?	
Is organ donation acceptable to you?	
Are you listed as a potential organ donor?	

Cultural assessment question	Comments
Would you consider having an organ transplant if needed?	
Are health-care services readily available to you?	
Do you have transportation problems accessing needed health-care services?	
Can you afford health care?	
Do you feel welcome when you see a health-care professional?	
What traditional health-care practices do you use? For example, mineral baths, sweating, acupuncture, acupressure, *cai gao*, coining, *moxibustion*, aromatherapy, etc.?	
What home difficulties do you have that might prevent you from receiving health care?	
Health-care practitioners	
What health-care providers do you see when you are ill? Physicians, nurses?	
Do you prefer a same-sex health-care provider for routine health problems? For intimate care?	
What healers do you use besides physicians and nurses?	
For what conditions do you use healers?	

Adapted from Purnell, L. (2014). Guide to Culturally Competent Health Care (3rd ed.) Philadelphia: F.A. Davis. Pp. 12–21. Reprinted with permission

References

Abdullahi AA (2011) Trends and challenges of traditional medicine in Africa. Afr J Tradit Complement Altern Med 8(5 Suppl):115–123

Al-Harthy M, Ohrbach R, Michelotti A, List T (2016) The effect of culture on pain sensitivity. J Oral Rehabil 43:81–88

Anderson NLR (2010). Culturally based health and illness beliefs and practices across the lifespan. In M Douglas and D Pacquiao. Eds. *Core Curriculum for Transcultural Nursing and Health Care [Supplement]. Journal of Transcultural Nursing,* 21 (Suppl.), pp. 152S – 235S.

Andrews MM, Boyle JS (2016) Transcultural concepts in nursing care, 7th edn. Wolters Kluwer, Philadelphia, pp A1–E4

Balaratnasingam S, Anderson L, Janca A, Lee J (2015) Towards culturally appropriate assessment of Aboriginal and Torres Strait Islander social and emotional well-being. Australas Psychiatry 23(6): 626–629. https://doi.org/10.1177/1039856215608283. Accessed 20 Nov 2017

Boerleider AW, Francke AL, van de Reep M, Manniën J, Wiegers TA, Deville WLJM (2014) "Being flexible and creative": a qualitative study on maternity care assistants' experiences with non-western immigrant women. PLoS One 9(3):e91843. https://doi.org/10.1371/journal.pone.0091843, pp 1–7. Accessed 20 Nov 2017

Braithwaite AC, Lemonde M (2017) Exploring health beliefs and practices of Caribbean immigrants in Ontario to prevent Type 2 Diabetes. J Transcult Nurs 28(1):15–23

Chen YC, Wei SH, Yeh KW, Chen MY (2013) Learning strengths from cultural differences: a comparative study of maternal health-related behaviors and infant care among Southern Asian immigrants and Taiwanese women. BMC Int Health Hum Rights 13(5):1–8. http://www.biomedcentral.com/1472-698X/13/5 or https://doi.org/10.1186/1472-698X-13-5. Accessed 18 Nov 2017

Douglas M, Rosenketter M, Pacquiao D, Clark Callister L, Hattar-Pollara M, Lauderdale J, Milsted J, Nardi D, Purnell L (2014) Guidelines for implementing culturally competent nursing care. J Transcult Nurs 25(2): 109–221. https://doi.org/10.1177/1043659614520998. Accessed 29 Oct 2017

El-Shawarby SA, Rymer J (2008) Female genital cutting. Obstet Gynaecol Reprod Med 18(9):253–255

Fishman C, Evans R, Jenks E (1988) Warm bodies, cool milk: conflicts in postpartum food choice for Indochinese women in California. Soc Sci Med 26(11):1125–1132

Gallagher RW, Polanin JR (2015) A meta-analysis of educational interventions designed to enhance cultural competence in professional nurses and nursing students. Nurs Educ 35(2):333–340. https://doi.org/10.1016/j.nedt.2014.10.021. Accessed 8 Dec 2017

Ghaedi F, Dehghan M, Salari M, Sheikhrabori A (2017) Complementary and alternative medicines: usage and its determinant factors among outpatients in Southeast of Iran [*sic*]. J Evid Based Complement Altern Med 22(2):210–215. https://doi.org/10.1177/2156587215621462. Accessed 15 Nov 2017

Giger JN, Davidhizar RE (2008) Transcultural nursing: assessment and intervention, 5th edn. Mosby Elsevier, St. Louis

Green CR, Anderson KO, Baker TA, Campbell LC, Decker S, Fillingim RB, Kaloukalani DA, Lasch KE, Myers C, Tait RC, Todd KH, Vallerand AH (2003) The unequal burden of pain: confronting racial and ethnic disparities in pain. Pain Med 4(3):277–294. https://doi.org/10.1046/j.1526-4637.2003.03034.x. Accessed 20 Nov 2017

Hadwiger MC, Hadwiger SC (2012) Filipina mothers' perceptions about childbirth at home. Int Nurs Rev 59:125–131

Haefeli WE, Carls A (2014) Drug interactions with phytotherapeutics in oncology. Expert Opin Drug Metab Toxicol 10(3):359–377. https://doi.org/10.1517/17425255.2014.873786. Accessed 11 Nov 2017

Hearst AA, Molnar AM (2013) Female genital cutting: an evidence-based approach to clinical management for the primary care physician. Mayo Clin Proc 88(6):618–629. https://doi.org/10.1016/j.mayocp.2013.04.004. Accessed 24 Nov 2017

Helman CG (2007) Culture, health and illness, 5th edn. Hodder Arnold, London, p 7

Jordan B (1980) Birth in four cultures: a cross-cultural investigation of childbirth in Yucatan, Holland, Sweden, and the United States. Eden Press Women's Publ, Montreal

Kim HJ, Yang GS, Greenspan JD, Downton KD, Griffith KA, Renn CL, Johantgen M, Dorsey SG (2017) Racial and ethnic differences in experimental pain sensitivity: systematic review and meta-analysis. Pain 158:194–211

Kooti W, Servatyari K, Behzadifar M, Asadi-Samani M, Sadeghi F, Nouri B, Marzouni HZ (2017) Effective medicinal plants in cancer treatment, part 2: review study. J Evid Based Complement Altern Med 22(4):982–995. https://doi.org/10.1177/2156587217696927. Accessed 4 May 2017

Kumar S, Dobos GJ, Rampp T (2017) The significance of Ayurvedic medicinal plants. J Evid Based Complement Altern Med 22(3):494–501

Lavin R, Park J (2014) A characterization of pain in racially and ethnically diverse older adults: a review of the literature. J Appl Gerontol 33(3):258–290

Leininger M (1979) Transcultural nursing. Masson, New York

MacDonald A (1984) Acupuncture. Allen and Unwin, St. Leonards

Mahjoub F, Salari R, Noras MR, Yousefi M (2017) Are traditional remedies useful in management of Fibromyalgia and Chronic Fatigue Syndrome? A review study. J Evid Based Complement Altern Med 22(4):1011–1016. https://doi.org/10.1177/2156587217712763. Accessed 1 Aug 2017

Manderson L (1981) Roasting, smoking and dieting in response to birth: Malay confinement in cross-cultural perspectives. Soc Sci Med 15B:509–520

Marinakis S, Van der Linden P, Tortora R, Massaut J, Pierrakos C, Wauthy P (2016) Outcomes from cardiac surgery in Jehovah's witness patients: experience over twenty-one years. J Cardiothorac Surg 11:67–78. https://doi.org/10.1186/s13019-016-0455-6. Accessed 1 Dec 2017

Marion L, Douglas M, Lavin M, Barr N, Gazaway S, Thomas L, Bickford C (2016) Implementing the new ANA Standard 8: culturally congruent practice. Online J Issues Nurs 22(1):1–9. https://doi.org/10.3912/OJIN.Vol22No01PPT20. Accessed 3 Dec 2017

Marrone SR (2016) Informed consent examined within the context of culturally congruent care: an interprofessional perspective. J Transcult Nurs 27(4):342–348

McCartney S, Guinn N, Roberson R, Boomer B, White W, Hill S (2014) Jehovah's witnesses and cardiac surgery: a single institution's experience. Transfusion 54:2745–2752. https://doi.org/10.1111/trf.12696. Accessed 30 Nov 2017

Meng Q, Liu K (2014) Pharmacokinetic interactions between herbal medicines and prescribed drugs: focus on drug metabolic enzymes and transporters. Curr Drug Metab 15(8):791–807. https://doi.org/10.2174/1389200216666150223152348. Accessed 10 Nov 2017

Momoh C, Ladhani S, Lochrie DP, Rymer J (2001) Female genital mutilation: analysis of the first twelve months of a Southeast London specialist clinic. Br J Obstet Gynecol 108(2):186–191

Morse JM (1989) Cultural variation in behavioral response to parturition: childbirth in Fiji. Med Anthropol 12(1):35–54. https://doi.org/10.1080/01459740.1989.9966010. Accessed 2 Dec 2017

Naser E, Mackey S, Arthur D, Klainen-Yobas P, Chen H, Creedy DK (2012) An exploratory study of traditional birthing practices of Chinese, Malay and Indian women in Singapore. Midwifery 28:e865–e871. https://doi.org/10.1016/j.midw.2011.10.003. Accessed 10 Nov 2017

Olaniran AA (2013) The relationship between female genital mutilation and HIV transmission in Sub-Saharan Africa. Afr J Reprod Health 17(4):156–160. http://www.bioline.org.br.ucsf.idm.oclc.org/abstract?id=rh13082&lang=en. https://www-ncbi-nlm-nih-gov.ucsf.idm.oclc.org/pubmed/24689327. Accessed 8 Dec 2017

Owiti JA, Ajaz A, Ascoli M, De Jongh B, Palinsky A, Bhui KS (2014) Cultural consultation as a model for training multidisciplinary mental healthcare professionals in cultural competence skills: preliminary results. J Psychiat Mental Health Nurs 21:814–826. https://doi.org/10.1111/jpm.12124. Accessed 30 Nov 2017

Purnell L (2014) Guide to culturally competent health care, 3rd edn. F.A. Davis, Philadelphia

Rahim-Williams B, Riley JL, Williams AKK, Filligim RB (2012) A quantitative review of ethnic group differences in experimental pain response: do biology, psychology, and culture matter? Pain Med 13:522–540

Rice PL, Manderson L (eds) (1996) Maternity and reproductive health in Asian societies. Harwood Academic Press, Amsterdam

Roberts SG, Warda M, Garbutt S, Curry K (2014) The use of high-fidelity simulation to teach cultural competence in the nursing curriculum. J Prof Nurs 30(3):259–265. https://doi.org/10.1016/j.profnurs.2013.09.012. Accessed 3 Dec 2017

Schiltenwolf M, Pogatzki-Zahn EM (2015) Schmerzmedizin au einer interkulturellen und geschlechterspezifischen perspektive [Pain medicine from intercultural and gender-related perspectives]. Der Schmerz 29(5):569–575. https://doi.org/10.1007/s00482-015-0038-9. Accessed 2 Nov 2017

Shahawy S, Deshpande NA, Nour NM (2015) Cross-cultural obstetric and gynecologic care of Muslim patients. Obstet Gynecol 126(5):969–973

Shewamene Z, Dune T, Smith CA (2017) The use of traditional medicine in maternity care among African women in Africa and the diaspora: a systematic review.

BMC Complement Altern Med 17:382–398. https://doi.org/10.1186/s12906-017-1886-x. Accessed 3 Nov 2017

Shokoohi R, Kianbakht S, Faramarzi M, Rahmanian M, Nabati F, Mehrzadi S, Huseini HF (2017) Effects of an herbal combination on glycemic control and lipid profile in diabetic women: a randomized, double-blind, placebo-controlled clinical trial. J Evid Based Complement Altern Med 22(4):1011–1016. https://doi.org/10.1177/2156587217737683. Accessed 4 Nov 2017

Small R, Rice PL, Yelland J, Lumley J (1999) Mothers in a new country: the role of culture and communication in Vietnamese, Turkish and Filipino women's experience of giving birth in Australia. Women Health 28(3):77–101. https://doi.org/10.1300/J013v28n03_06. Accessed 15 Nov 2017

Unger M (2013) Pharmacokinetic drug interactions involving ginkgo biloba. Drug Metab Rev 45(3):353–385. https://doi.org/10.3109/03602532.2013.815200. Accessed 4 Nov 2017

Upchurch DW, Rainisch BKW (2012) Racial and ethnic profiles of complementary and alternative medicine use among young adults in the United States: findings from the National Longitudinal Study of Adolescent Health. J Evid Based Complement Altern Med 17(3):172–179

van der Watt NG, Kola L, Appiah-Poku J, Othieno C, Harris B, Oladeji BD, Esan O, Makanjuola V, Price LN, Seedat S, Gureje O (2017) Collaboration between biomedical and complementary and alternative care providers: barriers and pathways. Qual Health Res 27(14):2177–2188. https://doi.org/10.1177/1049732317729342. Accessed 30 Sept 2017

Wandel M, Terragni L, Nguyen C, Lyngstad J, Amundsen M, de Paoli M (2016) Breastfeeding among Somali mothers living in Norway: attitudes, practices and challenges. Women Birth 29:487–493

World Health Organization (WHO) (1946) Constitution of the World Health Organization. http://www.who.int/about/mission/en/. Accessed 9 Dec 2017

World Health Organization (WHO) (2013) WHO traditional medicine strategy: 2014-2023. World Health Organization, Geneva. http://www.who.int/traditional-complementary-integrative-medicine/publications/trm_strategy14_23/en/. Accessed 25 Nov 2017

World Health Organization (WHO) (2017) International day of zero tolerance to female genital mutilation, February 3, 2017. http://www.unwomen.org/en/news/stories/2017/2/feature-international-day-of-zero-tolerance-to-female-genital-mutilation. Accessed 17 Nov 2017

Zborowski M (1952) Cultural components in the response to pain. J Soc Issues 8:16–30

Case Study: Perinatal Care for a Filipina Immigrant

20

Violeta Lopez

Francesca is a 19-year-old woman with a secondary education who, only a year ago, joined her American husband she met online. After 6 months of online communications, her husband decided to visit Francesca in the Philippines to personally meet her and to ask her parents' permission to marry her. Francesca comes from a small fishing village in the Philippines. Her father is a fisherman and her mother is a full-time housewife. She has four brothers and three sisters and she is the fifth child in the family. She did not pursue further studies due to the high cost of getting a university degree, like her brothers who also only completed secondary schooling. Her sisters are completing their primary and secondary schooling at a public school, which is 40 min by foot from their home. As the oldest child living with her parents, she helped her father sell fish in the local market. Her four brothers are already married and living in a nearby village.

After gaining her father's permission to marry, Francesca and her American husband moved to a small city in the southeast region of the USA. Her husband owns his own two-bedroom house. He is a divorced man with one 24-year-old son who is married with a 3-year-old daughter. Her husband

V. Lopez, Ph.D., R.N., FACN, FAAN
Alice Lee Centre for Nursing Studies,
Yong Loo Lin School of Medicine,
National University of Singapore,
Singapore, Singapore
e-mail: nurvl@nus.edu.sg

has worked as a primary school teacher for the past 20 years with an annual salary of US$34,390. In the area where they live, Asians comprise only about 2.6% of the population and has only a very small Filipino community. The closest Asian grocery store is 2 ½ hours drive from her home. The nearest public hospital is 3 miles away, but a specialist hospital is about 3 hours by car. There are, however, several health clinics near her home, which require appointments to see a doctor. There are a few walk-in clinics run by practical and auxiliary nurses and government-funded clinics for basic checkups for low-income women and children.

Francesca became pregnant soon after immigrating to the USA. Since she is isolated from her family and social support from home, and has not yet made friends or developed a social support network in their neighborhood, which is not representative of her culture, she is unaware of the available maternity services. Francesca has s a strong belief in family togetherness. Therefore, Francesca requested her husband pay for her mother's airfare to come to the USA to help her during her pregnancy and after delivery. Her mother arrived just 1 week before her delivery.

Her husband made an appointment for her to attend an antenatal clinic nearby, and once her mother arrived, she attended the clinic accompanied by her mother. At full term of her pregnancy, she was admitted to the hospital for her first delivery under the care of her obstetrician. She was very anxious, felt inexperienced, and was needing support from the nurses and most of all from her mother. Her husband was not present in the delivery. Although she can speak English well, at times of pain due to the contractions, she yelled in Tagalog (Filipino official language), which the nurses could not understand. This hospital situation was distinctly different from the practice in the Philippines where midwives are responsible for attending to the whole childbirth process in small hospitals and clinics. In the provinces, traditional birthing women (*hilot*) are used rather than midwives or obstetricians because of the expense associated with hospital delivery.

The delivery was uneventful and she delivered a healthy baby boy. Her mother asked the doctor if she could have the placenta to take home, but her request was refused. In the Philippines, especially in the area where Francesca was from, the placenta must be buried, as it signifies the end of labor pain, delivery, and blood loss. As for postpartum care, Francesca's mother insisted on following and obeying the rules set by her mother and grandmother and other elderly women in their home village out of respect and obedience to their traditional beliefs and practices.

20.1 Cultural Issues

A key concept of indigenous health is the balancing of the hot and cold of the body and of the food of postpartum women (McBride 2001). Childbirth is considered as a cold process and maintaining the body heat after childbirth is important. Drinking cold water or any cold liquids is forbidden as it is believed to cause relapse when one is ill or cause postpartum hemorrhage. After childbirth, the women must keep warm, wear heavy clothes or wrap themselves in blanket and always wear socks. They are not allowed to bathe or wash their hair for 10 days, as this will cause ill health and rheumatism in old age. They tightly bind their abdomen to prevent bleeding and help the uterus to contract. They can also receive healing massages with warm coconut oil, which is used to assist in expelling blood clots

from the uterus as well as in restoring the pelvic bones to their original position. Some traditional practices involve drying out of the womb, or "mother roasting", in which the woman lies beside a stove for 30 days, squats over a burning clay stove, or sits on a chair over a heated stone or a pot of steaming water with herbs. They are not even allowed to go out of the house for 40 days so as not to catch cold as keeping the body warm will hasten recuperation from childbirth.

After 10 days, the mother may have a sponge bath using warm water boiled with leaves of any citrus fruit trees, such as lemon, lime, or grapefruit. It is only after 40 days that the new mother is allowed to take a full bath, using warm water infused with citrus fruit leaves or warm boiled water with ginger to keep the body warm; at this time, she may also wash her hair with warm water infused with rosemary leaves (de Leon 2016).

Food and drinks are always served hot to a new mother. She is served herbal soups prepared with pork or chicken bones and boiled with sulfur-rich leaves such as watercress, morning glory, broccoli, cabbage, *malunggay* (moringa), and *saluyot* (no English translations). Cold foods such as turnips and cucumber are avoided as these will not help the uterus to contract. Sour foods such as tamarind and oranges are forbidden as this will cause the breast milk to curd or to stop breast milk production altogether.

Newborn babies are also sponged with warm water infused with herbs and not bathed fully submerged in water until 40 days, the same as the mother. A tight abdominal binder over the umbilical cord is also applied until the cord is dried and falls off. These practices are important to balance the hot and cold condition of the body. Breast feeding is adopted and encouraged immediately after birth as the most economical way to provide nutrition to the baby; nursing is maintained as long as 2 years and as long as there is sufficient breast milk.

Immunization is mandatory and provided free of charge by the Philippine government. Other than the mandatory immunization (BCG, DPT, Polio, Hepa-B, MMR) for infants after birth to 9 months (PFV 2016), school children from grades

1 to 7 are provided free immunization for measles, rubella, tetanus, and diphtheria every August each year and for females ages 9–10 years of age are vaccinated against HPV for free (PCHRD 2015). Hepatitis-B, H. influenza type B, and other types of influenza vaccinations may be determined by the Secretary of Health (Republic Act No. 10152 2010).

In the Filipino culture, pregnancy and delivery is a celebration, but care for the mother and baby must follow traditional beliefs, values, and practices. The mother and grandmother provide great support for the pregnant and postpartum women in the Philippines. This was especially important for Francesca's first childbirth, as her family beliefs play a role in health maintenance and maintaining health, and is viewed as a family responsibility (Darling et al. 2005).

As Francesca only recently arrived in the USA, she was newly exposed to a different culture. The long process of acculturation requires that she will need to adapt and possibly readjust her attitudes, beliefs, values, and mores about many issues, especially in pregnancy, giving birth, and health care after birth. Such acculturation can bring about psychological shock because it may be socially and culturally different from what she believes to be her customs and traditions in childbirth practices (Ea 2015). Adding to this stress, Filipino women living in Western countries have often been stigmatized because of their reputation as "mail-order brides," and as such, they have experienced social isolation from their family and lack the ability to develop important social support networks in their new adopted country (Kelaher et al. 2001).

20.2 Social Structural Factors

The Philippines is a country of 7107 islands located on the Pacific Rim of Southeast Asia, with a population of 103,406,752 as of April 2017, with 44.8% of the population living in urban areas. Moreover, there are approximately 10.2 million overseas Filipino workers (in United Arab Emirates, Qatar, Saudi Arabia, Japan, and Australia) in addition to over 3.5 million who

have settled permanently in the USA (World Population Review 2017). The Philippines consists of a diverse range of ethnic groups, with 81% practicing Roman Catholics, which is heavily influenced by its history as part of the Spanish empire for 377 years between 1521 and 1898 (Philippines History 2017). The official language is Filipino (or Tagalog). The Philippines is also composed of 110 ethnolinguistic tribes that speaks 70–80 dialects, such as Cebuano, Waray, Ilonggo, Ilocano, Bicolano, etc. More than half of Filipinos speak fluent English as this is the language used in colleges, universities, the courts, and the government. The Filipinos also use "Taglish" language which is a mixture of Filipino and English.

The literacy rate for adults 15 years and above is 95.4% (Unicef 2017). Filipinos regard education as the path to upward mobility, and education is compulsory until 12 years of age. A university degree is necessary to obtain positions that promise security and advancement in a profession. However, the Department of Education reports that children from the poorest 40% of the population do not even attend primary school, despite the compulsory requirement (Clarke 2015)

The Philippines is considered a low- to middle-income country, with a GDP of US$159.3 billion. Philippines GDP per capita averaged US$2753.30 in 2016 and is equivalent to 22% of the world's average. In the Philippines, 70% of resources and capital are held by the top 10% of the population, while 50.5% live below the poverty line. Among these 50.5%, 70% of the women live in poverty-like conditions. Unemployment rate as of January 2016 was 5.8%, and among the unemployed persons, 63.4% were males. The minimum wage is between P300 to P 500 per day (US$6 to US$10 per day) (Philippine Statistics Authority 2016).

Life expectancy in the Philippines is 70 years for females and 64 years for males. The Philippine Department of Health (2016) reports that heart disease is the leading cause of death followed by diseases of the vascular system (stroke), malignant neoplasms, pneumonia, and diabetes mellitus. Tuberculosis remains the sixth cause of death. As of 2016, the infant mortality rate was

21.9 deaths per thousand live births, and the five leading causes of infant mortality are bacterial sepsis, pneumonia, respiratory distress, congenital malformations of the heart and disorders related to short gestation and low birth weight. The maternal mortality rate was 114 per 100,000 live births; the most common causes of maternal deaths are hemorrhage, infection, obstructed labor, hypertensive disorders in pregnancy, and complications of unsafe abortion (Central Intelligence Agency 2017).

The national health-care law provides all citizens with basic health care at no cost through subsidies. Children received immunizations at no costs. Public hospitals and health centers provide services to everyone free of charge. Patients are allowed to have companions with them in the hospitals to assist with simple nursing chores, such as giving baths and getting food trays. The Traditional and Alternative Medicine Act was legislated to improve the quality and delivery of health-care services to the Filipino people through the development of traditional and complementary/alternative medicine (TCAM) and its integration into the national health-care delivery system (Romualdez et al. 2011).

Transnational marriages are an alternative to poverty. Foreign brides to Western men from the USA, Australia, and Canada usually come from Indonesia, Vietnam, Thailand, and the Philippines (Shu et al. 2011). Men using mail-order websites seeking foreign brides have expressed their disappointments with modern American women as they are more demanding and not willing to take on the responsibility of a "traditional" wife. Thus, they believe in marrying an Asian woman with the traditional values of obedience and subservience (Minervini and McAndrew 2006). The increasing prevalence of mail-order brides in the USA who were procured through web pages, although outlawed in the Philippines, continue to flourish. Women in the Philippines represent the largest marriage market for mail-order brides to foreign men (The Manila Times 2015). Many Filipino families are under desperate economic circumstances. Many parents of Filipino women view the USA as a land of opportunity and will support their daugh-

ters' wishes to seek a better life outside their current economic situation. Even though the gross domestic product (GDP) growth rate rose from 5.5% in the first half of 2015 to 6.9% in the first half of 2016 (World Bank 2016a, b), medium-term economic risks persist. Persistent vulnerability of the agricultural sector, unresolved constraints on private investment, a lack of competition in major sectors, and structural deficiencies in the business environment continue to suppress sufficient growth to inspire hope for those in dire poverty.

20.3 Culturally Competent Strategies Recommended

To address Francesca's concerns related to her postpartum care, nurses must utilize cross-cultural knowledge and culturally sensitive skills in implementing culturally congruent nursing care at three levels (Douglas et al. 2014). It is important to meet the diverse needs of patients and their families (Douglas et al. 2011).

20.3.1 Individual-/Family-Level Interventions

- Conduct a thorough assessment of the physical, psychological, and cultural factors that may affect Francesca's first childbirth experience.
- Identify the Filipino pregnant women's culture, which can include their values, beliefs, traditions, and practices in childbirth and puerperium.
- Respect the presence of her mother in the delivery room, and understand the significance associated with her wanting to take the placenta home with her.
- Ensure that culturally sensitive care is planned and implemented in collaboration with the multidisciplinary team and which is inclusive of the patient, her family, and their chosen cultural support networks.
- Whenever possible, foods should be chosen for Francesca that not only meet her meta-

bolic needs but also her cultural considerations. Recommended foods include shell fish (clams and mussels) as they are good for breast milk production and green leafy vegetables (moringa, spinach, watercress, morning glory, broccoli, etc.). Any sour foods (tamarind, oranges, turnip, etc.) are prohibited as they are believed to cause breast milk to curd or stop breast milk production altogether.

- Determine the patient and family's preferred language for verbal communication, making use of trained interpreters or qualified translators when necessary.

20.3.2 Organizational-Level Interventions

- Consider one's own culture, values, beliefs, and possible prejudices that may impact the provision of care. Set these aside to ensure equitable care for the immigrant pregnant woman.
- Midwives should possess appropriate knowledge, skills, and attributes to respect, advocate for, and effectively respond to the cultural needs of the Filipino pregnant women and their families.
- Analyze concerns and issues in providing transcultural care to individuals, families, groups, communities, and institutions. Antenatal interviews of Filipino women should include their beliefs and values and practices of childbirth including infant care, breastfeeding, and immunization.
- Provide ongoing educational workshops for nurses and midwives and other health professionals for effective cross-cultural practice.
- Organizational policies should include respecting the women's and family's vulnerability and the need for culturally sensitive care so as to establish trust.
- Health-care organizations should provide information booklets or brochures about Filipino health-care beliefs and practices including endorsed and prohibited foods during illness and childbirth.

20.3.3 Societal Level Interventions

- Midwifery education providers should ensure that cultural competence and cultural sensitivity is embedded within their curriculum framework.
- The local government could provide support to the Filipino community and support groups to hold workshops on Filipino culture in general and more specifically on health beliefs and practices.
- As there is no Filipino community where Francesca lives, collaborate with the Asian community to coordinate and provide parental- and child-care support.
- Collaborate with the medical clinics, pharmacies, and grocery stores to address the needs of their Asian constituents.

Conclusion

Childbirth should be a celebration, especially for the mother who has carried the pregnancy for nine months. For the immigrant and as a mail-order bride who may experience stigmatization, midwives and nurses should understand the sociocultural factors associated with the long process of acculturation to the new society and health-care practices. Respecting the women's beliefs and values, while integrating the woman's unique cultural practices into her care whenever possible, will ultimately assist in providing culturally competent care.

References

Central Intelligence Agency (2017) Maternal mortality rate. The World Fact Book. https://www.cia.gov/library/publications/the-worldfactbook/fields/2223.html. Accessed 12 July 2017

Clarke N (ed) (2015) Education in the Philippines. World education news and reviews, June 7, 2015. http://wenr.wes.org/2015/06/education-philippines. Accessed 3 Apr 2017

Darling N, Cumsille P, Peña-Alampay L (2005) Rules, legitimacy of parental authority and obligation to obey in Chili, the Philippines, and the United States. New Dir Child Adolesc Dev 108:47–60

De Leon RN (2016) Herbal remedies for beauty and health. S.G.E. Publishing Inc., Valenzuela City

Department of Health (2016) Philippine health picture 1993-2013. http://portal.doh.gov.ph/node/198.html. Accessed 12 July 2016

Douglas M, Pierce J, Rosenkoetter M, Pacquiao D, Callister L, Hattar-Pollara M, Purnell L (2011) Standards of practice for culturally competent nursing care: 2011 update. J Transcult Nurs 22(4):317–333

Douglas M, Rosenkoetter M, Pacquiao DF, Callister LC, Hattar-Pollara M, Lauderdale J, Milstead J, Nardi D, Purnell L (2014) Guidelines for implementing culturally competent nursing care. J Transcult Nurs 25:109–121

Ea E (2015) Acculturation, acculturative stress and health and health-related outcomes among Filipino Americans. Nurs Res 64:E29–E39

Kelaher M, Potts H, Manderson L (2001) Health issues among Filipino women in remote Queensland. Aust J Rural Health 9:150–157

McBride M (2001) Health and health care of Filipino American elders. http://stanford.edu/group/ethnoger. Accessed 21 March 2017

Minervini BP, McAndrew FT (2006) The mating strategies and male preferences of mail order brides. Cross Cult Resarch 40:111–129

Philippine Council for Health Research and Development (PCHRD) (2015) DOH Health launces nationwide school immunization program. http://www.pchrd.dost.gov.ph/index.php/news/library-health-news/4772-doh-launches-nationwide-school-immunization-program. Accessed 4 Aug 2017

Philippine Statistics Authority (2016) Employment rate in January 2016 is estimated at 94.2 percent. https://psa.gov.ph/content/employment-rate-january-2016-estimated-942-percent. Accessed 3 Apr 2017

Philippines Foundation for Vaccination (PFV) (2016) Childhood immunization schedule. http://www.phil-vaccine.org/vaccination-schedules/childhood-immunization-schedule. Accessed 4 Aug 2017

Philippines History (2017) Timeline of Philippines history. http://www.philippine-history.org/timeline.htm. Accessed 12 July 2017

Republic Act No. 10152 (2010) An Act providing for mandatory basic immunization services for infants and children, repealing for the purpose presidential decree No. 996. As amended. Official Gazette of the Philippines. Congress of the Philippines, Metro Manila, Philippines

Romualdez AG, dela Rosa JFE, Flavier JDA, Quimbo SLA, Hartigan-Go KY, Lagrada LP, David LC (2011) Health systems in transition. Philippines Health Rev 1(2):106–116

Shu B-C, Lung F-W, Chen C-H (2011) Mental health of female foreign spouses in transnational marriages in southern Taiwan. BMC Psychiatry 11:4. http://www.biomedcentral.com/1471-244X/11/4

The Manila Times (2015) Male order brides. http://www.manilatimes.net/male-order-brides/158083/. Accessed 12 July 2017

UNICEF (2017) As a glance: Philippines. https://www.unicef.org/infobycountry/philippines_statistics.html. Accessed 3 Apr 2017

World Bank (2016a) World development indicators. http://databank.worldbank.org/data/download/site-content/wdi-2016-highlights-featuring-sdgs-booklet.pdf. Accessed 3 Apr 2017

World Bank (2016b) Philippine economic update (October 2016): outperforming the region and managing the transition. http://www.worldbank.org/en/news/feature/2016/10/03/philippine-economic-update-october-2016-outperforming-the-region-and-managing-the-transition. Accessed 3 Apr 2017

World Population Review (2017) Philippines population 2017. http://worldpopulationreview.com/countries/philippines-population/. Accessed 3 Apr 2017

Case Study: Maternity Care for a Liberian Woman

21

Jody R. Lori

Bendu is a 33-year-old woman whose husband and two of her six children died during the Ebola crisis. Her husband was a subsistence farmer, and they lived in a rural, remote village in central Liberia. After her husband and children died, Bendu was unable to make enough money to care for herself and the rest of her family by working the farm. Her children had to stop attending school because she didn't have the money for books or school uniforms. Many of the villagers stigmatized her and her children as Ebola survivors and would not help the family. Neighboring families who once shared parenting responsibilities and supported one another shunned Bendu and her children. She was very isolated and alone. In addition, Bendu was pregnant when her husband died and is now nearing her seventh month gestation.

Her brother Steven helped arrange for Bendu and her remaining four children to join his family in the capital city of Monrovia. As the oldest boy in the family, Steven had been sent to attend secondary school in the capital. He now works as a waiter at a hotel in the city that caters to foreigners working in the country since the Ebola outbreak. Steven's wife, Martha, arranged a prenatal appointment for Bendu at the clinic where she received care during her own three pregnancies. Martha accompanies Bendu to her first visit. Bendu knows very little English as Kru was spoken in her rural village, and she only attended school through the fourth grade. Martha must serve as her interpreter when she is seen by the health-care provider.

Bendu gave birth to all six of her children at home with the help of a traditional midwife. Her younger sister died during childbirth after she was in labor for 3 days in the village and finally transferred to the district hospital 25 miles away. She underwent a cesarean section, but both she and the baby died within 24 h of admission. This has made Bendu suspicious of hospitals, and she believes that all they do is "cut on you" when you go to a hospital during labor.

21.1 Cultural Issues

All indigenous groups in Liberia are patrilineal and male dominated. Gender roles often place women in lower positions within the family and society, restricting women from educational and employment opportunities in favor of males in the family.

Children are highly valued, and most couples will have many children considering it "God's will." Having many children gives women a respected place in the society. The total fertility rate for Liberia is 4.7 children per woman with a

J. R. Lori, Ph.D., C.N.M., F.A.C.N.M., FAAN
PAHO/WHO Collaborating Center,
School of Nursing, University of Michigan,
Ann Arbor, MI, USA
e-mail: jrlori@umich.edu

© Springer International Publishing AG, part of Springer Nature 2018
M. Douglas et al. (eds.), *Global Applications of Culturally Competent Health Care: Guidelines for Practice*, https://doi.org/10.1007/978-3-319-69332-3_21

markedly higher rate (6.1 children per woman) among rural women (LISGIS et al. 2014). Households often consist of extended family members. It is not uncommon for children from rural areas to be sent away from parents to live with relatives in urban areas to attend school after primary school because of the lack of educational facilities in rural areas.

Secret societies, also known as bush schools, are prevalent throughout Liberia. These schools are part of Liberia's cultural heritage and attended by thousands of youngsters annually in rural Liberia. The Sande society, for girls, is the place where young girls learn domestic skills, such as how to cook, clean, care for their family and future husband, as well as moral lessons such as respecting elders and religious teachings. It is also the place where female genital mutilation (FGM) takes place. Initiation into the Sande society is an important social process for girls in Liberia. They are not considered part of the larger group in their village until they have attended the bush school and gone through the initiation of FGM. Undergoing FGM makes them a respected member of the society. Children usually attend these schools between the ages of 4 and 12 years old. Female genital mutilation can affect a woman's long-term health associated with childbearing. Women who have undergone FGM are at risk for multiple childbirth complications, such as obstructed labor, uterine rupture due to the obstructed labor, fistula formation, and incontinence of urine and stool.

Ritualistic cicatrization (scarification) is also often done to both women and men. These are intentional superficial cuttings on the face, back, and other areas of the body that takes place in the bush schools. They are considered body decoration that identify social origins. In West Africa they are used for identification of ethnic groups and families and also to express personal beauty. They are considered by some tribes as testimony that a woman will be able to withstand the pain of childbirth (Rand African Art 2002).

Men are not permitted to be present at the birth of their children, and women are not permitted to give birth inside the house when there are male children living in the household. To seek health care or assistance with a problem during pregnancy, women must obtain permission from their husband or a male elder. There is a distrust or disbelief in the benefits of the care received within the formalized health-care system, especially surrounding childbirth. Because women often seek care late for pregnancy-related problems, they present with more severe complications. Many rural Liberians believe if a woman goes to the hospital for childbirth, she will die (Lori and Boyle 2011).

There are many food taboos (foods to avoid during pregnancy) and special foods women eat during pregnancy. Women in rural Liberia often rely on the use of country medicine or herbs for health problems during pregnancy. There is an acceptance and comfort with traditional healers and indigenous practitioners who have long-standing legitimacy within communities.

There is also a strong belief that certain members of society enjoy supernatural powers not afforded by all humans. Anyone can have these powers and there is no way to identify who has them. These powers may be passed down from a family member, or a person may be part of a society that bestows supernatural powers to its members. These powers may be used to witch or bewitch another person, such as casting a spell on them to complicate their pregnancy, cause an illness or even death.

21.2 Social Structural Factors

Liberia, located in West Africa, has a total population of approximately 4.5 million (World Health Organization 2015). Liberia's social and health structures were devastated during 14 years of civil and rebel wars, which ended in a comprehensive peace agreement in 2003 (United States Institute of Peace 2003). Then, a decade later, the 2014–2015 Ebola outbreak further weakened an already failing health system. The World Health Organization (2016a, b) reports the total number of cases attributed to Ebola in West Africa surpassed 28,000 with the death toll over 11,000 in the three countries of Guinea, Liberia, and Sierra Leone.

Liberia was designated one of the "fragile" countries targeted by the Global Financing Facility (GFF) in 2015 and is ranked tenth in the world for maternal mortality. The maternal mortality rate is estimated at 1072 deaths per 100,000 live births, placing a woman's lifetime risk of dying from a pregnancy-related complication at 1 in 31.

In Liberian culture, women often have less personal autonomy, less freedom, and less access to information than their male counterparts. The literacy rate for females is 48% with 33% of women having no education (LISGIS et al. 2014).

Culture has a profound influence on childbirth. Liberian society has left Bendu with little authority or autonomy to advocate for herself. While biomedical knowledge is privileged over other ways of knowing in systems modeled on western medicine, it is not necessarily the authoritative knowledge (Jordan 1997) for childbearing women in Liberia.

21.3 Culturally Competent Strategies Recommended

Minority ethnic groups, used to traditional birth attendants caring for them during pregnancy, are likely to experience problems when presenting for perinatal care in the formalized health-care system A lack of understanding or experience with Western-modeled medicine often contributes to distrust of the health-care system (Lori and Boyle 2011). There are often conflicting beliefs, understandings, values, and expectations of both providers and pregnant women seeking care (Wojnar 2015). Navigating a formal system of health care for the first time can be challenging and frightening—especially for those fleeing from unstable or violent situations.

21.3.1 Individual-/Family-Level Interventions

- Providers need to be conscious of individual cultural differences in the populations they care for at the same time avoiding stereotyping. Become informed about nutritional practices and cultural traditions and when these conditions and practices can be harmful to the mother or fetus. Take a holistic, evidence-based approach to care.

- Develop a trusting relationship with the pregnant woman. Listen to her needs and fears— anticipate that this may take more time than with women who are familiar with the formal health-care system. Use terminology that is consistent with a client's educational level. Share decision-making.

- Obtain a careful health and obstetric history. Address her beliefs surrounding care for herself during pregnancy, labor, and delivery. Offer choices that do not conflict with her cultural beliefs whenever possible (Esegbona-Adeigbe 2011). Document the client's preferences in the medical record.

- Be familiar with managing the care of women with FGM (World Health Organization 2016b). Be prepared to provide appropriate care at the time of delivery to prevent and treat potential complications resulting from FGM.

- Provide continuity of care whenever possible, allowing the client to see the same provider throughout her pregnancy.

- Exercise self-reflection on your own cultural worldview.

21.3.2 Organizational Level

- Provide gender-aligned interpretation services whenever possible.

- Provide in-service training and educational workshops to providers and staff to become educated about the culture, beliefs, and health-care practices of all ethnic communities within the country.

- Provide in-service training and educational workshops for health-care providers and all staff regarding the care of women with FGM (World Health Organization 2016b).

- Develop simple, picture-focused educational materials for clients who do not read or understand English.

21.3.3 Societal Level

- Collaborate with community associations and social networks for women in the community (Dyer 2016). Become familiar with in-country programs related to FGM.

- Work with local, district, and ministry officials to ensure full coverage for pregnancy and childbirth to prevent barriers for women to use the formal health-care system.

Conclusion

Pervasive fear, distrust, and stigma surrounded Bendu's life prior to her move to the capital city of Monrovia. Her marginalization within her own community and her limited education are factors contributing to her vulnerability. Bendu's lack of individual rights, autonomy, and independence makes her especially vulnerable in advocating for her health-care needs.

To engage in culturally competent practice, providers must become familiar with the unique populations they care for with special attention to the political, social, and cultural context of childbirth including practices, beliefs, and traditions that influence health and illness. Cultural knowledge is critical to our understanding and care of minority ethnic groups during pregnancy and childbearing. Recognizing and respecting cultural diversity can have a lasting impact on a woman's life.

References

Dyer JM (2016) Women in migration: best practices in midwifery. In: Anderson BA, Rooks JP, Barroso R (eds) Best practices in midwifery: using the evidence to implement change. Springer, New York, pp 169–182

Esegbona-Adeigbe S (2011) Acquiring cultural competency in caring for black African women. Br J Midwifery 19(8):489–496

Jordan B (1997) Authoritative knowledge and its construction. In: Davis-Floyd RE, Sargent C (eds) Childbirth and authoritative knowledge: cross-cultural perspectives. University of California Press, Berkley, pp 55–79. ISBN: 9780520207851

Liberia Institute of Statistics and Geo-Information Services (LISGIS), Ministry of Health and Social Welfare [Liberia], National AIDS Control Program [Liberia], and ICF International (2014) Liberia demographic and health survey 2013. Liberia Institute of Statistics and Geo-Information Services (LISGIS) and ICF International, Monrovia

Lori JR, Boyle JS (2011) Cultural childbirth practices, beliefs, and traditions in postconflict Liberia. Health Care Women Int 32(6):454–473. https://doi.org/10.10 80/07399332.2011.555831

Rand African Art (2002) Scarification and cicatrisation among African cultures. Retrieved from http://www. randafricanart.com/Scarification_and_Cicatrisation_ among_African_cultures.html

United States Institute of Peace (2003). Peace agreements: Liberia. Retrieved from https://www.usip.org/ publications/2003/08/peace-agreements-liberia

Wojnar DM (2015) Perinatal experiences of Somali couples in the United States. J Obstet Gynecol Neonatal Nurs 44(3):358–369. https://doi.org/10.1111/1552-6909.12574

World Health Organization (2015) Liberia. Retrieved from http://www.who.int/countries/lbr/en/

World Health Organization (2016a) Ebola data and statistics. Retrieved from http://apps.who.int/gho/data/ view.ebola-sitrep.ebola-summary-latest?lang=en

World Health Organization (2016b) WHO guidelines on the management of health complications from female genital mutilation. Retrieved from http:// www.who.int/reproductivehealth/topics/fgm/ management-health-complications-fgm/en/

Case Study: Care of a Malay Muslim Woman in a Singaporean Hospital

Antoinette Sabapathy
and Asmah Binti Mohd Noor

Rosna, a 25-year-old Malay Muslim woman, is a marketing executive in a fairly large company located in Singapore. She enjoys her work and has been in the same company for the last 5 years. She is married to a 30-year-old technician. Her mother and mother-in-law take turns looking after her 4-year-old son while she is at work.

She is now 14 weeks pregnant with her second child. She was brought to the emergency department by her colleagues as she had vaginal bleeding. She appeared very anxious and had tears in her eyes as she was being examined. As she was obviously distressed, the nurse examining her asked her if she wanted to call her husband. Rosna became agitated and started to cry. On further probing, Rosna confided that she was afraid to call her husband as he and the family would accuse her of trying to miscarry. They had been asking her to have another child for the last 3 years.

She has not been using any birth control methods, but it still took her 3 years to conceive this pregnancy. However, her husband and family felt she was not trying hard enough and they would prefer her to stop working so that she could concentrate on being a wife and mother. Rosna enjoys her work and although she is willing to have the four children her husband wants, she would also like to continue working.

In view of the situation, the nurse decided to finish examining Rosna. She then arranged for Rosna to see her obstetrician before contacting Rosna's husband. An ultrasound was performed on Rosna and the fetus was viable. The obstetrician gave her a 7-day medical leave with an appointment to return in a week's time.

The nurse then contacted Rosna's husband to tell him that Rosna was ready to return home. The nurse also informed the husband that Rosna was rather anxious about her baby and was rather teary, and as such, having him to comfort her would be most helpful. The nurse also informed the husband that he could speak with the doctor to get more information if that would help him comfort his wife. The husband replied that he would consider it and said that he would come immediately. Rosna heard the conversation and was happy to hear what the nurse had to say.

While waiting for her husband to arrive, the nurse offered Rosna Milo, a hot chocolate malted milk drink that is popular among pregnant women as it is considered nutritious, and a chicken sandwich as Rosna had missed lunch. She assured Rosna that the sandwich was halal. Rosna appreciated the nurse's assurance regarding the halal food and accepted the snack gratefully because she was hungry.

A. Sabapathy, R.N., S.C.M., C.N.M, W.H.N.P. (✉)
Gleneagles Hospital, Singapore, Singapore

A. B. M. Noor, M.S.C., R.N., N.I.C.U.
Nanyang Polytechnic, Singapore, Singapore

22.1 Cultural Issues

The Malay Muslim culture views the husband as head of the family and although the Malay Muslim woman is respected and has made significant progress, as a wife, she is still expected to respect the husband and submit to him. As Ramadan (2017) says "It is as though the aspirations of the female were implicitly the same as those of the men". And according to Maqsood (2008) "… even if she is more intelligent, more educated, or more spiritually and morally gifted than him, she must agree to obey him". Additionally, Imam Ali Ibrahim (2014) states that "The Jihad of a woman is to take care of her husband well". Therefore, in the majority of Muslim homes, the husband's aspirations take precedence over the wife's.

In Singapore, the Malay Muslim women are free to work outside the home and move around unaccompanied by a male relative. She can choose not to wear the tudong and the burqa prior to marriage. Many women tend to wear the tudong with secular clothes. The Majlis Ugama Islam Singapura (MUIS), a statutory board, tasked with seeing to the interests of the Muslims and to advise the president on Muslim matters, states that "It is compulsory for Muslim women to wear the Hijab" and advised that the woman should take a job that enables her to wear the tudong (2015).

Usually, after marriage, the husband's preference takes precedence. The Muslim husbands do take an active role in the woman's health and are involved in the final decision-making. So the adoption of the Muslim rules and regulations is very much dependent on individual preference.

Many of the beliefs about prenatal care are passed on from mothers to daughters. Pregnant women are exhorted to stay indoors after sunset. It is believed that there are unclean spirits that prey on pregnant women after sunset. Pregnant women must ensure that their activities do not put their unborn child at risk. They do go for prenatal care and will take supplements as long as the contents do not contain lecithin from animals for example pigs.

Pregnant women may break their fast if they feel it poses a danger to themselves or their unborn child. If breastfeeding, they can also break their fast if it impacts the breastfeeding process. They can then make up the lost days when they are well (Ramadan 2017) in addition to making religious donations (MUIS 2015a, b).

Unlike the Chinese, there is no balancing of Yin and Yang for the Malay Muslims. However, Asian women tend to avoid cold drinks during pregnancy and this applies to Muslim women too. Hot drinks are considered soothing and do not induce cramps.

The Muslims believe that babies are gifts from God; this belief has remained unchanged to the present day (Maqsood 2008). The Muslim religion encourages its followers to marry and to populate the earth (Majlis Ugama Islam Singapura (MUIS) 2017). This is demonstrated in the differences of the average number of children born by ethnic groups. In 2015, the Malay Muslims had an average of 2.64 children, while the Chinese had 1.23 children and the Indians had 1.94 children. Abortions are not allowed and considered sinful in the Muslim religion.

Healthcare personnel should also be aware of the dietary restrictions when caring for the Muslim patients. The food should be free of pork and be certified halal (Elnakib 2017). Foods are considered "HALAL" if it does not contain any components or products of animals that are considered non-halal by Syariah law or animals that are not slaughtered according to Syariah law; foods must be processed or manufactured using equipment and facilities that are free from contamination or from forbidden ingredients, such as alcohol. Additionally, the crockery and cutlery must be differentiated from those used for non-Muslims.

There are some types of food, e.g., mutton, cuttlefish, and pineapples, that Muslim pregnant women tend to avoid as they believe that these foods cause harm to the fetus. They believe that eating mutton may result in the baby having seizures (A. Mohamad Noor, personal communication, April 27, 2017).

22.2 Social Structural Factors

Singapore is an island in the heart of Southeast Asia, between Malaysia and Indonesia, with a population of more than 5.7 million as of 2016.

Its population comprises 74.2% Chinese, 13.3% Malay, 9.1% Indian, and 3.3% other ethnicities (Singapore Demographics Profile 2016). Corresponding to the different ethnic groups, it has four official languages, namely, English, Malay, Mandarin, and Tamil. Most Singaporeans are bilingual in English and a second language, commonly Mandarin, Tamil, or Malay (Singapore Demographics Profile 2016).

Despite being in the minority, the Malay population is well regarded and favored. Their progress reflects the island's progress. The average household income for the Malays has increased from a total of $3151 in 2000 to $4575 in 2010. At a recent rally of the ruling People's Action Party, the Minister of State for Defense and National Development, Mr. Mohamad Maliki Osman, stated that the "Malay community's tremendous progress over the years is a reflection of Singapore's success" as the Malays "have excelled academically, with more Malays these days graduating with first-class honours" (2015).

The Muslim religious beliefs and practices are well protected and upheld in Singapore. There are 71 mosques to meet the needs of the Muslims all over the island (MUIS 2015a, b). Any disrespect shown to Muslims is punishable by law.

22.3 Culturally Competent Strategies Recommended

The Malay Muslim community is well established in Singapore and is valued. Their religious beliefs and practices are respected and upheld. As such, all healthcare personnel must be competent and are expected to be competent in providing culturally appropriate and effective care. Nursing students are taught culturally appropriate care from the first year of their program. They are taught that the father will pray into the ear of his newborn immediately after birth, and as part of providing culturally appropriate care, nurses should facilitate this religious practice. Muslims also bury their dead on the same day and last rites are expedited. Each hospital also has a list of religious personnel appropriate for the religion of their patients that they can contact, e.g., the ustaz

for the Muslim patients. Each room also has an arrow on the ceiling indicating the direction they should face while praying. The direction faces Mecca and they are praying toward the Kaaba in Mecca, the holiest place for the Muslims.

22.3.1 Individual-/Family-Level Interventions

- On admission, if unfamiliar with the patient's cultural identity and religious status, conduct an in-depth cultural assessment.
- Respect the person's view of family and procreation.
- Provide interventions to unite the family regardless of personal beliefs.
- Provide education of early pregnancy precautions and possible complications.
- Ensure dietary requirements, such as halal food, are met.

22.3.2 Organizational-Level Interventions

- Provide signage, educational information materials in the major languages.
- Printed information should take into account the religious sensitivities of the Muslim population.
- Provide training for staff to ensure they are familiar with the Muslim cultural and religious practices.
- Provide interpreters as necessary.
- Ensure kitchen premises has an area that is "HALAL" certified and manned by Muslims.

22.3.3 Community Societal Level Interventions

- Collaborate with the religious committees so that the hospital can access their knowledge and expertise.
- Advocate for community and federal legislation that mandates maternity care is delivered in a culturally appropriate manner and that allows culturally specific practices and taboos be respected whenever it is safe and practical.

Conclusion

In the Malay Muslim community, healthcare personnel must remember that the males are the head of the household and regardless of their own beliefs, decisions regarding the women's health must be made in collaboration with their husbands. The women will consult their husbands with regard to treatments, and obtaining the husbands' support from the beginning will facilitate the treatment process. This knowledge and acceptance of the Malay Muslim culture will result in the husband's support of his wife, maintain family harmony and encourage the use of the healthcare facilities.

References

Elnakib S (2017) Understanding the diverse culinary traditions of Islam. Retrieved from http://www.eatrightpro.org/resource/news-center/in-practice/dietetics-in-action/understanding-the-diverse-culinary-traditions-of-islam

Ibrahim A (2014) Principles of marriage and family ethics. Lulu Press, Raleigh. Retrieved from https://www.al-islam.org/principles-marriage-family-ethics-ayatullah-ibrahim-amini

Majlis Ugama Islam Singapura (MUIS) (2015a) Frequently asked questions on Ramadan. Retrieved from http://www.muis.gov.sg/officeofthemufti/documents/FAQ%20english%20ramadan.pdf

Majlis Ugama Islam Singapura (MUIS) (2015b) Strengthening institutions, empowering community: annual report 2015. Retrieved from http://www.muis.gov.sg/documents/Annual_Reports/MUIS_AR_2015-Full-FA-LR.pdf

Majlis Ugama Islam Singapura (MUIS) (2017) Guidelines to preparation & handling of halal food. Retrieved from http://www.muis.gov.sg/halal/Consumer/guide-to-halal-food-preparation.html

Maqsood RW (2008) Islam : understand the religion behind the headlines. HarperCollins, London

Progress of Malays reflects S'pore's success. Retrieved from http://www.straitstimes.com/politics/progress-of-malays-reflects-spores-success

Ramadan T (2017) Islam: the essentials. Penguin Random House, London

Singapore Demographics Profile (2016). Retrieved from http://www.indexmundi.com/singapore/demographics_profile.html

Part VI

Guideline: Cultural Competence in Health Care Systems and Organizations

Building an Organizational Environment of Cultural Competence

23

Marilyn "Marty" Douglas

Guideline: *Healthcare organizations should provide the structure and resources necessary to evaluate and meet the cultural and language needs of their diverse clients.*

23.1 Introduction

An individual cannot stay healthy solely through personal effort but rather needs the support system of family and friends, fresh foods, safe streets, and clean air and water to maintain health. Similarly, healthcare providers cannot provide culturally competent care without an organizational infrastructure that provides the framework and tools to implement that care. Healthcare organizations and agencies are responsible for providing that infrastructure so healthcare professional can deliver safe, culturally congruent, and compassionate care to all who seek its services.

More than 15 years ago, the Institute of Medicine in the United States published the report *Unequal: Confronting Racial and Ethnic Disparities in Health Care* (Smedley et al. 2003). The IOM committee reviewed more than 100 studies that investigated the quality of care delivered to racial and ethnic minorities. Despite the fact that many variables were controlled,

such as insurance status, patient income, severity of disease, comorbid illnesses, age, gender, and where the care was provided, the majority of studies found that minorities were less likely to receive the care they needed, including clinically necessary procedures. These inequalities were found across illnesses as varied as cancer, mental illness, cardiovascular disease, diabetes, and HIV/AIDS as well as routine treatments for common health problems. Ultimately, this inequality of care results in disparities in healthcare outcomes between Whites and minority populations that persist to the present day (AHRQ 2016).

The IOM Report identifies three main categories of causes of these racial and ethnic minority health disparities. The first are patient-level variables, which, other than access-related factors, include mistrust, a misunderstanding of provider's instructions, a poor cultural match between the minority patient and provider, poor prior interaction with the healthcare system, or just a lack of knowledge of how to use the healthcare system. In the second category are provider-level variables, including provider bias against minorities, provider's uncertainty when interacting with minorities, and provider stereotypes about the health beliefs, behaviors, and

M. Douglas, Ph.D., R.N., FAAN
School of Nursing, University of California,
San Francisco, San Francisco, CA, USA
e-mail: martydoug@comcast.net,
marilyn.douglas@nursing.ucsf.edu

© Springer International Publishing AG, part of Springer Nature 2018
M. Douglas et al. (eds.), *Global Applications of Culturally Competent Health Care: Guidelines for Practice*, https://doi.org/10.1007/978-3-319-69332-3_23

health of minority groups. The final category of causes of disparities in healthcare include healthcare system level variables, such as the availability and financing of services, language barriers, and the location and times of service delivery. The first two categories have been addressed in previous chapters. This chapter will concentrate on the healthcare system variables and what measures can be taken to construct an environment in which cultural competence can be practiced.

dures that are trusted by the providers, and (5) training that is meaningful and that explains how to deal with cross-cultural situations. After the IOM report was published, a number of professional organizations and governmental agencies developed toolkits and standards to guide organizations in becoming culturally competent. Table 23.1 provides web addresses to access some of these toolkits. In addition, the CLAS Standards provide a blueprint for organizations to implement culturally competent care (US Department of Health and Human Services 2013).

23.2 Strategies for Building a Culturally Competent Healthcare System

In order to effect a sustained change at the organizational level, several key elements are needed: (1) leadership from the top, (2) demonstrated accountability, (3) policies in place that are communicated to employees, (4) proce-

23.2.1 Organizational Structure

23.2.1.1 Leadership
Commitment from the executive leadership of a healthcare institution or agency is the essential first step to integrating health equity and health disparities focus into organizational practices.

Table 23.1 Toolkit for designing a culturally competent organization

Organization/agency	Title	Source
American Hospital Association	Equity of Care: A Toolkit for Eliminating Health Care Disparities	http://www.hpoe.org/resources/ahahret-guides/1788 or http://www.hpoe.org/Reports-HPOE/equity-of-care-toolkit.pdf
Association of American Medical Colleges	Assessing Institutional Culture and Climate	https://www.aamc.org/initiatives/diversity/learningseries/335954/cultureclimatewebcast.html
Center for Medicare and Medicaid Services	A Practical Guide to Implementing the National CLAS Standards: For Racial and Ethnic and Linguistic Minorities, People with Disabilities and Sexual and Gender Minorities	https://www.cms.gov/About-CMS/Agency-Information/OMH/Downloads/CLAS-Toolkit-12-7-16.pdf
Health Research and Educational Trust	Improving Health Equity Through Data Collection and Use: A Guide for Hospital Leaders	http://www.hret.org/health-equity/index.shtml and http://www.hretdisparities.org
Massachusetts General Hospital, The Disparities Solution Center	Improving Quality and Achieving Equity: A Guide for Hospital Leaders	https://mghdisparitiessolutions.files.wordpress.com/2015/12/improving-quality-safety-guide-hospital-leaders.pdf
US Department of Health and Human Services (HHS). Office of Minority Healths	HHS Action Plan to Reduce Racial and Ethnic Health Disparities, A Nation Frees of Disparities in Health and Health Care	https://minorityhealth.hhs.gov/npa/files/plans/hhs/hhs_plan_complete.pdf

It is the responsibility of the leadership to incorporate these principles into the mission and vision of the organization. The board of directors should reflect the diversity of the population served so that the healthcare needs of vulnerable groups within their geographic area can be identified and addressed by programs designed and funded by the leadership. It is also the responsibility of the leadership for developing and implementing policies and procedures assuring quality of care is delivered to culturally diverse populations and that these policies are integrated throughout the organization (Weech-Maldonado et al. 2018). These include policies that address discrimination and bias of the institution as a whole and staff in particular.

23.2.1.2 Central Diversity Committee

The creation of a multidisciplinary committee directly accountable to chief executive is needed to coordinate and direct all activities related to the delivery of culturally competent care. Its functions are to assess what is being done, address disparities, address data collection, coordinate diversity activities, and develop a strategic plan.

23.2.1.3 Organizational Self-Assessment

A first step in developing a strategic plan for cultural competence is to assess the current level of services. An organizational self-assessment will give the organization the information it needs to understand its capacity for offering effective communication that meets the needs of individuals accessing the organization's services. One example of such an organizational assessment tool is provided below in Appendix 1 Cultural Assessment of an Organization, Institution, or Agency (Andrews 2016). Another source of guidelines to assess organizational cultural competence in the areas of administration, human resources, education, nursing department, and dietary services is provided by Purnell et al. (2011).

23.2.1.4 Care Delivery

Depending on the nature of the diverse population served, some departments may need to expand options for care delivery. For example, clinic hours may need to be expanded to evenings and weekends if it is found that many of the minority patients hold multiple jobs with limited opportunity to take time off during regular business hours. Community outreach clinics within ethnic neighborhoods may be needed to facilitate access to healthcare services. Dietary services may need to expand their options for food choices, for example, kosher foods, more vegetarian options, and ethnic foods. Maternity services may need to incorporate new procedures to accommodate traditional practices for labor and delivery. Examples of institutional barriers to access of maternity services in China (Kyei-Nimakoh et al. 2017), sub-Saharan Africa (Listyowardojo et al. 2017), Indonesia (Kurniati et al. 2017), and Australia (Hughson et al. 2017) illustrate this need to review policies and procedures in the way care is delivered. The general wards and intensive care units may need to be more flexible with visiting hours because some cultures require all family members to accompany an ill family member. Each institution and agency needs to address its own policies and procedures for its services depending on the findings of their institutional assessment.

23.2.2 Data Collection

23.2.2.1 Demographic Data

In order to determine whether disparities of care exist within both the institution and the community it serves, healthcare organizations need to collect the racial and ethnic affiliations of their patients and citizens as well as their primary language and literacy capabilities. According to the American College of Physicians position paper on racial and ethnic disparities in healthcare, "an ongoing dialogue with surrounding communities can help a healthcare organization integrate cultural beliefs and perspectives into healthcare practices and health promotion activities" (American College of Physicians 2010). While most hospitals do collect basic race and ethnicity data on their own patients and a large majority collect data on their patients' primary language, there is a lack of standardization of what is collected. For example, they may have a racial category of Black, but this would include African Americans, Caribbean Blacks, and refugees of a number of African countries. Similarly, a category of Whites would include Irish, German, and Eastern Europeans and not differentiate between multigeneration Americans and new immigrants. All have unique cultural needs. The toolkit developed by the Health Research and Educational Disparities Trust, as listed on Table 23.1, is particularly useful in delineating the specifics of data collection for identifying disparities in care (Hasnain-Wynia et al. 2007).

23.2.2.2 Health Outcome Data

Collecting the racial and ethnic demographic data is only the first step. Correlating these with the health outcomes of the population served is vital to assessing the healthcare needs of the community. Combining the demographic and health outcome data of their community will guide the healthcare organization in planning for new programs to address the disparities in health outcomes. It will also help in identifying key quality indicators that need to be measured and then stratifying them according to race and ethnicity.

23.2.2.3 Patient Satisfaction Data

In order to determine whether the services that the organization is providing are appropriate and effective, patient satisfaction survey data should be stratified and analyzed according to racial and ethnic populations. These results can be correlated with health outcome data on these populations to identify areas that can be improved and determine which new programs need to be designed to meet the needs of this population. These data can be used by the patient ombudsman to guide future interactions with persons from these populations.

23.2.2.4 Electronic Health Records (EHR) or Medical Record

In addition to demographic racial and ethnic data, other cultural variables should be included in the medical record. For example, depending on the population served, the following items could be included in an intake or admission assessment: primary language spoken, facility with dominant language, preferred greeting, principal decision-maker, preferred food and beverage choices, the use of herbal teas, or other alternative or complementary therapies. Other traditional practices can be integrated into the electronic health record. For example, many persons of Asian heritage prefer warm beverages rather than cold ones when ill. Therefore, hot/warm teas are preferred over cold drinks both with and between meals. Having the person's preferences recorded on admission assists the healthcare provider design an individualized plan of care.

23.2.3 Communication

23.2.3.1 Interpreter Services

Using family members as ad hoc interpreters when a patient does not speak the dominant language is ill-advised. The patient may not wish to divulge sensitive health information to the family member acting as an interpreter, who may be a young child or an abusive spouse. And the family member interpreter may not wish to convey information from the healthcare provider to the patient, such as a diagnosis of cancer or other terminal diagnosis. Instead, certified interpreters are recommended, whether they are face-to-face or through phone or other technologies. Chapter 14 provides a more extensive discussion on the use of interpreters and other technologies that can be used to bridge the language barrier between patients and healthcare providers.

In a systematic review of culturally appropriate interventions in a population of culturally and linguistically diverse (CALD) communities,

Henderson et al. (2011) found that in the experimental group using full-time, trained interpreters who were available 24 h per day, there was a significant increase in clinical service usage, in the number of prescriptions written and rectal exams performed as compared to the control group in which family member interpreters were used. From the results of this study, they concluded that there is an increase in health services when an interpreter service is used for CALD communities. However, more studies comparing the use of interpreter services are needed to confirm their conclusion.

23.2.3.2 Signage

Negotiating the numerous hallways of a large healthcare organization is difficult enough if a person speaks the dominant language. It is so much more difficult if a person and family members are not only less familiar with medical terms but also have limited proficiency in the dominant language. Therefore, the signage throughout the organization should be in as many languages as the populations they serve. To assure adequate communication, the language on the signs should be verified by members in the community so that the dialect is accurate.

23.2.3.3 Patient Education

Another function of the interpreter services is to translate patient education materials into the languages of the population served. These may be any written information, consent forms for medical treatments, tests and research, diets, discharge instructions, and even clarifying prescriptions. For example, the word "*once*" in Spanish means 11, in English it means 1. The difference in dosage taken can be catastrophic. Patient education videos should also be translated and include actors of similar race and ethnicity of the populations served.

23.2.4 Multicultural Workforce

23.2.4.1 Recruitment and Retention

One way to reduce institutional barriers to cultural competence is to recruit healthcare professionals, administrators, and policy-makers

drawn from the minority communities in the geographic area they serve. They may be helpful in designing programs and services that are more culturally appropriate to the diverse community they serve. One example would be to assess the value of expanding the types of acceptable signatures for consent forms to include the family decision-maker; in many cultures, the individual does not make such a major decision as surgery by themselves but rather requires consultation and approval of the family decision-maker. In Chap. 31, the advantages and challenges of a multicultural workforce are described, as well as strategies for building a workforce composed of multiethnic members of the population it serves.

23.2.4.2 Performance Evaluations

In order to integrate cultural competency into all levels of service, the institution needs to assure the accountability of all its staff to its mission and vision. At both the organizational and individual level, cultural competence requirements and performance measures should be included in job descriptions, functional statements, performance evaluations, and promotion criteria. These performance measures should be included for all staff, from the upper levels of management to all professional care givers and to the nonprofessional staff who have contact with patients.

23.2.5 Cultural Competency Education

Regardless of the type or amount of patient-employee contact, an awareness of cultural beliefs and attitudes can create either a welcoming or negative environment. Cultural competency education helps healthcare providers be responsive to diverse cultural beliefs and practices, preferred languages, literacy levels, and other patient needs. All employees, including the professional clinical staff, nonprofessional staff who have contact with patients or families, and even executive staff, should have cultural competency training. Educational sessions can be adapted to each group. For example, for the professional clinical staff who obviously will have the most in-depth interactions with diverse populations, content should be more comprehensive. An example of key concepts to be included in cultural competence training for professional staff are given below in Appendix 2. In Chap. 6, a more thorough discussion of the content of cultural competence training is provided.

The executive level managers also would benefit from cultural competency training. Knowledge of the degree of racial and ethnic disparities in health outcomes, on a national level and particularly in the area served by the institution, would provide rationale for program planning and budget allocations. In addition, it would guide the plan for data collection on the diverse populations served and assist in the strategic planning process.

Cultural competence training should also be provided for nonprofessional staff, e.g., admission and ward clerks, unlicensed assistive care providers, food service personnel, cashiers, or those performing housekeeping services on the wards. Their orientation training should at a minimum include elements of cultural awareness exercises and basic communication styles, such as forms of address, spatial distance when speaking with others, the use of eye contact, the use of gestures, etc.

Orientation and continuing education sessions should be face-to-face and interactive, with role-playing using patient vignettes of real situations and time for group discussions that augment the didactic portions of the classes. Simply completing an online module is insufficient to preparing staff for real cross-cultural encounters. Recently, there has been a trend to shift from using the term "diversity" training to naming it "unconscious bias" training, where the emphasis is placed on learning strategies to recognize and neutralize prejudices (Lipman 2018).

23.2.6 Fiscal Resource Allocation

Building a culturally competent organization requires not only specific personnel but also fiscal resources. Budget allocations need to be allocated for hiring of interpreters, cultural competence training for all staff, production of multilingual written materials and videos for patient education, consent forms and patient satisfaction surveys, adding multilingual signage throughout the institution, and supplemental recruitment of diverse staff, among others. In a culturally competent organization, these costs can be offset by improved health outcomes for members of racial and ethnic minority and reflected in such high-cost quality measures as reduced hospital length of stay, reduced emergency department length-of-stay for treatment-and-release patients, reduced 30-day readmissions, and reduced 72-h revisits to the emergency department. On balance, it is not only morally and ethically responsible for an organization to provide culturally competent care, but it is also fiscally responsible to do so.

23.2.7 Community and Cross-Sector Collaboration

Healthcare institutions exist to serve the people in its community. Therefore, community engagement can accomplish at least four goals: to build trust between community members and the healthcare providers, to assess the needs of the community, to design ways to enable access to healthcare, and to meet the healthcare needs of the community. Members of the community need to be seen as equal partners in assuring a healthy society. They should be recruited to serve on the organization's board of directors and participate with full membership in such groups as the "Diversity" Committee, Patient Education Committee, Research Committee, Nutrition Committee, Ethics Committee, and others with relevance to cultural differences in healthcare delivery. They can assist with cultural competency curriculum development and in delivering the training sessions. They can collaborate in analyzing patient satisfaction surveys and in identifying the rationale for both positive and negative comments made by the community members.

Enlisting the help from community health workers has been found to be beneficial when working with culturally and linguistically diverse populations (Henderson et al. 2011). For example, these community health workers can serve as a healthcare resource for the population, as well as assist discharged patients with implementing their plan of care, or collaborate with the organization to operate an off-site clinic.

Besides collaborating with the local community, organizations must unite with other community groups with similar priorities to have greater political power to make policy changes to help reduce racial and ethnic disparities in healthcare. By forming stakeholder coalitions of many institutions and agencies with similar goals, they can build leadership capacity across sectors, share best practices for reducing health disparities, collaborate to assure consistency in data collection and survey results, and share technical support (Espinoza et al. 2017). By establishing a cohesive partnership of such organizations, they can serve as a forum for sharing information and resources, as well as undertaking collaborative projects designed to reduce health disparities and yield more generalizable results than solely the community in which a single organization provides care. Considering that the causes of health disparities are complex and, in many cases, are embedded in social determinants of health, coalitions of many sectors are needed to develop strategies to eventually eliminate health disparities and achieve equity.

Conclusion

Quality of care must be equivalent to equity of care. In order for healthcare providers to deliver culturally competent care, they must be able practice within an environment that enables and facilitates healthcare delivery to diverse populations. Without this support, the healthcare provider will be unable to adequately deliver culturally competent care at the point-of-care level. Healthcare organizations are responsible for providing this structure.

Despite the initial expenses of building a culturally competent organization, the business case can be made that these strategies yield a greater benefits-to-costs ratio. Besides greater patient satisfaction survey results from diverse populations, culturally competent care yields decreased hospital readmissions, decreased length of stay in both the emergency department and hospital, decreased emergency department revisits within 72 h, and improved health outcomes. Those benefits far outweigh the costs of investment in training of the workforce, hiring interpreters, and adding multilingual signage. Healthcare organizations, regardless of size, are responsible for providing services that are respectful of and responsive to all individuals' cultural health beliefs and practices, preferred languages, health literacy, and communication needs. By building a structure of cultural competence, the organization is meeting these needs.

Appendix 1: Cultural Assessment of an Organization, Institution, or Agency

Demographic/Descriptive Data

- What types of cultural diversity are represented by clients, families, visitors, and others significant to the clients? Indicate approximate numbers and percentages according to the conventional system used for reporting census data.
- What types of cultural diversity are represented? What types of diversity are present among patients, physicians, nurses, X-ray technicians, and other staff? Indicate approximate numbers and percentages by department and discipline.
- How is the organization, institution, or agency structured? Who is in charge? How do the administrators support cultural diversity and interventions to foster multiculturalism?
- How many key leaders/decision-makers within the organization, institution, or agency come from culturally diverse backgrounds?
- What languages are spoken by patients, family members or significant others, and staff?

Assessment of Strengths

- What are the cultural strengths or positive characteristics and qualities?
- What institutional resources (fiscal, human) are available to support multiculturalism?
- What goals and needs related to cultural diversity already have been expressed?
- What successes in making services accessible and culturally appropriate have occurred to date? Highlight goals, programs, and activities that have been successful.
- What positive comments have been given by clients and significant others from culturally diverse backgrounds about their experiences with the organization, institution, or agency?

Assessment of Community Resources

- What efforts are made to use multicultural community-based resources (e.g., community organizations for ethnic or religious groups, anthropology and foreign language faculty and students from area colleges and universities, and similar resources)?
- To what extent are leaders from racial, ethnic, and religious communities involved with the institution (e.g., invited to serve on boards and advisory committees)?
- To what extent is there political and economic support for multicultural programs and projects?

Assessment of Weakness/Areas for Continued Growth

- What are the organization's weaknesses, limitations, and areas for continued growth?
- What could be done to better promote multiculturalism?

Assessment from the Perspective of Clients and Families

- How do clients (and families/significant others) evaluate the multicultural aspects of the organization, institution, or agency? Do patient satisfaction data indicate that clients from various cultural backgrounds are satisfied or dissatisfied with care? How are the quality outcomes the same or different for individuals of various races and ethnicities?
- How adequate is the system for translation and interpretation? What materials are available in the client's primary language (in written and in other forms, such as audiocassettes, videotapes, computer programs)? How is the literacy level of clients assessed?
- Are educational programs available in the languages spoken by clients?
- Are cultural and religious calendars used in determining scheduling for preadmission testing, procedures, educational programs, follow-up visits, or other appointments?
- Are cultural considerations given to the acceptability of certain medical and surgical procedures (e.g., amputations, blood transfusions, disposal of body parts, and handling of various types of human tissue)?
- Are cultural considerations a factor in administering medicines? How familiar are nurses, physicians, and pharmacists with current research in ethnopharmacology?
- If a client dies, what cultural considerations are given during post-mortem care? How are cultural needs associated with dying addressed with the family and others significant to the deceased? Does the roster of religious representatives available to the nursing staff include traditional spiritual healers such as shamans and medicine men/women as well as rabbis, priests, elders, and others?

Assessment from an Institutional Perspective

- To what extent do the philosophy and mission statement support, foster, and promote multiculturalism and respect for cultural diversity? Is there congruence between philosophy/mission statement and reality? How is this evident?

- To what extent is there administrative support for multiculturalism? In what ways is support present or absent? Provide evidence to support this.
- Are data being gathered to provide documentation concerning multicultural issues? Are there missing data? Are data disseminated to appropriate decision-makers and leaders within the institution? How are these data used?
- Are opportunities for continuing professional education and development in topics pertaining to multiculturalism provided for nurses and other staff?
- Are there racial, ethnic, religious, or other tensions evident within the institution? If so, objectively and nonjudgmentally assess their origins and nature in as much detail as possible.
- Are adequate resources being allocated for the purpose of promoting a harmonious multicultural healthcare environment? If not, indicate areas in which additional resources are needed.
- What multicultural library resources and audiovisual and computer software are available for use by nurses and other staff?
- What efforts are made to recruit and retain nurses and other staff from racially, ethnically, and religiously diverse backgrounds? What other types of diversity (e.g., sexual orientation) are fostered or discouraged?
- How would you describe the cultural climate of the institution? Are ethnic/racial/religious jokes prevalent? Are negative remarks or comments about certain cultural groups permitted? Who is doing the talking and who is listening to negative comments/jokes?
- Are human resources initiatives pertaining to advertising, hiring, promotion, and performance evaluation free from discrimination?
- Are cultural and religious considerations reflected in staff scheduling policies for nursing and other departments?
- Are policies and procedures appropriate from a multicultural perspective? What process is used for reviewing them for cultural appropriateness and relevance?

Assessment of Need and Readiness for Change

- Is there a need for change? If so, indicate who, what, when, where, why and how.
- Who is in favor of change? Who is against it?
- What are the anticipated obstacles to change?
- What financial and human resources would be necessary to bring about the recommended changes?

Source: Andrews MM. (2016) Cultural Diversity in the Health Care Workforce. In: M Andrews & J Boyle, eds., *Transcultural Concepts in Nursing Care*, 7th ed. Philadelphia, PA: Wolters Kluwer. pg. 383. Reprinted with Permission.

Appendix 2: Key Concepts for Organizational Orientation and Continuing Education Training in Cultural Competence for Professional Clinical Staff

- Definition of culture, ethnicity, cultural sensitivity and culturally competent care
- Critical reflection
  (a) Exercises to identify one's own heritage and unconscious biases
  (b) Stereotyping versus generalizing
  (c) Ethnocentrism
  (d) Assimilation into dominant culture
- Cultural variations in modes of communication
  (a) Differences in greetings, e.g., formal versus informal
  (b) Verbal language
  (c) Non-verbal language, i.e., body language
  (d) Interpreters versus translators
- Cultural differences in health beliefs and practices
  (a) Select examples from ethnic populations most frequently served
  (b) Select examples of health problems of ethnic populations most frequently served
  (c) Select beliefs and practices applicable to specific clinical area, e.g., maternity
  (d) Provide clinical experiences with ethnic populations

- Biological variations among racial and ethnic populations
  - (a) Assessment of skin conditions in different racial populations
  - (b) Assessment of cyanosis and jaundice in different racial populations
- Dietary practices among various ethnic populations
  - (a) For example, kosher foods for Jewish patients
  - (b) For example, no pork for Muslim patients
  - (c) Balance of "hot" and "cold" for many Asian groups
- Use of traditional remedies (complementary and alternative medicines)
  - (a) Select examples from ethnic populations most frequently served
  - (b) Interactions with prescription medicines (ethnopharmacology)
- Small group discussion of case studies that integrate principles of cultural competence
  - (a) Identify cultural conflict
  - (b) Develop a plan of care or solutions to conflict
  - (c) Present plan to whole group

References

Agency for Healthcare Research and Quality (AHRQ) (2016) 2015 National Healthcare Quality and Disparities report and 5th anniversary update on the National Quality Strategy. U.S. Department of Health and Human Services, Rockville, May 2015. AHRQ Publication No. 16-0015. https://www.ahrq.gov/sites/default/files/wysiwyg/research/findings/nhqrdr/nhqdr15/2015nhqdr.pdf. Accessed 16 Jan 2018

American College of Physicians (2010) Racial and ethnic disparities in health care, updated 2010. American College of Physicians, Philadelphia. https://www.acponline.org/system/files/documents/advocacy//current_policy_papers/assests/racial_disparities.pdf. Accessed 26 Jan 2018

American Hospital Association (2015) Equity of care: a toolkit for eliminating health care disparities. http://www.hpoe.org/resources/ahahret-guides/1788. Accessed 23 Jan 2018

Andrews MM (2016) Cultural diversity in the health care workforce. In: Andrews M, Boyle J (eds) Transcultural concepts in nursing care, 7th edn. Wolters Kluwer, Philadelphia, p 383

Association of American Medical Colleges. Assessing institutional culture and climate. https://www.aamc.org/initiatives/diversity/learningseries/335954/cultureclimatewebcast.html. Accessed 21 Jan 2018

Center for Medicare and Medicaid Services (2016) A practical guide to implementing the National CLAS Standards: for racial and ethnic and linguistic minorities, people with disabilities and sexual and gender minorities. https://www.cms.gov/About-CMS/Agency-Information/OMH/Downloads/CLAS-Toolkit-12-7-16.pdf. Accessed 16 Jan 2018

Espinoza O, Coffee-Borden B, Bakos AS, Nweke O (2017) Implementation of the National Partnership for Action to End Health Disparities: a three-year retrospective. J Health Dispar Res Pract 9(OMH Special Issue 6):20–36

Hasnain-Wynia, R, Pierce D, Haque A, Hedges Greising C, Prince V, Reiter J (2007) Health research and educational trust disparities toolkit. http://www.hretdisparities.org. Accessed 23 Jan 2018

Health Research and Educational Trust (2011) Improving health equity through data collection and use: a guide for hospital leaders. Health Research & Educational Trust, Chicago. http://www.hret.org/health-equity/index.shtml. Accessed 23 Jan 2018

Henderson S, Kendall E, See L (2011) The effectiveness of culturally appropriate interventions to manage or prevent chronic disease in culturally and linguistically diverse communities: a systematic literature review. Health Soc Care Community 19(3):225–249

Hughson JA, Marshall F, Daly JO, Woodward-Kron R, Hajek J, Story D (2017) Health professionals' views on health literacy issues for culturally and linguistically diverse women in maternity care: Barriers, enablers and the need for an integrated approach. Aust Health Rev 30:2017. https://doi.org/10.1071/AH17067

Kurniati A, Chen CM, Efendi F, Berliana SM (2017) Factors Influencing Indonesian Women's Use of Maternal Health Care Services. Health Care Women Int 20:2017. https://doi.org/10.1080/07399332.2017.1393077

Kyei-Nimakoh M, Carolan-Olan M, McCann TV (2017) Access barriers to obstetric care at health facilities in sub-Saharan Africa-a systematic review. Syst Rev 6:110–126. https://doi.org/10.1186/s13643-017-0503-x

Lipman J (2018) How diversity training infuriates men and fails women. TIME Magazine, 5 Feb 2018, vol 191, no 4, pp 17–19. TIME Inc., New York

Listyowardojo TA, Yan Z, Leyshon S, Ray-Sannerud B, Yu XY, Zheng K, Duan T (2017) A safety culture assessment by mixed methods at a public maternity and infant hospital in China. J Multidiscip Healthc 10:253–262

Massachusetts General Hospital (2015) Improving quality and achieving equity: a guide for hospital leaders. https://mghdisparitiessolutions.files.wordpress.com/2015/12/improving-quality-safety-guide-hospital-leaders.pdf. Accessed 23 Jan 2018

Purnell L, Davidhizar RE, Giger JN, Strickland OL, Fishman D, Allison DM (2011) A guide to developing a culturally competent organization. J Transcult Nurs 23(1):7–14

Smedley BD, Stith AY, Nelson AR (eds), Committee on Understanding and Eliminating Racial and Ethnic Disparities in Health Care, Board on Health Sciences Policy, Institute of Medicine (2003) Unequal treatment: confronting racial and ethnic disparities in health care. National Academies Press, Washington, DC. https://doi.org/10.17226/10260. https://www.nap.edu/download/10260; https://www.ncbi.nlm.nih.gov/books/NBK220358/. Accessed 4 Jan 2018

U.S. Department of Health and Human Services (HHS), Office of Minority Health (2013) National Culturally and Linguistically Appropriate Services (CLAS) standards. https://www.thinkculturalhealth.hhs.gov/clas/standards. Accessed 3 Jan 2018

U.S. Department of Health and Human Services (HHS). Office of Minority Health. HHS action plan to reduce racial and ethnic health disparities, a nation frees of disparities in health and health care. https://minorityhealth.hhs.gov/npa/files/plans/hhs/hhs_plan_complete.pdf. Accessed 15 Jan 2018

Weech-Maldonado R, Dreachslin JL, Epané JP, Gail J, Gupta S, Wainio JA (2018) Hospital cultural competency as a systematic organizational intervention: key findings from national center for healthcare leadership diversity demonstration project. Health Care Manag Rev 43(1):30–41

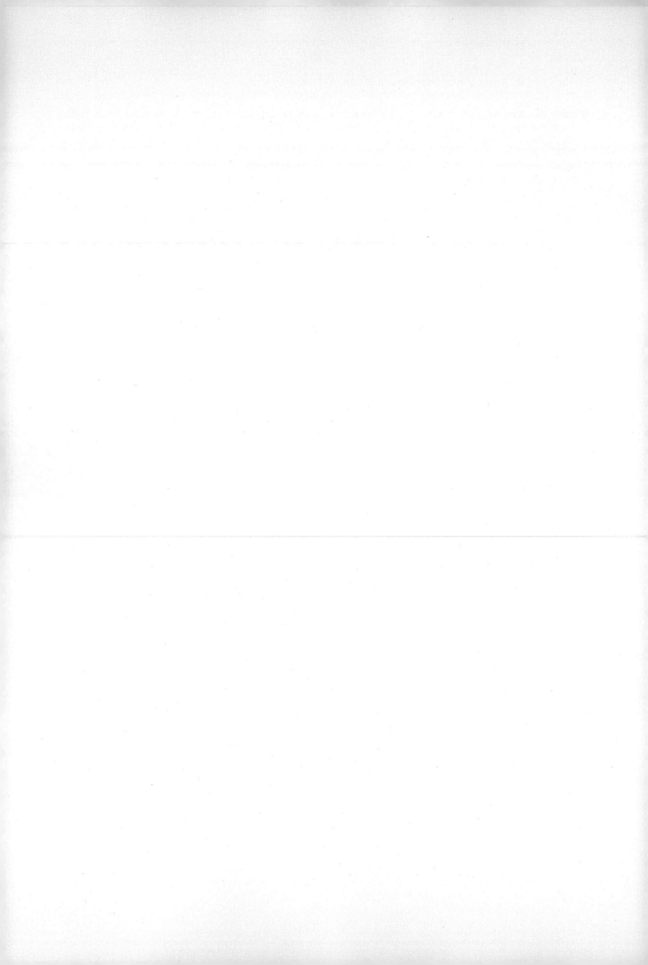

Case Study: Culturally Competent Strategies Toward Living Well with Dementia on the Mediterranean Coast

24

Manuel Lillo-Crespo and Jorge Riquelme-Galindo

Barbara is a 65-year-old Scottish woman who arrived in Spain with her husband John and two pet dogs. They planned to permanently live in a rural area on the Mediterranean Coast, which has been traditionally selected by the retired elderly population from Central and Northern European countries as a place to live when they are still active and healthy. The Scottish middle-income couple were retired in an urban Scottish area for 1 year before relocating. They then decided to move to the sunny coastal area of Southeast Spain, investing their life savings in a country house in the village where they vacationed every year. For them Spain was an affordable country where their savings would be worth more; it had a lower cost of living and a higher quality of life and was perceived as a safe place to live. They had even heard from other expats that healthcare costs were assumed by the Spanish government, and healthcare was considered as high quality as any in Europe. They settled in the countryside with their pets, in a rural area with 1100 inhabitants, with widely separated properties. There were no other foreign residents living nearby.

M. Lillo-Crespo, Ph.D., M Anthro, M.S.N., R.N. (✉)
Department of Nursing, Faculty of Health Sciences, University of Alicante, Alicante, Spain

Clinica Vistahermosa Hospital, Alicante, Spain
e-mail: Manuel.Lillo@ua.es

J. Riquelme-Galindo, M.S.N, R.N.
Department of Nursing, Faculty of Health Sciences, University of Alicante, Alicante, Spain

The nearest British Community was in a big town by the sea where the only British Expats' Association was located.

Six months after being settled in their new home, the couple experienced a medical crisis. Barbara had gone missing for 6 h. Her husband John finally found her, completely disoriented and standing in the middle of a field. John decided to take her to the nearest public health center, where the staff recommended they go to the nearest Spanish public hospital, 20 km away. When they arrived at the hospital, they were told she did not qualify for care because her condition was not seen as an emergency, and she did not have either the Spanish public insurance card or the insurance plan provided by the European Union for European population mobility.

John was given the option to pay cash for the healthcare services in the meantime. But John refused to do so, recalling that he had a contract with an international health insurance, which he set up years ago when they started visiting Spain on vacations. Now, however, he also realized that he could neither speak Spanish fluently enough to explain Barbara's situation to the staff nor could he sufficiently understand what he was being told. Complicating matters, the Spanish staff could not speak English well enough to communicate adequately with John and Barbara. John barely managed to understand the hospital staff's explanation about the steps to take toward receiving any type of public healthcare in Spain.

Being in this crossroads situation, John felt alone and overwhelmed. He called the telephone number written on the back of the private health insurance card to ask where they qualified to receive a professional assessment for Barbara. He then drove another 10 km to the private healthcare center approved by their insurance company. After Barbara was examined by a physician, the staff explained that their insurance coverage had some limitations; that is, neurological conditions were excluded due to their age and their family's medical history that they reported when they contracted the insurance 3 years ago. Therefore they were responsible for 100% payment for Barbara's consultation. She was diagnosed with presumed dementia, onset of unspecified type. More tests would be needed to be more specific.

Being confused and unsure, John decided to go home and assume a "watch and wait" strategy to see how Barbara progressed. Over the next 6 months, Barbara experienced progressively more episodes of memory loss. She was eventually diagnosed with Alzheimer's disease at the same private hospital as her original visit, despite the fact that John was responsible for payment for all scans and other tests.

Meanwhile, John began to explore the process for obtaining a Spanish public healthcare insurance and other possible sources of support. However, the political situation of the United Kingdom breaking away from the European Union (Brexit) and the restrictive financial situation in Spain posed additional barriers and challenges to obtain health insurance. At the same time, Barbara's disease was worsening. They were hardly able to pay their bills every month, and they could see how their Spanish dream was vanishing. She was prescribed a medication to decrease the progression of the disease, which was not covered by any insurance or support. John even searched for different types of support at the Public Health Centre nearby and from the Town Council, but he was denied because such funding support was restricted to use by the Spanish population.

Barbara had a lot of insight into her condition. She was aware that she was losing track of time as well as finding it difficult to tell time, which resulted in her being confused about times for appointments and activities. She found this upsetting at times, and sometimes made her reluctant to go out with her husband and participate in the activities planned by the retired foreigners' community. She begun to use timetables and reminders and became more reliant on John to prompt her.

From the beginning, the couple decided not to communicate Barbara's diagnosis to their son and daughter, both who were living in Scotland. This decision consequently caused an increased sense of isolation. She complained that they lived very far away from other people and that she could not even practice her Anglican faith as most churches in Spain were Catholic. Moreover, the Spanish economic recession made it difficult for them to sell their property and move to an area with better access to healthcare.

24.1 Cultural Issues

Dementia is a major public health concern across Europe, and the number of people with dementia is predicted to increase from 9.95 million in 2010 to 18.65 million by 2050 (Prince et al. 2013; Wortmann 2012). The Scottish culture is considered to be more of an individualistic culture as compared to the family-centered Spanish culture in which caring is traditionally a female responsibility, although Scotland is one of the European regions where more policies and rules regarding dementia have been developed, including the so-called dementia-friendly communities. On the other hand, in Spain, care of the elderly, even of those with neurodegenerative diseases, has traditionally been considered as a family issue until very recently. In fact, just 11 of the 28-member countries of the European Union have national dementia plans that address dementia awareness raising, education, diagnosis and treatment, and home, institutional, and residential care (Alzheimer Europe 2014). Spain is not one of these countries with such a national plan.

The Palliare Project Policy Review, which studied seven countries, including Scotland and Spain, revealed that Finland and Scotland had the most established and comprehensive national dementia action plans in Europe (Tolson et al. 2016).

Moreover, Spanish culture has traditionally promoted that the elderly remain in their homes, surrounded by their beloved ones (Cox and Monk 1993). In contrast, those who do not care for their elderly relatives are not well regarded in Spain. Consequently, the Spanish government historically has not assumed this responsibility. Furthermore, some authors have stated that family or home care seems to decrease the disease progression, promoting the person's routine and stabilization, making the person feel comfortable in their own known environment (Fratiglioni et al. 2004; Dawson et al. 2015).

The Spanish Institute for the Elderly and Social Services (IMSERSO), a division of the Ministry of Health, reported in 2016 that 8.7 million of the country's total population were over the age of 64 (Instituto Nacional de Estadística de España 2016a). However, those statistics do not include the high rates of elderly foreign population settled on the Mediterranean Coast. The southeastern province, where Barbara and John decided to retire, has the highest percentage of elderly foreigners who emigrate mainly from Central and Northern Europe (Instituto Nacional de Estadística de España 2016b). Furthermore, among the elderly living in their homes, the incidences of isolation and the previously unseen phenomenon of elderly abandonment are also increasing. Since care of the elderly is a family obligation, and not the government's responsibility, the Spain's Primary Health System is not directly focused on this problem, and in Barbara's case, the differences between her individualistic culture and the family-centered Spanish culture make living with dementia much more difficult. Whereas Spanish patients living with dementia rely on their families for care and do not expect government services for assistance, Barbara and John are left with little or no resources.

24.2 Social Structural Factors

The recently implemented Dependency Law in Spain (de Estado 2006) fully funds home-based care services or financial support for Spanish citizens who receive a minimum pension. Those with an income twice the minimum pension or more are responsible for full payment for these services, whereas the costs are prorated for those with an intermediary income.

There is no current nationwide law covering the provision of any primary social service specifically for persons with dementia. Each of Spain's 17 autonomous regions has developed its own laws based on the National Dependency Law's framework. Because decrees and regulations concerning social services are established by each autonomous region and further interpreted by town councils, there is a lack of uniformity in the policies regarding care of the elderly. Consequently, Spanish citizens do not have a legally established constitutional right to social services regarding elder care. Support for the elderly is only understood under a proven dependency situation and is determined by the person's income level. Thus, the Public National Health Service in Spain does not cover social and community care since these services are regarded as the family's responsibility. Only a primary healthcare service that includes home visits, which is not comparable to the Community Nursing Services provided in other countries such as the United Kingdom, is available and only for people with Spanish nationality. The limited range of these services underscores the traditional emphasis on treatment based on pathology but excludes prevention and health promotion policies. Moreover, the Spanish healthcare and social welfare systems are independent in their decision-making process. The National Health and Social Systems provide users with a wide yet insufficient range of services. Funding and regulations from the national Dependency Law allowed local councils to provide the following services: care homes for low-income and high-dependent populations, additional training and resources for hospital-based professionals caring for patients in the acute stages of dementia, and respite home care, which provides nonprofessional caregiver's support in the form of domestic chores in the homes of middle-stage dementia dependent populations. In the case of Barbara, she did not qualify for any of these services because she lacked Spanish citizenship, and her private health insurance did not fully cover all of her needs.

24.3 Culturally Competent Strategies Recommended

Elderly Central and Northern European retirees living on the Mediterranean Coast in Spain could be considered as potentially at risk for the onset of neurodegenerative diseases and their consequences but without access to the health services they require. Because the Spanish Health System considers elder care a family responsibility, foreign retirees who are separated from the families are left without the services they would have expected in their native countries. The following are recommendations to enable the development of strategies that are culturally appropriate, adequate, and effective in the case of Barbara and John, who represent a current situation of retirees living on the Mediterranean Coast, by following the guidelines for implementing culturally competent nursing care (Douglas et al. 2014).

24.3.1 Individual-/Family-/Caregiver-Level Interventions

- Before diagnosis and on admission to the healthcare systems: conduct an in-depth assessment of the person's cultural identity, linguistic preferences, environmental, occupational, socioeconomic, background, and educational status, including family roles and a gender-based scope.
- Before diagnosis and on admission to the healthcare systems: conduct an in-depth assessment of the main caregiver's identity, linguistic preferences, and their experience and background regarding the disease.
- Once a diagnosis is made: provide patient and main caregiver/s with information about the services provided for patients with that diagnosis at different levels (national, regional, local, and community). Include the procedures and the required documentation needed to apply for such services.
- Be aware of the social stigma of the diagnosis and the effect on the person, the patient's family, and the community.

- Provide support after the diagnosis is made with an appropriate and personalized care plan, which is integrated and multidisciplinary, including the evaluation for home adaptation.
- Provide as much personal control as possible, enabling those with dementia and their caregivers to exert control over their own care and their lives, even in advanced stages, including at the end of life.
- Provide patient with information about social and religious support and associated networks in the community nearby.
- Secure a referral to health and social services to help Barbara and John apply for health insurance and other social programs and aids regarding dementia.
- Provide education on active and healthy habits related to basic needs and according to her disease progression in the preferred language and considering her preferences.
- Provide persons diagnosed of dementia and their caregivers with a positive practice approach and guidelines, such as the European Palliare Best Practice Statement (Homerova et al. 2016).

24.3.2 Organizational-Level Interventions

- Prevent potential risks, errors, complications, and harmful events for the person affected and caregivers by assigning a managerial-level task force to oversee diversity-related issues within the organization.
- Provide high-quality and compassionate culturally congruent care in all the contexts and organizations ensuring that mission and organizational policies reflect respect and values related to diversity and inclusivity.
- Include cultural competence as a compulsory requirement in the organization's job descriptions, performance evaluations, and management and quality improvement indicators.
- Provide persons with dementia with flexible, appropriate, timely, and evidence-based care monitored by skilled staff whether at home, in hospital, or in a care home.

- Promote social impact research (stated below) by including professionals from different fields and cultures to improve the relevancy, availability, and quality of data on dementia care and support.
- Establish organization-wide committees to address the promotion of culturally competent care delivery to all patients, especially of those persons from other cultures who reside in the organization's service area.
- Enlist community members from diverse cultures to participate in the organization's program planning and decision-making.
- Allocate financial resources to fund certified interpreters in the major languages of the populations served.
- Provide a certified interpreter when the patient has limited language proficiency in the language that is different from the healthcare providers.
- Provide signage and printed materials on multiple conditions in the major languages of the populations served.
- Partner with local associations and international health agencies to exchange and provide information on dementia care and its relevance.
- Design interprofessional higher education modules on dementia care, including experiential learning with patients from different cultures.
- Measure the impact and patient satisfaction of the strategies developed to determine the appropriateness and effectiveness of services.

24.3.3 Community- and Societal-Level Interventions

- Establish a partnership with the Retired European Associations to assist with health education regarding dementia, including potential risk populations and caregivers.
- Collaborate with the retired European community living in the area to organize workshops and sessions about living with dementia.
- Collaborate with the retired European community in working toward an environment that fosters healthy and active lifestyles.

- Expand dementia education and training for health and social care staff who should be made aware of the signs of dementia and how best to support persons with the condition and their families and caregivers, thus establishing dementia-friendly communities and societies.
- Design education modules that make use of modern technology, communication, and networking to support learning in a virtual environment through membership of a facilitated virtual international community of practice, such as the Palliare Community of Practice (University of the West of Scotland 2015).
- Collect demographic, socioeconomic, and health data, including morbidity and mortality, of the Central and Northern European populations settled in the Mediterranean Coast.

Conclusion

Several social structural factors and important cultural differences and issues had enormous impact on Barbara's health and illness experience and also on her main caregiver John. In addition, this case illuminates a current situation that is evolving in Spain today. Both Barbara and John lacked the services for the elderly that they were accustomed to in their native country. Complicating the situation were the inconsistencies perceived in services and a lack of social support and aids because of their cultural background and expectancies. All these factors create cumulative risks and vulnerability as well as increase Barbara's dependence on others. In order to promote her health, strategies should be focused on creating a positive society where people can live well with dementia, respecting the context and culture, and on fostering a greater global collaboration and leadership among healthcare professional to improve the lives of those affected.

References

Alzheimer Europe (2014) National policies covering the care and support of people with dementia and their carers-Sweden, Dementia in Europe Yearbook as part of Alzheimer Europe's 2013 Work Plan. [online] Available at: http://www.alzheimer-europe.

org/Policy-in-Practice2/Country-comparisons/ National-policies-coveringthe-care-and-support-of-people-with-dementia-andtheir-carers/Sweden. Accessed 15 April 2017

Cox C, Monk A (1993) Hispanic culture and family care of Alzheimer's patients. Health & Social Work 18(2):92–100

Dawson A, Bowes A, Kelly F, Velzke K, Ward R (2015) Evidence of what works to support and sustain care at home for people with dementia: a literature review with a systematic approach. BMC Geriatr 15(1):59

de Estado J (2006) Ley 39/2006, de 14 de diciembre, de Promoción de la Autonomía Personal y Atención a las personas en situación de dependencia. Boletín Oficial del Estado 299:15

Douglas MK, Rosenkoetter M, Pacquiao DF, Callister LC, Hattar-Pollara M, Lauderdale J, Purnell L (2014) Guidelines for implementing culturally competent nursing care. J Transcult Nurs 25(2):109–121

Fratiglioni L, Paillard-Borg S, Winblad B (2004) An active and socially integrated lifestyle in late life might protect against dementia. Lancet Neurol 3(6):343–353

Homerova I, Waugh A, Macrae R, Sandvide A, Hanson E, Jackson G, Watchman K, Tolson D (2016) Dementia palliare best practice statement. University of the West of Scotland. Available at: http://dementia. uws.ac.uk/ documents/2015/12/dementia-palliarebest-practice-statement-web.pdf. Accessed 15 April 2017

Instituto Nacional de Estadística de España (2016a) Basic demographic indicators. Available at: http://www.ine. es/dynt3/inebase/index.htm?padre=1365. Accessed 15 April 2017

Instituto Nacional de Estadística de España (2016b) Población Extranjera según nacionalidad en la provincia de Alicante, 2016. Available at: http://www. ine.es/jaxi/Datos.htm?path=/t20/e245/p04/provi/ l0/&file=0ccaa002.px. Accessed 15 April 2017

Prince M, Bryce R, Albanese E, Wimo A, Ribeiro W, Ferri CP (2013) The global prevalence of dementia: a systematic review and metaanalysis. Alzheimers Dement 9(1):63–75. https://doi.org/10.1016/j.jalz. 2012.1.9.0072

Tolson D, Fleming A, Hanson E, Abreu W, Crespo ML, Macrae R, Jackson G, Hvalič S, Routasalo P, Holmerová I (2016) Achieving prudent dementia care (palliare): an international policy and practice imperative. Int J Integr Care 16(4):18

University of the West of Scotland (2015) Palliare project 2015. Available at: http://www.uws.ac.uk/palliareproject/. Accessed 15 April 2017

Wortmann M (2012) Dementia: a global health priority-highlights from an ADI and World Health Organization report. Alzheimers Res Ther 4(5):40

Case Study: Culturally Competent Healthcare Organizations for Arab Muslims

25

Stephen R. Marrone

Mustafa is a 55-year-old man who emigrated from a small desert city in the eastern province of the Kingdom of Saudi Arabia 20 years ago to a metropolitan area of the United States that has a large Arab Muslim population. He is a smoker with a history of hypertension, obesity, and type 2 diabetes. As such, Mustafa emigrated to the United States in order to seek better healthcare, to provide his children with a good education, and for the family to enjoy a more relaxed lifestyle.

Mustafa lives with his wife in a predominantly Arab Muslim community in the Midwestern United States that has a population of almost 100,000, where more than 40% of the people are of Middle Eastern ancestries. The racial and ethnic composition of the community is approximately 85% Caucasian, 4% Black/African-American, 0.5% Native American, 2% Asian, 0.5% non-Hispanics of some other race, 5.0% reporting two or more races, and 3.4% Hispanic or Latino. Approximately, half of the Caucasian population claim Irish, German, Polish, or Maltese ancestry. The small African-American population includes those whose ancestors came from the rural South. Middle Eastern ancestries include immigrants primarily

from Lebanon, Syria, Yemen, Iraq, and Palestine, the more recent immigrants fleeing war in their countries. The dominant languages spoken in the general community are English, Arabic, Spanish, and Polish (Pew Research Center 2013; U.S. Census Bureau 2015).

The median annual household income in the region is just under US$50,000; however, about 30% of the population lives in poverty. In spite of the median household income being higher than that of the region, the number of people living in poverty also exceeds that of the geographic levels of the region (Pew Research Center 2013; U.S. Census Bureau 2015). Like Mustafa and his wife, many Arabs and Arab Muslims who emigrated to this region 15–20 years ago have established themselves within the community over time and currently benefit from annual incomes that are higher than the median for the region. Yet, more recent immigrants who are on the upward economic trajectory live either in or at borderline poverty levels.

Mustafa and his wife have three children, two sons and one daughter, all of whom live nearby. As the eldest male of the family, Mustafa is considered the patriarch and primary decision-maker. The children were born in Saudi Arabia and were 16, 13, and 12 years old, respectively, when they emigrated to the United States. To prepare the children for life in America, Mustafa and his wife hired an English language tutor for them so that, by the time the children arrived in the United

S. R. Marrone, Ed.D., R.N.-B.C., N.E.A.-B.C., C.T.N.-A.
Harriet Rothkoft Heilbrunn School of Nursing, Long Island University of Nursing, Brooklyn, NY, USA
e-mail: stephen.marrone@liu.edu

States, they had basic English speaking, reading, and writing skills.

Mustafa and his wife have a primary school education and can speak, read, and write in Arabic. However, they do not speak, read, or write English fluently. They require an Arabic language interpreter and translated English to Arabic written materials in order to actively participate in the decision-making process. However, their children are university educated, employed, and speak English fluently.

Mustafa's family is well-respected in the community for their strong Muslim faith, sense of family values, and generosity. However, due to limited English proficiency, Mustafa and his wife have been marginalized within the larger community, thus relying primarily on traditional lifeways to navigate safely through their day-to-day activities.

Many Arabs in the community own and operate businesses that provide services in both English and Arabic and offer foods and merchandise that appeal to Arab Muslims. Grocery stores offer fresh and packaged products that reflect the diverse demographics of the community at large. Fresh produce and meats are readily available, and there are many stores that cater exclusively to the needs of the Arab community.

The community is considered to be safe even though its crime rate is slightly above the national average. Although the property crime rate is higher than the national average, there is little reported use of force against victims (Sperling 2017). The neighborhood has adequate education, transportation, and healthcare services.

Two years ago, Mustafa suffered a stroke that resulted in residual left-sided hemiparesis, impaired cognition, and slurred speech resulting in his reluctance to be seen in public due to his limited physical and cognitive abilities. These changes disrupted the family's social dynamic and decision-making structure as his eldest son Faisal must now serve as head of the family by proxy.

Mustafa is being admitted to the hospital with a diagnosis of pneumonia. Due to his limited ability to verbally express himself, he acknowledged his eldest son Faisal as the key decision-maker of the family. Because of his limited English proficiency, Mustafa was offered interpreter services, but he refused for fear that the interpreter would discuss his condition with the larger community. Thus, Mustafa relied on family members to interpret for him.

Mustafa seeks care at this hospital in particular because he feels that his culture care needs are met and respected. For example, the hospital's governance structure, as evidenced by its mission, vision, values, and strategic plan, supports diversity and inclusion among its consumers and within the healthcare team.

To diversify all levels of its workforce that reflects the demographics of the service area, from the frontline to the boardroom, the hospital actively recruits Arabs, Muslims, Irish, Polish, Maltese, Black/African-Americans, Hispanics, and Native Americans. For instance, in addition to mainstream nursing and healthcare organizations and journals, nursing recruitment and networking efforts target organizations and their respective journals, such as the National Arab American Nurses Association, the National Black Nurses Association, the National Association of Hispanic Nurses, the Association of Men in Nursing, and advertisements in *Minority Nurse*.

Through signage and written materials available at all points of entry into the hospital, consumers are informed of the language services that are offered and how to access them. Language services, both interpreter and translation services, reflect the major languages of the service area, Arabic, Spanish, Polish, and Maltese. To ensure that programs and services meet the consumers' needs, respect for diversity and inclusion are integrated into the hospital's shared governance infrastructure and critical decision-making teams such as the ethics committee, patient education committee, and human resource practices that address conflict management and resolution.

Specific to the Arab Muslim population, during the holy month of Ramadan, when Muslims fast from dawn until sunset, clinic hours, medication administration times, and visiting hours are adjusted to reflect the change in eating and sleep/wake patterns. Halal meals are also available at all times for Muslim patients, families, and staff, and an imam is available to advise staff on the care of Muslims and minister to the spiritual needs of Muslim patients and staff.

Prior to his illness, Mustafa owned and operated a Middle Eastern clothing and textile shop that catered to customers from both the Arab and general communities. To meet the customer's needs, Mustafa employed Arabic-English-speaking friends to translate for non-Arabic-speaking customers. Whenever possible, Mustafa's sons would also help out in the shop. However, consistent with fundamental Saudi tradition, Mustafa's wife did not work outside of the home, and his daughter did not help out in the shop.

Although Mustafa is presently unemployed due to his illness, he does have adequate private health insurance coverage that he purchased for himself and his family when self-employed. Coordinated by the hospital case manager and social worker, Mustafa receives hospital-based home care from a team that includes Arabic-speaking nurses, home health aides, physical and occupational therapists, and a social worker, all of whom are male. Mustafa and his family also receive help and support from the local stroke support group (National Stroke Association 2017) and the Imam, a Muslim religious leader, in the community.

25.1 Cultural Issues

Arab culture is recognized as a high-context culture whereby the needs of the group or community are valued over those of the individual. Consequences of the actions of individual family members will have consequences, positive and negative, for the entire family and, in the Arab community, typically influence the family's honor, respect, reputation, social status, esteem, and shame within the community.

Family honor, respect, and reputation are paramount and based on attributes, such as faith, modesty, protecting family, social stability, material security, obedience, and ambition (Miller and Feinberg 2002). Since typical Arab worldviews stipulate that males serve as family guardians, the eldest male is characteristically the key decision-maker who assumes responsibility for communicating information to the rest of the family (Kulwicki and Ballout 2013). When the eldest male of the family is no longer able to ensure family stability and security and function as the key decision-maker, individual and family dishonor may ensue.

Modesty is one of the core values in Islam. Visiting the sick is considered a communal obligation and fervently practiced by Arab Muslims (Islam Questions and Answers 2017; Kulwicki and Ballout 2013; McFarland and Wehbe-Alamah 2015). The family and the patient would be embarrassed and feel shame if visitors were not permitted or asked to leave.

As a fatalistic culture, Arab Muslims have strong belief that all things depend on Allah's will (*In Sha"llah*) and stipulates that only Allah can predict the future. Prayer is performed five times each day. As the second pillar of Islam, prayer is a fundamental requirement of all Muslims. Although there are no *official* exceptions excusing adult Muslims from performing daily prayers, people who are ill or traveling, for example, may modify the prayer rituals as described below.

Hygiene is an intrinsic value of Islamic law whereby the left hand is considered dirty, while the right hand is considered clean. *Wudu*, the ritual washing of the hands, mouth, nasal cavity, face, forearms, hair, and feet before prayers, is performed before each prayer. Muslims who cannot perform *Wudu* may substitute *Tayammum*, the rubbing of sand with both palms and sweeping it over the face and back of the hands. People who are unable to perform *Tayammum* are exempted and can still perform prayers (Kulwicki and Ballout 2013; McFarland and Wehbe-Alamah 2015). Muslims are also expected to face Mecca when performing prayer. If this is not possible, Muslims will also ask for privacy and quiet in order to perform the prayer rituals.

25.2   Social Structural Factors

In the US, the majority of Arabs reside in Los Angeles, Detroit, New York, New Jersey, Chicago, and Washington D.C. (Arab American Institute 2012). As a result of the September 11, 2001 attacks in the United States, public attitudes toward Arabs typically blur the distinctions among Arabs, Muslims, Islamists, and terrorists, regarding them as one and the same (Middle East Report, 2004) and often in a manner that openly advocates the de facto criminalization of all Arabs (Middle East Report, 2004). As a result, Arab Muslims in the United States are one of the populations most at risk for being victims of verbal and physical assault, discrimination, and ethnic profiling.

Saudi Arabia is consistently ranked among one of the richest countries in the world (Sharma 2017), with a more sedentary lifestyle as one consequence. Diabetes, hypertension, hypercholesterolemia, smoking, and obesity are among the leading health issues affecting Saudis. The prevalence of diabetes is 14.8% for males and 11.7% for females; for hypertension, it is 17.7% for males and 12.5% for females; and for hypercholesterolemia, it is 9.5% for males and 7.3% for females (IHME 2017). Despite the increased awareness of the hazards of smoking, smoking is also increasing in the Arab community. Overall, 21.5% of men currently smoke, of which 20.9% smoke shisha, an aromatic tobacco smoked using a hookah, a stemmed device used for smoking tobacco. Obesity in the Arab community is also related to the cultural value equating overweight with prosperity, with almost half of women and 23% of men reported being physically inactive (Daoud et al. 2015; IHME 2017).

The Arab Muslim community where Mustafa resides illustrates the environmental and socioeconomic issues that contribute to the vulnerability of this population. Although Mustafa does not live in poverty, he can understand basic health information; has access to healthcare services, insurance coverage, and healthy foods; and lives within a supportive family and social structure. However, he does live in a large metropolitan area where pollution, crime, and discrimination feature as significant social determinants of health. Nevertheless, Saudi/Arab culture and sedentary lifestyle pose substantial challenges to health and well-being and require support from the broader society and healthcare systems.

25.3   Culturally Competent Strategies Recommended

To provide culturally congruent care to Mustafa and his family, the following recommendations are offered (Kulwicki and Ballout 2013; OMH 2013).

25.3.1 Individual-/Family-Level Interventions

- On admission, conduct a comprehensive cultural health assessment that includes cultural health beliefs and practices, preferred language, health literacy, faith-based needs, and preferred communication and decision-making practices.
- Offer Arabic language assistance services at all points of care that ensure privacy and confidentiality.
- Offer the services of an imam upon admission and throughout the hospitalization.
- Recognize the potential stigma attached to Mustafa, as the eldest male, who can no longer serve as key decision-maker for the family.
- Assign only male nursing staff to care for Mustafa, if possible, especially for intimate procedures.
- If male nursing staff are not available, alternatives may include the following: (1) a female nurse may provide care that does not involve physical contact such as administering medications or hourly rounding, (2) a male staff member such as a unit clerk or patient care technician may accompany and assist the female nurse in providing care that includes physical contact, and (3) Mustafa can arrange for a male private duty nurse or certified nursing assistant to assist with intimate care needs.

- Relax visiting hour restrictions to accommodate the Arab Muslim need to visit the sick.
- Consider the right-handed preference when providing care to Arab Muslims.
- Provide education to Mustafa and his family on stroke, obesity, hypertension, diabetes, hypercholesterolemia, and the hazards of a sedentary lifestyle provided by the National Center on Health, Physical Activity, and Disability (NCHPAD, 2017).
- Provide privacy and support for Mustafa and his family to complete daily prayer rituals.
- Maintain communication with the home health agency to support a smooth transition from inpatient to home care upon discharge.
- Offer caregiver support and resources to the family to relieve caregiver burden and compassion fatigue.

25.3.2 Organizational-Level Interventions

- Create and sustain an organizational governance and leadership infrastructure that promotes the provision of culturally and linguistically appropriate healthcare services as evidenced by mission and vision statements, values, and strategic plans, which support diversity and inclusion among its consumers, within the healthcare team, and for students and faculty.
- Integrate culturally and linguistically appropriate goals; standard operating procedures, policies, and practices; and management accountability into the organization's operational strategic plans, outcomes measurements, and continuous quality improvement initiatives.
- Educate governance, leadership, and the workforce in culturally and linguistically appropriate practices. Principles and practices of cultural competence and language assistance services must be integrated into initial orientation and ongoing education programs for all levels of staff. Workshops that address the culture care needs of the dominant cultural and linguistic populations within the service area should be offered on an ongoing basis. The design of such programs should include

input from members of the respective communities. Leadership development workshops should emphasize the requisite knowledge and skills for leading interprofessional, multicultural teams.

- Evaluate cultural competence of all levels of staff during, orientation, and periodically, at least annually, throughout the terms of employment. Provide remediation, as needed.
- Collect and maintain demographic data to monitor and evaluate the impact of culturally and linguistically appropriate services on health equity and outcomes and to inform service delivery.
- Partner with the community to design, implement, and evaluate policies, practices, and services to ensure cultural and linguistic appropriateness.
- Include cultural and language competencies in the job descriptions and performance evaluations of into all levels of staff from frontline to executive.
- Plan special events to increase awareness of the customs, values, beliefs, and culture care needs of the dominate groups within the service area. Events should coincide with special days for each group such as Ramadan, Eid al-Fitr, and Eid al-Adha for Muslims, Cinco de Mayo for people of Mexican descent, Black History Month, St. Patricks' Day for people of Irish heritage, and Polish American Heritage Day.
- Review and revise policies and procedures related to visiting and visiting hours, medication administration practices, religious services and practices, and language assistance services that reflect the needs of the demographics of the service area and the healthcare team. Human resource policies must also include strategies that address culturally related conflict management and resolution.
- Incorporate diversity and inclusion strategies into the organization's shared governance infrastructure and interprofessional decision-making teams such as the ethics committee, patient education committee, and human resource practices that address conflict management and resolution.

- Ensure the initial and ongoing competence of individuals providing language assistance services that reflect the preferred languages of the population in the service area.
- Allocate resources to support a diverse governance, leadership, and workforce that reflect the population in the service area. For example, to meet the needs of Arab Muslims, partner with the National Arab American Nurses Association and the Association of Men in Nursing to recruit Arab, Muslim, Arabic-speaking, and men into the nursing workforce.
- Establish an interprofessional Diversity and Inclusion Council to address and monitor the delivery and outcomes of the provision of culturally competent care that includes members who reflect the population of the service area: Arabs, Muslims, Irish, Polish, Maltese, Black/African-American, Hispanic, and Native American.
- Provide signage, printed, and multimedia materials on common health conditions and support services in the major languages of the population served, namely, Arabic, Spanish, Polish, and Maltese.
- Include items on patient satisfaction surveys to determine if the care provided was perceived as culturally sensitive and in the patient's preferred language. Include items on staff satisfaction surveys that address if the practice environment is inclusive.
- Partner with local Arab Muslim community centers, mosques, hookah lounges, markets, businesses, and local, regional, and national media to provide information in English and Arabic on the dangers of sedentary lifestyles.
- Ensure the 24/7 availability of an imam who can advise and minister to the spiritual care and dietary needs of Muslim patients, families, and staff.

25.3.3 Community Societal-Level Interventions

- Conduct regular assessments of the community's health outcomes and population-based social determinants of health to plan and implement services that respond to the diversity in the service area.
- Establish a partnership with the Arab American Institute in order to support healthcare policy and program development for Arab Muslims at the national level.
- Partner with the Arab Muslim community to organize health fairs to address lifestyle issues that affect the Arab Muslim population.
- Collaborate with the Arab Muslim community to develop programs and services that promote healthy lifestyles.
- Communicate the organization's culturally and linguistically appropriate programs and services to key internal and external stakeholders via print, visual, oral, and social media.

Conclusion

Several cultural and social structural factors influence Mustafa's health and illness experience. Mustafa has a primary school education, a limited English proficiency, a sedentary lifestyle, and multiple comorbidities that resulted in stroke. These limited his ability to fully participate in his care, hindered his being involved in the larger metropolitan community, and prevented him from working and being fully engaged in family decision-making. The stigma associated with no longer being the key decision-maker for the family can potentially isolate Mustafa from his family and the Arab Muslim community. This stigma may also extend to his family as well.

In aggregate, these factors create risks to Mustafa's health and well-being. Culturally competent care strategies should emphasize holistic care related to managing Mustafa's medical condition as well as the cultural and social determinants of health and lifestyle issues. These can impact his condition, prevent hazards of immobility, maximize his ability to contribute to the family decision-making, and access and use of organizational and societal resources to minimize his marginalization from the Arab Muslim community and within his family.

References

Arab American Institute [AAI] (2012) Arab American demographics. Retrieved from http://www.aaiusa.org/demographics/

Daoud N, Hayek S, Muhammad AS, Abu-Saad K, Osman A, Thrasher JF, Kalter-Leibovici O (2015) Stages of change of the readiness to quit smoking among a random sample of minority Arab-male smokers in Israel. BMC Public Health. 15:672. https://doi.org/10.1186/s12889-015-1950-8

Institute for Health Metrics and Evaluation [IHME] (2017) Saudi health interview survey finds high rates of chronic diseases in the Kingdom of Saudi Arabia. Retrieved from http://www.healthdata.org/news-release/saudi-health-interview-survey-finds-high-rates-chronic-diseases-kingdom-saudi-arabia

Islam Questions and Answers (2017) Visiting the sick: some etiquettes. Retrieved from https://islamqa.info/en/71968

Kulwicki AD, Ballout S (2013) People of Arab heritage. In: Purnell LD (ed) Transcultural heath care: a culturally competent approach, 4th edn. PA Davis, Philadelphia, pp 159–177

McFarland MR, Wehbe-Alamah HB (2015) Leininger's culture care diversity and universality: a worldwide nursing theory, 3rd edn. McGraw-Hill, New York

Miller TAW, Feinberg DG (2002) Culture clash. Public Perspective, March/April, pp 6–9

National Center on Health, Physical Activity and Disability [NCHPAD] (2017) Building Healthy Inclusive Communities through the National Center on Health, Physical Activity and Disability. Retrieved from http://www.nchpad.org/403/2216/Sedentary~Lifestyle~is~Dangerous~to~Your~Health

National Stroke Association (2017) Stroke support groups. Retrieved from http://www.stroke.org/stroke-resources/stroke-support-groups

Office of Minority Health [OMH] (2013) The national standards for culturally and linguistically appropriate services in health and health care. Retrieved from http://minorityhealth.hhs.gov/omh/browse.aspx?lvl=2&lvlid=53

Pew Research Center (2013) World's Muslim population more widespread than you might think. Retrieved from http://www.pewresearch.org/fact-tank/2013/06/07/worlds-muslim-population-more-widespread-than-you-might-think/

Sharma R (2017) Top 10 richest Arab countries. Retrieved from http://www.trendingtopmost.com/worlds-popular-list-top-10/2017-2018-2019-2020-2021/travelling/richest-arab-countries-best-famous-beautiful-amazing-wonderful/

Sperling (2017) Sperling's best place. Dearborn, Michigan. http://www.bestplaces.net/crime/city/michigan/dearborn

United States Census Bureau (2015) US and World Population Clock. Retrieved from https://www.census.gov/popclock/?intcmp=home_pop

Case Study: A Lebanese Immigrant Family Copes with a Terminal Diagnosis

26

Anahid Kulwicki

Samira, an 18-year-old female, has been complaining from extreme lethargy, loss of weight, and spiking temperature with unknown cause.

Samira's parents do not have health insurance as Mr. Habib, Samira's father, who was a store owner in his home country, could not find a job in the United States. The only employment he was able to secure was working as a dishwasher in a local restaurant, which paid him minimum wage. He has no health insurance. Concerned about taking Samira to the doctor due to their financial condition, Samira's parents were hoping that with the help of home remedies and some over-the-counter medications, Samira's condition will improve.

However, despite all their efforts, Samira's condition was getting worse. Finally, Samira's parents decided to borrow money from an uncle, Mr. Khalil, and take Samira to a local pediatrician. After examining Samira and reviewing her blood test results, the pediatrician asked the parents to take Samira to the nearby children's hospital emergency room for further tests. He suspected Samira's condition was serious due to the very high white blood cell count. Samira's

parents, with the help of her uncle who has good English conversational skills, took her to the hospital for further evaluation.

After a series of tests, the pediatrician at the medical center emergency department recommended that Samira be admitted to the hospital for further evaluation as he suspected her life was in danger. After 3 days of hospitalization and several tests, Samira was diagnosed with acute lymphocytic leukemia (ALL).

The physician informed Mr. Khalil about Samira's diagnosis and asked that he explain to the parents, who did not speak English, about Samira's health status. Mr. Khalil was alarmed with the news and did not have the courage to inform his sister and brother-in-law about Samira's diagnosis. He thought if he told his sister and brother-in-law that Samira has cancer, the family will not be able to cope with the news as in his culture cancer is believed to be terminal disease. Instead, he told his sister and brother-in-law that Samira had a severe infection and that she needs to stay in the hospital to be treated for a little while longer.

After a week of hospitalization, Samira's parents asked Mr. Khalil as to why their daughter was not getting better. Mr. Khalil informed Mr. Habib in private that Samira was diagnosed with "that disease." Mr. Khalil explained that according to Samira's doctor, Samira may die within 3 months due to the severity of her condition.

A. Kulwicki, Ph.D., R.N., FAAN
School of Nursing, Byblos Campus, Lebanese American University, Byblos, Lebanon
e-mail: anahid.kulwicki@lau.edu.lb

© Springer International Publishing AG, part of Springer Nature 2018
M. Douglas et al. (eds.), *Global Applications of Culturally Competent Health Care: Guidelines for Practice*, https://doi.org/10.1007/978-3-319-69332-3_26

Mr. Habib was very distraught about the news. He asked Mr. Khalil not to tell his wife about Samira's diagnosis for fear that she will not take the news well. Mr. Habib was very upset when he heard that Samira's doctor was acting as God by indicating that Samira had 3 months to live. He insisted to find another doctor to treat his daughter because he did not trust a doctor who acted as God, hoping that another doctor will be more compassionate and more optimistic about the condition of his daughter. Mr. Khalil tried to comfort Mr. Habib by stating that his daughter was in the best medical center cared by the best doctors and changing doctors will not change the prognosis of his daughter. He explained to him that Samira's mother should be informed. Mr. Habib insisted that neither Samira nor anyone in the family should know about Samira's condition. He thought giving such bad news to his daughter and wife will probably kill them both from grief. He wanted Samira and his wife to be hopeful that Samira's condition will be better. He believed only God can determine when his daughter will die and that he should help her and his wife to stay upbeat and not give up hope.

A week has gone by, and all tests results indicated that Samira was not responding to the treatment as her condition was much more advanced than what was initially thought by the medical team. Mr. Habib and Mr. Khalil finally decided to tell Mrs. Habib about Samira's condition, while Samira was taken from her room for additional tests. Mr. Habib explained to his wife that Samira had "that disease." When Mrs. Habib heard the news, she started screaming and beating on her chest and asking for God's help in curing Samira from "that disease." She blamed herself for bringing the problem on by putting her family through immigration as she heard that stress can cause "that disease."

Samira, who had limited English-speaking skills, became more and more concerned as she started losing her hair and feel weaker. She asked the nurse whether she would ever get out of the hospital. The nurse was alarmed that Samira was not informed about her condition and asked Samira's uncle to request the family let Samira

know. Samira's mother insisted that Samira not know about her disease. She explained that Samira will be depressed, and lose hope and will to live if she knew she had cancer. The nurse informed the doctor about her conversation with Samira's mother. The doctor and the nurse both decided to contact the social worker who is familiar with the Arab culture to help Samira and her family deal with her illness. The nurse was aware that Samira belonged to the Muslim religion and contacted the imam to visit Samira's family for spiritual support. In addition, the nurse, the physician, along with the social worker and the imam met with the hospital ethics committee to discuss the ethical considerations in caring for Samira and her family.

26.1 Cultural Issues

In the Arab culture, as in many other cultures, the family is the fundamental unit in society. Immediate and extended family members are closely engaged in family matters especially when facing difficult situations (Kulwicki and Ballout 2013). Collective decision-making is the norm rather than individuals making their own decision as in the United States (Kulwicki and Ballout 2013). Although the family structure among Arab immigrants is changing from that of an extended family to nuclear family where decisions are jointly made by males and females in the family, patriarchal family structure continues to be common where males are primarily breadwinners and females are the caregivers or nurturers. Gender roles are clearly defined and regarded as complementary division of labor (Kulwicki and Ballout 2013). Decisions are primarily made by men, and the responsibility for family members' well-being usually rests with men. Women and children are considered emotionally fragile and are protected from emotional stress and spared from being informed about bad news, such as the diagnosis of a terminal disease or death. Although Muslims accept death as being inevitable, the timing of death is considered to be the will of God, and individuals are expected not to give up hope (Kulwicki 2011). In the healthcare context, family members collectively make decisions about patient's treatment (Kulwicki and Ballout 2013; Ahmad 2004). Spiritual support is readily accepted by Muslim patients and is considered desirable by most patients (Lawrence and Rozmus 2001). Most Arab health-care providers and families do not consider disclosure of serious health conditions acceptable, especially in cases of terminal illness. Many believe that such disclosure is unnecessary and inhumane to the patients' emotional well-being and withhold such information out of concern for patient beneficence (Pentheny O'kelly et al. 2011). Such bad news can only lead to patients' depression and facilitate death, as they may lose hope to live.

Opposing views regarding disclosure of a patient's diagnosis and prognosis can cause conflict between health-care providers and the families of patients with terminal diseases in the Arab culture. In the United States, American healthcare values are based on the Patient Self-Determination Act (1990) that protects individual rights to be informed about their health condition, make informed decisions, and determine their treatment choices. Individualism is one of the core values of the American culture, whereas collectivism is a core value of the Arab culture. In a culture where collectivism is the norm, the decision of disclosure of patient's terminal illness rests with the family (Hassouneh and Kulwicki 2009). These differing views can create friction between health-care providers and patients and their families. It is important that health-care providers understand cultural norms regarding disclosure of a patient's illness to avoid undue stress for the families and to the patients under their care. Culturally sensitive communication strategies in informing their terminally ill patients and their families need to be developed and implemented (Doumit and Abu-Saad 2008; Chittem and Butow 2015).

26.2 Social Structure Factors

Although most Arab immigrants are successful in the United States and high educational attainment is more prevalent among Arabs (Arab

American Institute 2010) than among many other immigrant groups, many new immigrants who come from lower socioeconomic backgrounds and war-torn countries may not have the educational preparation, English language skills, health literacy, and access to quality health-care services. Consequently, their cultural beliefs, norms, and practices may be substantially different than those of the Americans, American health-care providers, and even to some extent to the more acculturated Arab American immigrants (Hassouneh and Kulwicki 2007).

Although medical care is excellent in the major cities in Lebanon where Samira's parents were raised, access to medical care in the rural areas is difficult both financially and geographically. Health insurance is available for individuals who work for private and Lebanese governmental agencies. Individuals who do not have health insurance and are unable to pay for health care are cared for by the governmental health-care system. However, the process of eligibility for care may be difficult. Patients are required to pay a portion of the cost.

Patients who do not have the financial means usually wait until their health condition becomes severe. In the case of cancer, most patients are in advanced stages of the disease when admitted to the hospital. Hence, among the poor and illiterate populations, the diagnosis of cancer is considered a terminal disease. Therefore, the mere use of the word cancer invokes fear in people. For this reason, many avoid using the word cancer and instead refer to it as "that disease" or "the bad disease" or use the phrase "God keep you away from that disease."

In the culture where Samira's parents came from, doctors often make decisions about treatment for a patient's condition. Families and patients depend on the doctor's expertise and defer all treatment modalities to the physician (Kulwicki 2008a, b). Decisions about disclosure of illness are made by the family, and doctors often respect the family's decision and defer disclosure of a terminal illness to the family members.

For new immigrants in the United States, the socioeconomic conditions of Arabs are similar to those in their country of origin. Most do not have health insurance due to unemployment or under-employment. There are several community agencies available in highly populated Arab immigrant communities where primary health care and social services are available, but in areas where the number of Arab immigrants is few, accessing quality and culturally competent care may be a challenge.

26.3 Culturally Competent Strategies Recommended

Arab immigrants like many other immigrants in the United States are considered a vulnerable population due to their lack of economic resources, experiences of war prior to immigration, lack of health literacy, inability to speak English, and difference in cultural norms and religious beliefs between the American mainstream culture and Arab culture that create barriers in health-care utilization (Kulwicki et al. 2010). It is important that health-care professionals understand the culture and develop appropriate interventions to avoid further disparities in access and quality of health care for this population (Kulwicki et al. 2000). Because Arab Americans come from 22 different countries with diverse socioeconomic, cultural, religious, and health-care experiences, it is important that the health-care providers be sensitive to intra-ethnic differences while planning and implementing culturally competent services for Arab American immigrants in the United States. Health-care providers are urged to consider the following recommendations when caring for Arab American patients:

26.3.1 Individual-Level Interventions

- Complete a thorough assessment of the cultural norms, social structure, educational preparation, and spiritual beliefs of each patient and their families.
- Assess the family structure and gender role differences.
- Assess patients and their families' preferences in the decision-making process related to care.

- Avoid generalizations as each patient is unique and some cultural norms, social structure, gender differences, spiritual beliefs, and views about life and death may be different between individuals of the same culture.
- Assess communication styles of the patient and their families.
- Be informed that there may be intra-ethnic differences as Arabs come from different countries with different expectations from health-care system.
- Be sensitive to areas of conflicts between the culture of the health-care provider and the culture of the patient and avoid them by a thorough assessment.
- Establish a trusting relationship with the patient and their families through open communication.
- Make sure that a social worker who speaks the language of the patient and understands the culture is available when needed.
- Assess the spiritual needs of the patient and their families and ask if they would like the help of a spiritual leader at times of need.
- Assess patient's norms, rituals, beliefs, and practices about death and dying.
- Assess the patient's family structure. Ask who makes decisions for the family.
- Assess patients and patient's family experiences and expectations from the health-care providers.
- Make sure an interpreter is available when needed.
- Provide audiovisual materials in the language of the patient if available and if the patient does not speak English or is illiterate in their own language.
- Provide written materials that may familiarize patients and the family members to better understand the rules and policies of the health-care system.
- Provide written materials about the resources that are available to them, and make sure that the patient and family are aware how to access those services.
- Assess issues surrounding confidentiality. Some patients or patient's families may not

want to discuss their health conditions with individuals from their own culture for fear that information may be shared with community members.

- Make sure that patients and their families understand that everything they say is held confidential and is not shared with anyone except with individuals caring for them.
- Provide educational materials to the patient regarding the diagnosis of the patient after making sure that the family members are comfortable with the information shared.
- Check with patient and their families to make sure they understand the information given to them or if they have questions.

26.3.2 Organizational-Level Interventions

- Partner with community service organizations that provide health care to the Arab immigrants. If none exists in the immediate geographic vicinity, partner with national organization(s).
- Partner with American Arab Nurses Association and Arab American Medical Association to access community health professionals when needed.
- Develop a resource guide for services that can be shared with the patients.
- Develop audiovisual materials or use library resources in obtaining materials for patients who do not read in English and Arabic languages.
- Conduct training programs for health professions.
- Include Arab community leaders on the hospital advisory board.
- Provide a certified interpreter.
- Establish a list of Arab health professionals within the hospital and within the community for referral.
- Include an Arab American cultural expert on the hospital ethics committee.
- Employ Arab American health-care providers such as nurses, doctors, receptionists, and social workers from the communities served.

26.3.3 Community- and Societal- Level Interventions

- Establish a collaborative relationship with Arab community health centers if available.
- Plan, develop, and implement community health fairs in partnership with community leaders.
- Provide online or include health information resources on hospital website.
- Have hospital representative on health advisory committees or coalitions serving Arab American population.
- Include community leadership on the advisory board of the hospital.
- Provide consistent culturally tailored health promotion materials to the communities with a large number of Arab American immigrants.
- Employ community members in the hospitals and/or health-care centers.

Conclusion

It is important for health-care providers to be aware that culture is dynamic and that cultural norms and beliefs continuously change and evolve as the context in which cultural groups live, work, and age. What may be true in a given cultural group 10 years ago may not be applicable in the current situation. It is therefore imperative that health-care providers continuously learn the social determinants of health and its impact on a given population. A recent study regarding truth telling or disclosure of cancer diagnosis indicated that a majority of the surveyed population preferred that such information be shared with the patient directly rather than having family members make that decision (Farhat et al. 2015). This was attributed to the availability of public awareness about cancer. Changes were also reported in the attitudes and practices of physician in truth telling and disclosure. The study pointed out that younger or recent graduates were more open to disclosing the diagnosis to the patient compared to the older physicians (Naji et al. 2015). Similar changes have been reported in the literature where individuals are more aware of their health and health-care services than previous generations due to greater efforts made in educating the public.

Organizational and community level efforts in educating vulnerable populations about cancer, signs and symptoms, treatment modalities, and cancer survival rate can help dispel myths about the deadliness of the disease and promote early detection and treatment. In addition, organizational and public education efforts in care of terminally ill patients, implications of disclosure, and truth telling can assist patients and families to better cope with terminal illness and facilitate quality of life for cancer patients.

It is important that health-care professionals develop expertise in preparing educational materials that are tailored to the cultural, linguistic, and literacy levels of the populations they serve using a variety of educational approaches such as written, oral, digital, or audiovisual materials that can serve the needs of a diverse population. Promoting health literacy in immigrant populations is imperative to avoid conflict between health-care providers and patients from cultures other than their own.

Research indicates that disclosure and truth telling is becoming more common in the Arab world than decades ago. However, it is essential that health-care providers understand that in some cultures, disclosure of illness may still be controversial (Bou Khalil 2013) and that health-care professionals must take into consideration the social determinants of health of their patients before they make decisions that may be detrimental to their patients' well-being. In the case of Samira, it was important that the health-care professionals assess the social structure of the patient, understand the family dynamics, and consider their socioeconomic conditions, their health beliefs, perceptions, and experiences before they impose American health-care values on their patients. Truth telling and disclosure of terminal illness can be accomplished if there is open communication, understanding and apprecia-

tion of the patient's backgrounds, and the ability of health-care providers to address the disclosure in a culturally skilled manner. By doing so, the quality of the health-care services for ethnically vulnerable populations can be improved, and disparities in health status and access to care can be significantly reduced.

References

Ahmad NM (2004) Arab-American culture and health care. http://www.case.edu/med/epidbio/mphp439/Arab-Americans.html. Accessed 15 Jan 2007

Arab American Institute (2010) Demographics. http://www.aaiusa.org/arab-americans/22/demographics. Accessed 15 Nov 2010

Bou Khalil R (2013) Attitudes, beliefs and perceptions regarding truth disclosure of cancer-related information in the Middle East: a review. Palliat Support Care 11(1):69–78

Chittem M, Butow P (2015) Responding to family requests for nondisclosure. The impact of the oncologist' cultural background. J Can Res Ther 11:174–180

Doumit MA, Abu-Saad HH (2008) Lebanese cancer patients: communication and truth-telling preferences. Contemp Nurse 28:74–82

Farhat F, Othman A, El Baba G, Kattan J (2015) Revealing a cancer diagnosis to patients: attitudes of patients, families, friends, nurses, and physicians in Lebanon-results of a cross sectional study. Curr Oncol 22(4):e264–e272

Hassouneh DM, Kulwicki A (2007) Mental health, discrimination, and trauma in Arab Muslim women living in the US: a pilot study. Ment Health Relig Cul 10(3):257–262

Hassouneh P, Kulwicki A (2009) Family privacy as protection village: a qualitative pilot study of mental illness in Arab-American Muslim women. In: Piedmont R, Village A (eds) Research in the social scientific study of religion. Brill, Boston, pp 195–216

Kulwicki A (2008a) Culture and ethnicity. In: Potter P, Perry A (eds) Fundamentals in nursing, 7th edn. CV. Mosby, St. Louis, pp 106–120

Kulwicki A (2008b) Patient education. In: Nasir LS, Abdul-Haq AK (eds) Caring for Arab patients: a biopsychosocial approach. Radcliffe Publishing, Oxford, pp 235–246

Kulwicki A (2011) Islam's influence on health in the family. In: Craft-Rosenberg M, Pehler S (eds) Encyclopedia of family health. Sage, Thousand Oaks, pp 676–678. https://doi.org/10.4135/9781412994071.n225

Kulwicki A, Ballout S (2013) People of Arab heritage. In: Purnell L, Paulanka B (eds) Transcultural health care, 3rd edn. F. A. Davis, Philadelphia

Kulwicki A, Miller J, Schim S (2000) Collaborative partnership for culture care: Enhancing health services for the Arab community. J Transcult Nurs 11(1):31–39

Kulwicki A, Aswad B, Carmona T, Ballout S (2010) Barriers in the utilization of domestic violence services among Arab immigrant women: perceptions of professionals, service providers & community leaders. J Fam Viol 25(8):727–735

Lawrence P, Rozmus C (2001) Culturally sensitive care of the Muslim patient. J Transcult Nurs 12:228–233

Naji F, Hamadeh G, Hlais S, Adib S (2015) Truth disclosure to cancer patients: shifting attitudes and practices of Lebanese physicians. AJOB Empir Bioeth 6(3):41–49

Pentheny O'kelly C, Urch C, Brown E (2011) The impact of culture and religion on truth telling at end of life. Nephrol Dial Transplant 26(12):3838–3842

Part VII

Guideline: Patient Advocacy and Empowerment

Advocacy and Empowerment of Individuals, Families and Communities

27

Dula Pacquiao

Guideline: *Nurses shall recognize the effect of healthcare policies, delivery systems, and resources on their patient populations and shall empower and advocate for their patients as indicated. Nurses shall advocate for the inclusion of their patient's cultural beliefs and practices in all dimensions of their healthcare when possible.*

Douglas et al. (2014: 113)

27.1 Introduction

In 1948, the UN General Assembly proclaimed the Universal Declaration of Human Rights (UDHR) in order to achieve peace in the world. *Human rights* are deemed as fundamental, universal, and inalienable rights of all people that need to be protected. UDHR upholds the inherent equality in dignity and rights of all human beings (Article 1) and protection from discrimination based on ascribed and acquired statuses (Article 2). The right to security, economic, and social and cultural rights are considered indispensable for development of human potential (Article 22). Article 25 proclaims the rights of individuals and their families to a standard of living adequate for health and well-being (e.g., food, clothing, housing, medical care, and necessary social services) and security in the event of unemployment, sickness, disability, widowhood, old age, or other circumstances beyond their control. Other articles have implications in the provision of care such as the right to privacy, education, and freedom of movement (UNHRC 1948).

Eleanor Roosevelt, who chaired the UN Commission that drafted the document, emphasized the ubiquity of the need for human rights protection in all places, such as home, school, work, and neighborhood, "such are the places where every man, woman, and child seeks equal justice, equal opportunity, and equal dignity without discrimination. Unless these rights have meaning there, they have little meaning anywhere." She underscored the responsibility of everyone for protecting these rights, "without concerted citizen action to uphold them close to home, we shall look in vain for progress in the larger world" (Roosevelt 1958).

27.2 Need for Advocacy

UDHR was the impetus for advocacy embodied in the definition of nursing and its code of ethics. The fundamental responsibilities of nursing to promote and optimize health, prevent illness and injury, and alleviate suffering are prescribed by the International Council of Nurses (ICN 2012) and the American Nurses Association (ANA 2010). The Preamble to ICN's Code of Ethics for Nurses states, "Inherent in nursing is a respect for human rights, including cultural rights, the right to life and choice, to dignity and to be treated with respect [regardless] of age, colour, creed, culture, disability or illness, gender,

D. Pacquiao, Ed.D., R.N., C.T.N-.A., T.N.S.
School of Nursing, Rutgers University, Newark, NJ, USA

School of Nursing, University of Hawaii, Hilo, Hilo, HI, USA

© Springer International Publishing AG, part of Springer Nature 2018
M. Douglas et al. (eds.), *Global Applications of Culturally Competent Health Care: Guidelines for Practice*, https://doi.org/10.1007/978-3-319-69332-3_27

sexual orientation, nationality, politics, race or social status" (ICN 2012: 2). It sets the obligation for nurses to advocate for equity and social justice in resource allocation, access to healthcare, and other social and economic services (ICN 2012). The American Nurses Association Code of Ethics (2015) stipulates that the nurse promotes, advocates for, and strives to protect the health, safety, and rights of the patient (Proposition 3) (Winland-Brown et al. 2015).

The need for advocacy is inherent in humans as social beings whose identities, shared meanings, and life experiences are shaped by the social arrangements of power and statuses (Rose 1990). Advocacy is needed as one's ability to compete, negotiate, and secure one's "place" in society is differentially structured by the social structural conditions. A particular individual's or group's "place" within the social order is patterned by factors such as race, gender, ethnicity, and socioeconomic status. These factors impact growth, development, and life chances not only of the present but also of future generations. Hence, one's "place" in society determines the degree of exposure to risks and social privileges one can enjoy.

There is ample evidence of health inequities attributed to social inequalities that create cumulative disadvantages in populations within local, national, and global contexts (see Chap. 1). Causes and effects of social inequalities in health maybe located mainly in the social structure and the environment or within the individual, but both are closely linked with each other. Individualistic explanations of health inequalities in terms of unhealthy lifestyles and choices continue to exist, but there is increasing evidence on the harmful impact on health of poverty, deprivation, and social exclusion at both individual and population levels (Wilkinson 1996; Davey Smith et al. 1999).

27.2.1 Definitions of Advocacy

Advocacy is a process of acting for or on behalf of others who are unable to do so for themselves (Bennett 1999). To advocate is to plead or sup-port a cause or position (Oxford Dictionary 2017). Central to advocacy is the concept of vulnerability or circumstances threatening a person's autonomy. Vulnerability can exist in an individual, families, communities, and populations. Although the role of patient advocate is often ascribed to helping professions such as nursing and social work involved in caring for the sick and vulnerable individuals, patient advocacy also includes the work of policymakers, legal professionals, and activists to improve healthcare for people marginalized by socially stigmatizing illnesses (Gilkey and Earp 2009).

27.2.1.1 Patient and Health Advocacy

In nursing, patient advocacy can be on behalf of an individual, family, community, group, or population (ICN 2012; Winland-Brown et al. 2015). Patient advocacy has evolved toward *health advocacy* to protect people who are vulnerable or discriminated against and empower those who need a stronger voice by enabling them to express their needs and make their own decisions (Carlisle 2000). According to the World Health Organization (1995), *advocacy for health* is a combination of individual and social actions to gain political commitment, policy support, social acceptance, and systems support for a particular health goal or program. Such action may be taken on behalf of individuals and groups to create life conditions conducive to health and the achievement of healthy lifestyles (Nutbeam 1998). Health promotion may be carried out without the intended recipient or recipients asking for it (Seedhouse 2004).

Health advocacy encompasses direct service to the individual or family as well as activities that promote health and access to healthcare in communities and the larger public. Advocates support and promote the rights of the patient in healthcare, help build capacity to improve community health, and enhance health policy initiatives focused on available, safe, and quality care. Health advocates are best suited to address the challenge of patient-centered care in our complex healthcare system. Today, advocates for the well-being of populations are needed. Health advocates are found working in a wide range of agencies and sectors striving to improve health of entire populations, defined communities or groups, and single individuals.

According to Rees (1991), health advocacy aims for protection of the vulnerable (representational advocacy) and empowerment of the disadvantaged (facilitational advocacy). *Representational advocacy* can take place at the level of both cases and causes. *Case advocacy* encompasses activities to represent the underprivileged, disadvantaged, or sick to promote their rights or redress power imbalances. *Cause advocacy* addresses the structural determinants of health inequities and barriers to health beyond the control of individuals. *Facilitational* advocacy promotes community participation and development as well as empowerment of disadvantaged individuals or groups to represent themselves and lobby for their own health needs (Rees 1991). Health advocacy may include challenging powerful anti-health interests such as the tobacco lobby; acting as a channel for mediating and negotiating between opposing forces in the interests of positive health; and forming coalitions to develop a common agenda and find mutually achievable goals.

27.2.1.2 Ethical and Moral Foundation of Advocacy

As discussed earlier, UDHR was influential in creating the movement for advocacy across disciplines and institutions. *Rights-based care* stems from the tenets of human rights emphasizing health as a basic right and access to quality and safe healthcare services. Healthcare providers are obligated to promote patient autonomy and the right to make informed choices (Entwistle et al. 2010). Advocacy has its roots in the *ethics of care* emphasizing interpersonal relationships and care or benevolence as central to moral action. Developed by feminists, this ethical theory also known as *care-focused feminism* is based on the assumptions that persons have varying degrees of dependence and interdependence on one another; the vulnerable deserve extra consideration based on their vulnerability; and the need to examine the situational contexts to safeguard and protect

the vulnerable (Gilligan 2008; Noddings 1984). Tronto (2012) identifies the four elements of ethical care as attentiveness, responsibility, competence, and responsiveness. Advocacy is built on a caring interpersonal relationship and a sense of obligation to care for others. It requires careful attention to the power relationships that influence the individual's well-being and affirmation of the responsiveness of care by the individual. Since the time of Florence Nightingale, the nursing profession has maintained its advocacy for providing a safe and caring environment that promotes the patient's health and well-being (Selanders and Crane 2012).

Advocacy is also founded on the principle of *justice* and *fairness* by ensuring that each person is given his or her due. Justice and fairness are closely related and often used interchangeably. Individuals should be treated the same, unless they differ in ways that are relevant to the situation in which they are involved (Velasquez et al. 1990). According to John Rawls (1971), the stability of a society depends upon the extent to which the members feel that they are being treated justly. Lack of fairness and unequal treatment have led to social unrest, disturbances, and strife.

Social justice is the fair and just relation between the individual and society. The principles of social justice provide a way of assigning rights and duties in the basic institutions of society and define the appropriate distribution of benefits and burdens of social cooperation (Rawls 1971). Social justice is measured by the distribution of wealth, opportunities, and social privileges as well as risks and disadvantages. The current global trend in social justice emphasizes breaking barriers to social mobility, creating safety nets, and economic and environmental justice. The movement from patient advocacy to health advocacy reflects the growing recognition that health equity is achieved through social structural changes and social justice to ameliorate the causes of cumulative disadvantages and vulnerability.

Presumably the outcome of advocacy is *beneficence* as it seeks remedies or solutions to promote health and well-being. However, Gadow (1989) argues for the difference between beneficence and advocacy. While both seem to establish their goal of promoting the patient's best interest, the practice of beneficence assumes that the professional knows with a greater accuracy and certainty what is in the patient's best interest. It is assumed that patients' subjective ability to define their own good is replaced by the professional's objective view. While in certain situations, some patients might prefer to trust the nurse to provide the most appropriate care when they feel unable to make informed decisions and feel empowered by trusting the care providers. But patients' autonomy may be threatened when they are unable or prevented from expressing their subjective views. There are concerns with advocates who assume a paternalistic role in constructing people as uninformed, ill-educated, and in need of the services of interventionists who know better (Carlisle 2000).

The risk of fostering dependency, alienation, and decreased autonomy among those advocated for is more likely to occur when the advocate assumes that decisions are for the patient's good without a full opportunity for a genuine relationship to develop that can foster mutuality and reciprocity of perspectives and goals. A paternalistic stance is tantamount to cultural imposition or imperialism. *Cultural imperialism* is the practice of promoting and imposing a culture, usually that of a politically powerful nation over a less powerful society, or by a dominant individual or group over others and subcultures (Lechner and Boli 2012). According to Leininger (1996) *cultural imposition* in patient care occurs when the values of the care provider are forced onto patients and their families. *Cultural hegemony* objectifies and disregards the subjective experiences of patients by medical professionals such as with vulnerable patients suffering from mental illness (Foucault 1980).

The paternalistic attitude of healthcare workers may exist because of limitations imposed by the setting and work constraints, and, thus, solutions are chosen for expedience and conflict avoidance. Power differences secondary to age, knowledge, and socioeconomic and cultural differences between the advocate and the patient can hinder development of trust and meaningful interactions (Murgic et al. 2015). Feminist theory and relational ethics emphasize that the nature of

the caring process should not only aim to prevent harm (*non-maleficence*) but more importantly transform life conditions to benefit the care recipient (*beneficence*). The latter is only possible when patients and populations are actively engaged in the process, allowing their own thoughts, emotions, and experiences to be fully integrated in the process and outcome of care.

27.3 Evolution of Empowerment

The concept of empowerment is associated with the work of the Brazilian philosopher and educator, Paulo Freire who advocated for *emancipatory education* to liberate the peasants from the shackles of poverty and oppression (Shor and Freire 1987). He viewed education as instrumental in transforming individuals and society. Freire proposed *critical pedagogy* as the process that allows active participation of learners in uncovering social inequalities and how these impact their lives. The development of *critical consciousness* (concientization) through education enables individuals to identify, examine, and act on the root causes of their oppression (Carroll and Minkler 2000). The role of the teacher is to engage students in active dialogue in order to question existing norms and power structure and critically examine how they create oppression. In *participatory education* students are not objects or passive recipients of knowledge from authorities but rather as authors and creators of knowledge. This state of critical consciousness allows students to engage in active dialogue and participate in identifying problems and innovative solutions to change oppressive circumstances. The role of the teacher is not a giver of facts to be memorized by students but rather as a facilitator for awakening students' consciousness and enable them to critically examine facts in light of their own experiences and observations. Critical consciousness is prerequisite to *praxis* or practices that can transform their lives and society. Individual empowerment can only flourish when one's feelings of liberation is shared by others in society. Freire emphasized the need for individual and community empowerment (Carroll and Minkler 2000).

Empowerment in health has been given impetus by the Ottawa Charter for Health Promotion (WHO 1986). *Health promotion* is defined as the process of enabling people to increase their control over and to improve their health. *Health* is viewed as a resource for everyday life emphasizing social and personal resources, as well as physical capacities. To reach a state of complete physical and social well-being, an individual or group must be able to identify and realize their aspirations, satisfy their needs, and change or cope with their environment.

The Ottawa Charter (WHO 1986) identified the three major strategies for health promotion: (1) advocacy for resources favorable to health including political, economic, social, cultural, and environmental resources as well as behavioral and biological changes; (2) enablement or empowerment of individuals and groups to control the determinants that affect their health in order to reach the highest attainable quality of life; and (3) mediation through multisectoral and multilevel collaboration by all sectors of government, organizations, and communities. In other words, *empowerment* is the process through which an individual or people gain greater control over decisions and actions affecting their health; it is both an individual and a community process (WHO 2009).

Seedhouse (2004) differentiates medical from social health promotion. *Medical health promotion* seeks to prevent or ameliorate disease, illness, and injury based on scientific evidence. By contrast, *social health promotion* seeks to change the world and challenge the injustices that cause ill-health by improving the lives of the least well-off members of society. Seedhouse recommends using a variety of approaches as well as flexibility in using different strategies to promote health.

Unlike advocacy that tends to be more aligned with the health provider or advocate, empowerment is more oriented toward the patient's point of view (WHO 2009), thus more patient-centered. Empowerment is both a process and an outcome; it is considered an outcome of advocacy. Since empowerment involves active engagement and participation by individuals and communities, they achieve greater autonomy, capacity, and self-efficacy in improving their health and well-

being. There is greater likelihood for sustainable outcomes through empowerment because it builds individual and community capacity for health achievement. According to Rappaport (1984), empowerment links individual strengths and competencies, support systems, and proactive behaviors to social policy and social change.

27.3.1 Types of Empowerment

27.3.1.1 Patient Empowerment

Patient empowerment is a process in which patients understand their role and are given the knowledge and skills by their healthcare provider to perform a task in an environment that recognizes community and cultural differences and encourages patient participation (WHO 2009). Patient empowerment puts the patient in the heart of services. It is about designing and delivering health and social care services in a way that is inclusive and enables citizens to take control of their healthcare needs (European Network on Patient Empowerment/ENOPE 2014). Patient empowerment is a process designed to facilitate self-directed behavior change (Anderson and Funnell 2010).

Kaldoudi and Makris (2015) describe patient empowerment as a cognitive process with three levels. At the first level, patients need to develop awareness of their health status, health-related risks, and measures to stay healthy and prevent illness. The second level is the stage of active participation characterized by active engagement in the healthcare process, seeking feedback, managing illness and comorbidities, and accessing appropriate resources. At the third level, patients are able to control their health by collaborating in decision-making with healthcare providers, participating in shared decision-making, and reframing mind-sets to adapt to new situations.

There are four components fundamental to the process of patient empowerment: (1) understanding by patients of their role, (2) acquisition by patients of sufficient knowledge to be able to engage with their healthcare provider, (3) acquisition of relevant skills such as managing illness, and (4) presence of a facilitating environment (WHO 2009).

27.3.1.2 Community Empowerment

Wallerstein and Bernstein (1994) prefer *community empowerment* because it is a social action process by which interactions occur in the social context of human relationships at home, communities, and institutions. Community empowerment is both a process and an outcome in which individuals and groups act to gain mastery over their lives in the context of changing their social and political environment. Institutions and communities become transformed as people who participate in changing them become transformed. Rather than putting individuals against community and overall societal needs, community empowerment focuses on both individual and community change. Community empowerment is a basis for healthcare reform as individuals are connected and engage with others in the community to identify common problems, goals, and strategies for personal and social capacity building to transform their lives (Wallerstein and Bernstein 1994). The Ottawa Charter for Health Promotion (WHO 1986) recognizes the significance of patient and community empowerment in transforming health of individuals and populations.

27.3.2 Challenges in Advocacy and Empowerment

There are issues and challenges in community empowerment. Individual autonomy maybe threatened when efforts are focused on what benefits the group or community. In mixed groups, less powerful individuals may have less autonomy than dominant groups. Different perspectives must be represented, and individuals should be allowed to fully express their opinions during interactions. Health workers should promote open dialogue and foster mutual trust and reciprocity among participants. Individual contributions should be recognized along with the group's accomplishments.

Health workers may not be prepared for effective advocacy and empowerment that requires training and expertise. Advocates should have knowledge of the community, history of the problem and the people, relevant policies and programs, decision-making infrastructure, and potential resources and partners. Advocacy requires a set of skills including problem-solving, communication, influencing, and collaboration needed to successfully support a cause or interest on one's own behalf or that of another (Tomajan 2012).

Existing power differences can impair open dialogue and individual expression. Power differences may exist among family members, between patients and health workers, between genders, and among community members. Health workers should be aware of their own social status and influence on the social hierarchy of the group. Culturally appropriate mediation and negotiation should be applied to create a more equitable distribution of power and allow the vulnerable to be heard. Coalitions among groups seeking similar remedies may be formed to counterbalance more powerful individuals and groups.

Sustaining long-term commitment and engagement of participants is problematic as social problems are not likely to have immediate solutions. Developing mutual trust, consensus, and commitment among diverse individuals and groups takes time. The leadership role of facilitators and advocates is important in developing realistic goals that can be implemented, keeping participants on track, and maintaining communication and interest in the project. Adequate resources are needed to support group participation and engagement over time.

27.3.3 Studies on Patient Empowerment

Studies on patient empowerment use a variety of related terms such as patient engagement, self-management, activation, participation, confidence, and shared decision-making. Several studies have noted the lack of consensus on the concept of empowerment and how it is operationalized (McAllister et al. 2012). Although a number of guiding principles and values of empowerment exist, there is no well-articulated theory of empowerment (Aujoulat et al. 2006). Empowerment studies are difficult to compare because of the ambiguity in the outcomes being measured which also limits the development of valid and reliable instruments (Barr et al. 2015; Salmon and Hall 2004). However, there is substantial evidence to support the development of core constructs and strategies of empowerment (Coulter and Ellins 2007). Studies have also shown that it is both a process and an outcome with a range of possible outcomes to be a viable public health strategy (Wallerstein 2006).

27.3.3.1 Patient Empowerment Process and Outcomes

Several studies revealed that increased patient participation in the health process was associated with patients' favorable judgments about the hospital and the quality of care they received. Patient participation was associated with reduced risk of adverse events among patients (Weingart et al. 2011). Significant changes in the provision of care across different care settings were attributed to increased participation (Crawford et al. 2002). Nygardh et al. (2012) found that shared decision-making between providers and patients improved healthcare quality and patient satisfaction.

When patients are given good-quality decision aids, they are more informed and participate more in decision-making (O'Connor et al. 2009). Patient education programs teaching self-management skills are more effective in improving clinical outcomes than giving only information (Bodenheimer et al. 2002). When patients gain knowledge about their health, they gain more confidence (Ludman et al. 2013), become more motivated and self-determined, and communicate more freely their health concerns and preferences with their providers (Chen et al. 2014). Improving patient health literacy and engagement enables them to select treatments, manage chronic conditions, increase drug safety and infection control, enhance utilization of health services, and improve health outcomes (Coulter and Ellins 2007). The use of prompts and reminders to perform specific tasks related to care is associated with significant improvement in illness control by patients (Weingarten et al. 2002).

Effective self-management skills can improve patient self-efficacy and reduce healthcare costs (Wallerstein 2006) because of fewer outpatient visits and hospital admissions (Holman and Lorig

2004; Muenchberger and Kendall 2010). Patients with chronic illness who have greater capacity for self-care are more likely to adhere to the therapeutic regimen, maintain healthy behaviors, monitor their symptoms, make self-care decisions, manage their emotions, and improve their communication with their healthcare provider (Inglis et al. 2010; Peytremann-Bridevaux et al. 2015). Studies of patient empowerment to improve chronic disease care management in general practice and primary care have revealed increased satisfaction of both patients and professionals, greater adherence to treatment guidelines, and improved clinical outcomes (Collins and Rochfort 2016; Mola 2013). Self-care interventions for long-term conditions improve mental health, care provider-patient communication, healthy eating, and patient self-efficacy (Lorig et al. 2009).

27.3.3.2 Barriers and Facilitators of Patient Empowerment

Patient participation is codetermined by the patient and the healthcare provider and occurs only through reciprocal dialogue and shared decision-making (Thompson 2006). Patient-provider communication characterized by open communication and collaborative treatment goal setting significantly improves patient engagement (Hearld and Alexander 2012). Provider-related factors that affect patient participation include patient-provider relationship, recognition of patients' knowledge, and allocation of sufficient time for interaction with the patient. Patient-related factors include level of knowledge, physical and cognitive ability, emotional connections with provider, and differences in beliefs, values, and experiences with healthcare (Vahdat et al. 2014).

Henderson (2003) found unwillingness by nurses to delegate power and control to their patients. Control can be exerted by asking closed-ended questions, limiting depth of information shared, fostering patient uncertainty, using authoritative and condescending language, or being untruthful (Johnson et al. 2007). Nurses in an Iranian hospital identified the following barriers to patient advocacy: their subordinate status in the organizational and social hierarchy resulting in feelings of powerlessness, lack of support from administrators and physicians, laws, code of ethics, limited communication, insufficient time, and risks associated with advocacy (Negarandeh et al. 2006). Physicians' reluctance to encourage patient participation may be due to fear of losing power and control or losing their identity (Ford et al. 2002; O'Flynn and Britten 2006). Primary care physicians tend to allow more patient participation than other specialists (Bettes et al. 2007).

A significant factor in improving patient outcomes is maximizing patient self-management. Other factors include increasing clinician's expertise and skill in educating and supporting patients, team-based care delivery, and effective use of technology (Renders et al. 2001). Health professional training in empowerment is associated with better acceptance, implementation, and effectiveness of patient self-management programs (Lawn and Schoo 2010).

27.3.3.3 Empowerment of Racially/ Ethnically Diverse Patients

Patient engagement levels differ by race and ethnicity. African Americans and Latinos have lower level of engagement than Whites (Cunningham et al. 2011) which impact engagement in wellness and prevention (IOM 2002). Compared to Whites, racial and ethnic minorities assume a relatively passive role in healthcare and are less willing to participate in care decisions (Sandman et al. 2012).

Racial and ethnic minorities are more likely to experience stress from unemployment, poverty, limited healthcare access, or single parenthood (Macartney et al. 2013). Latinos' lower activation and empowerment may reflect their limited access to healthcare (Cunningham et al. 2011) and type of health insurance (Hibbard et al. 2008). Out-of-pocket cost sharing with health insurance can influence a patient's willingness to seek treatment and adhere to the plan of care (Carman et al. 2013; Korda and Eldridge 2012). In addition to adequate insurance coverage (Vargas-Bustamante and Chen 2011), the feeling of being valued in the interaction (James 2013) can increase patients' confidence and empowerment (Cunningham et al. 2011).

Latinos and African Americans report worse patient-provider relationships and communication and are less likely to initiate health behaviors and adhere to treatment than Whites (Wang et al. 2003). Minority patients are less likely to have opportunities to ask questions during provider visits, receive less information on their treatments, and are less likely to be consulted for their preferences in treatment decisions (Link and Phelan 1995). Compared to Whites, African Americans have significantly smaller social networks (Shaw and Krause 2001). Many racial and ethnic minorities reside in neighborhoods with limited social and public services and facilities with high prevalence of violence and poverty. Residents suffer from chronic stress of everyday life that impacts their level of motivation and belief in achieving a healthy life (Williams et al. 2012). Racial and language concordance can promote trusting relationship between patients and providers (Vargas-Bustamante and Chen 2011). Culturally tailored community-based patient education (Alegría et al. 2009) and programs reducing language barriers can effectively engage minorities in their care (Flores 2006).

27.3.4 Studies on Community Empowerment

Wallerstein (2006) cites outcomes of global initiatives of WHO on empowerment in some countries in Latin America, Africa, and Asia. Youth empowerment has strengthened self and collective efficacy and improved mental health and school performance. In addition, there is stronger group bonding, formation of suitable youth groups, and increased youth participation in structured activities for social action and policy changes. Empowerment of HIV/AIDS-affected populations has addressed disease prevention and improved capacity of women and their families to manage the illness. Women empowerment has created movement toward gender equality and initiatives integrating economic, educational, and political empowerment for environmental and policy changes.

Souliotis et al. (2016) examined participation by patient associations in Cyprus and found that they had greater involvement in consultations with health-related organizations and policy reforms and the Ministry of Health. However, they were much less involved with health institutions such as hospitals, ethics committees, clinical trials, and health technology assessment.

27.4 Culturally Competent Empowerment

Healthcare reforms and health promotion require transformation of individuals and society. Empowered individuals are key to transforming populations and communities (Freire 2000); sustainable institutionalized reforms require broad efforts through multisectoral and multilevel collaboration among different sectors of government, organizations, individuals, and communities (WHO 1986). According to Leininger, *culturally congruent and competent care* is a culturally meaningful way to support, facilitate, or enable patients to regain health or help them face disability or death (McFarland and Wehbe-Alamah 2015). Human beings are social beings; hence, empowerment should be informed by the social and cultural contexts of people's lives.

Rose and Black (1985) described the process of empowerment based on three principles. The principles are apropos to understanding the process of culturally competent empowerment. The first principle, *contextualization*, aims to understand the individual's reality by unraveling perceptions, feelings, and interpretations of their experiences. The role of health workers is to engage them to describe their experiences within the context of their interactions, relationships, and other events. Through empathic listening and keen observations, individuals are supported in externalizing their problem by linking their experiences with factors such as poverty, discrimination, environmental deprivation, cul-

tural taboos, etc. Externalization allows the discovery of the root cause of the problem outside of one's biology and behaviors.

The second principle, *empowerment*, encourages individuals to identify a range of possible solutions to the problem. Contradictory solutions are likely to emerge and healthcare workers should welcome them as a problem can have different solutions. Social problems generally have no permanent solutions (Rappaport 1981). The role of the healthcare provider is to engage them to critically examine these remedies to determine the benefits, likelihood of success, and other resources needed to achieve them. Healthcare providers should validate individuals' identity by affirming their ideas, strengths, and abilities.

The third principle, *collectivity*, focuses on defining the sociocultural basis of individuals' identity and experiences to reduce feelings of fear, isolation, powerlessness, and hopelessness. Social networks are developed by connecting individuals with support groups in the community. Socialization with others who have similar experiences can lead to identification of more effective solutions and group-oriented actions for change. The role of healthcare providers is to foster horizontal interdependence focused on concrete needs such as housing, food, medical care, and emotional support and encourage individuals to critically reflect on common and contrasting experiences. Collectivity fosters social development that can bring about social change and transformation (Rose and Black 1985).

27.4.1 Culturally Competent Advocacy and Empowerment Strategies

Table 27.1 presents selected strategies using the principles outlined by Rose and Black (1985). Selected strategies are organized according to the different levels of advocacy and empowerment, which include individual/family, organizational/ institutional, and community levels.

Table 27.1 Culturally competent advocacy and empowerment strategies

Principle	Individual/family level	Organizational level	Community level
Contextualization	• Introduce yourself and the purpose of the interaction, emphasizing the importance of the individual/family's participation in the entire process. • Engage in dialogue to determine the individual/family's goals, perceptions, and shared meanings about the problems. • Demonstrate respect and genuineness in interactions (not rushing, listening, using appropriate distance, communicating empathy, etc.). • Observe influence of family social hierarchy on individual decision-making and behaviors. • Promote awareness of the problem using culturally and linguistically appropriate communication and learning strategies. • Facilitate individual/family assessment of social and cultural factors that contribute to the problem (income, education, housing, environment, kinship, literacy, language, race, ethnicity, religion, gender, age, ethnohistory, etc.). • Facilitate assessment by individual and family of existing resources and support systems.	• Promote employee awareness of the population and community being served (ethnohistory, SES, and cultural values and practices relevant to health and caring). • Increase staff awareness of social and cultural factors that hamper healthcare delivery and health promotion for the population. • Assess organizational capacity for addressing needs of the population (religious, language, signage, telephone answering system, educational materials, social services, gender and age specific, dietary, visiting policies, schedule of services, community outreach, navigators, advocates, etc.). • Assess degree of representation of community and population groups in organizational decisions. • Assess accessibility and affordability of services to disadvantaged groups.	• Identify community leaders and gatekeepers for potential partnership and collaboration. • Engage community leaders and stakeholders in identifying health-related issues. • Ensure fair representation of population groups in health assessment. • Collaborate with scientific and academic community to identify impact of local, regional, and federal policies/programs on population health. • Promote awareness of social and cultural issues that influence population health. • Increase awareness of community of common health issues and factors contributing to the problems. • Promote community awareness of how decisions are made in the community and the people responsible for services they need (senior housing, garbage collection, recreation, police, schools, hospitals, etc.).
Empowerment	• Work with established family hierarchy in developing priority goals and plan of action. • Use cultural mediation/negotiation to ensure that individual members' ideas and aspirations are considered by the group. • Use culturally and linguistically appropriate (*congruent may not be appropriate but appropriate includes congruent*) teaching strategies to promote knowledge and skills of the individual and family. • Use available technology and teaching materials at the level of understanding and capacity of the individual/family. • Link individual and family with resources and support systems in the community (ethnic associations, ethnic grocery stores, churches, legal advocates, social services, support groups, ethnic health practitioners etc.).	• Provide training for multidisciplinary staff and leadership on culturally competent care, social determinants of health, and vulnerable population health. • Restructure services to enhance access and utilization of services by disadvantaged populations (language services, dietary menus, etc.). • Establish incentives for culturally competent care delivery. • Create staff champions to assist other personnel in culturally competent care. • Ensure representation of disadvantaged populations in organizational governance.	• Organize community collaboratives and partnerships to work on specific initiatives. • Identify potential leaders who will organize and coordinate efforts for change. • Seek experts to provide information and talking points to be presented to policy makers. • Provide training on a variety of possible actions targeting specific causes. • Provide information on specific persons, offices, and leaders to present proposals for change. • Seek funding from community stakeholders and public and private organizations.

	• Seek community members with similar background to assist the individual and family in navigating the healthcare system. • Facilitate access to community resources by the individual and family (carpooling, senior transport, handicap transport services, bus and train schedule, etc.). • Provide training to improve individual/family capacity to access services in the community (using phones, internet, EHRs, etc.).	• Establish systems for evaluating outcomes of culturally competent care delivery. • Establish a dedicated structure/personnel for advocacy and empowerment of vulnerable patients and families.	• Develop a schedule of events, activities, and media coverage of community initiatives.
Collectivity	• Connect individuals and family with community groups with similar interests and engaged in seeking solutions to similar problems (churches, ethnic organization, workers' union, and local politicians and bureaucrats interested in their cause). • Provide contact information of community members with specific expertise and resources for dealing with certain problems. • Provide contact information of specific service providers and organizations in the community. • Improve capacity of individuals and families in reaching out to community members and services (police, emergency services, local media, medical providers, hospitals, etc.).	• Establish incentives for employee engagement in community health promotion. • Develop initiatives for health promotion in vulnerable communities such as health fairs, mobile clinics, health education in community settings, etc. • Restructure services to maximize access by vulnerable populations to outpatient clinics using more user-friendly scheduling. • Recruit and train potential interpreters and translators from the community. • Ensure availability of language support at all times. • Develop partnerships with local community groups working on health initiatives.	• Seek multisectoral and multilevel representation of public and private organization along with community members in health promotion. • Promote sustained commitment by maintaining communication with the community, leaders, partners, and collaborators. • Use community gatekeepers and ethnic leaders to maintain enthusiasm of their members. • Disseminate progress and outcomes of initiatives through local and ethnic media as well as places frequently visited by community members. • Create a systematic and permanent structure for coordinating activities from start to finish.

Source: Rose SM, Black BL (1985) Advocacy and empowerment: Mental health care in the community. London: Routledge & Kegan Paul Ltd.

Conclusion

Advocacy and empowerment are used together in this chapter. Both are processes aimed to amplify the voices of individuals, families, and communities into the health process in order to assure their participation and engagement in their health and well-being. While empowerment is an outcome of advocacy, empowerment is both a process and an outcome. Among vulnerable populations, it is critical that advocacy and empowerment for individuals and families are linked with social reforms. Social determinants of poor health are addressed at the macrosocial level through policies. Advocacy for health in every policy will more effectively minimize health inequity.

The challenge for culturally competent advocacy and empowerment is bridging the gap in between individuals and society. The disadvantaged and most vulnerable populations in society tend to be those who belong to subcultures or minority groups. Empowerment starts with increasing awareness of the close links between individual level vulnerability and societal arrangements of power and distribution of resources. When power is limited at the individual, family, and community levels, advocacy and empowerment must occur through broad-based coalitions and commitments for the same cause. While diversity is a virtue, coalitions are founded on the finding a common ground, common understanding, and commitment to the cause. Externalization and contextualization of the individual's experiences can foster a common understanding of the root cause of vulnerability across different groups. Right to health and access to quality care for all can only occur when sustained empowerment and mutual respect for human dignity can generate health and social reforms.

Advocacy and empowerment are built on an emotional attachment to the moral obligation of justice and fairness. We need to build knowledge of the similarities and differences between ourselves and others. Knowing the other more fully allows us to uncover the pathway between social inequality and health inequity, and to understand how we can harness cultural diversity to strengthen bonds and interdependence among people, and comprehend the broader social and cultural contexts in which we live and work. Advocacy and empowerment require a set of skills communication, problem-solving, motivating others, leadership, change process, coalition building, maintaining sustainable collaborations, policy making, etc. Most significantly is nurturing an attitude of empathy, other centeredness, care, and respect for others.

References

Alegría M, Scribney W, Perez D et al (2009) The role of patient activation on patient provider communication and quality of care for US and foreign born Latino patients. J Intern Med 24:534–541

ANA (2010) Scope and standards of practice. In: Code of ethics for nurses with interpretive statements, 2nd edn. Author, Silver Spring

ANA (2015) Code of ethics for nurses with interpretive statements. Nursesbooks.org, Silver Spring

Anderson RM, Funnell MM (2010) Patient empowerment: myths and misconceptions. Patient Educ Couns 79(3):277–282. https://doi.org/10.1016/j.pec.2009.07.025

Aujoulat I, d'Hoore W, Deccache A (2006) Patient empowerment in theory and practice: polysemy or cacophony? Patient Educ Couns. https://doi.org/10.1016/j.pec.2006.09.008

Barr PJ, Scholl I, Bravo P et al (2015) Assessment of patient empowerment – a systematic review of measures. PLoS One 10(5):e0126553. https://doi.org/10.1371/journal.pone.0126553

Bennett O (1999) Advocacy in nursing. Nurs Stand 14(11):40–41

Bettes BA, Coleman VH, Zinberg S et al (2007) Cesarean delivery on maternal request: obstetrician-gynecologists' knowledge, perception, and practice patterns. Obstet Gynecol 109(1):57–66

Bodenheimer T, Lorig K, Holman H et al (2002) Patient self-management of chronic disease in primary care. JAMA 288(19):2469–2475

Carlisle S (2000) Health promotion, advocacy and health inequalities: a conceptual framework. Health Promot Int 15(4):369–376

Carman KL, Dardess P, Maurer M et al (2013) Patient and family engagement: a framework for understanding the elements and developing interventions and policies. Health Aff 32:223–231. [PubMed: 23381514]

Carroll J, Minkler M (2000) Freire's message for social workers: looking back, looking ahead. J Commun Pract 8(1):21–36

Chen J, Mortensen K, Bloodworth R (2014) Exploring contextual factors and patient activation: evidence from a nationally representative sample of patients with depression. Health Educ Behav 41:614–624. [PubMed: 24786791]

Collins C, Rochfort A (2016) Promoting self-management and patient empowerment in primary care. In: Capelli O (ed) Primary care in practice-integration is needed. INTECHOpen.com, Croatia, pp 27–42. https://doi.org/10.5772/62763

Coulter A, Ellins J (2007) Effectiveness of strategies for informing, educating, and involving patients. BMJ 335:24–27

Crawford D, Rutter MJ, Manley C et al (2002) Systematic review of involving patients in the planning and development of health care. BMJ 325:1–5

Cunningham P, Hibbard J, Gibbons C (2011) Raising low 'patient activation' rates among Hispanic immigrants may equal expanded coverage in reducing access disparities. Health Aff 30:1888–1894. [PubMed: 21976331]

Davey Smith G, Dorling D, Gordon D et al (1999) The widening health gap: what are the solutions? Crit Public Health 9(2):151–170

Douglas MK, Rosenkotter M, Pacquiao DF, Callister LC, Hattar-Pollara M, Lauderdale J, Milstead J, Nardi D, and Purnell L (2014) Guidelines for implemenbting culturally competent nursing care. J Transcult Nurs 25(2):109–121. https://doi.org/1177/1043659614520998

Entwistle VA, Carter SM, Crib A et al (2010) Supporting autonomy: the importance of clinician-patient relationships. J Gen Intern Med 25(7):741–745

European Network on Patient Empowerment (ENOPE) (2014) About patient empowerment. Available at http://www.enope.eu/patient-empowerment.aspx

Flores G (2006) Language barriers to health care in the United States. N Engl J Med 355:229–231. [PubMed: 16855260]

Ford S, Schofield T, Hope T (2002) Barriers to the evidence-based patient choice (EBPC) consultation. Patient Educ Couns 47(2):179–185

Foucault M (1980) Power/knowledge: selected interviews and other writings, 1962-1977. Knopf Doubleday, New York

Freire P (2000) Pedagogy of the oppressed, 30th edn. Bloomsbury Academic, New York

Gadow S (1989) Clinical subjectivity. Advocacy with silent patients. Nurs Clin North Am 24(2):535–541

Gilkey MB, Earp JA (2009) Defining patient advocacy in the post-quality chasm era. N C Med J 70(2):120–124

Gilligan C (2008) Moral orientation and moral development. In: Bailey A, Cuomo CJ (eds) The feminist philosophy reader. McGraw Hill, Boston, pp 463–466

Hearld LR, Alexander JA (2012) Patient-centered care and emergency department utilization a path analysis of the mediating effects of care coordination and delays in care. Med Care Res Rev 69:560–580. [PubMed: 22813721]

Henderson S (2003) Power imbalance between nurses and patients: a potential inhibitor of partnership in care. J Clin Nurs 12(4):501–508

Hibbard JH, Greene J, Becker ER et al (2008) Racial/ethnic disparities and consumer activation in health. Health Aff 27:1442–1453. [PubMed: 18780935]

Holman H, Lorig K (2004) Patient self-management: a key to effectiveness and efficiency in care of chronic disease. Public Health Rep 119(3):239–243

Inglis S, Clark R, Mcalister FA et al (2010) Structured telephone support or telemonitoring programmes for patients with chronic heart failure. Cochrane Database Syst Rev. https://doi.org/10.1002/14651858.CD007228.pub2

Institute of Medicine/IOM (2002) Unequal treatment: confronting racial and ethnic disparities in health care. National Academies Press, Washington, DC

International Council for Nurses (ICN) (2012) The ICN code of ethics for nurses. Author, Geneva. Available at: http://jimbergmd.com/Way%20of%20Barefoot%20Doctoring/WEB%20way%20of%20bfd/nurses%20code%20of%20ethics.pdf

James J (2013) Patient engagement. People actively involved in their health and health care tend to have better outcomes—and, some evidence suggests, lower costs. Health Affairs, pp 1–6

Johnson M, Haigh C, Yates-Bolton N (2007) Valuing of altruism and honesty in nursing students: a two-decade replication study. J Adv Nurs 57(4):366–374

Kaldoudi E, Makris N (2015) Patient empowerment as a cognitive process. In: Verdier C, Bienkiewicz M, Fred A, et al (eds) The proceedings of HealthInf 2015: 8th international conference on health informatics, Lisbon, Portugal, pp 605–610. ISBN: 978-989-758-068-0

Korda H, Eldridge GN (2012) Payment incentives and integrated care delivery: levers for health system reform and cost containment. Inquiry 48:277–287. [PubMed: 22397058]

Lawn S, Schoo A (2010) Supporting self-management of chronic health conditions: common approaches. Patient Educ Couns 80(2):205–211. https://doi.org/10.1016/j.pec.2009.10.006

Lechner FJ, Boli J (2012) The globalization reader, 5th edn. Routledge, London

Leininger M (1996) Culture care theory, research, and practice. Nurs Sci Q 9(2):71–78

Link BG, Phelan J (1995) Social conditions as fundamental causes of disease. Journal of Health and Social Behavior, Extra Issue, pp 80–94

Lorig K, Ritter PL, Villa FJ et al (2009) Community-based peer-led diabetes self-management: a randomized trial. Diabetes Educ 35:641–651. https://doi.org/10.1177/0145721709335006. PMID: 19407333

Ludman E, Peterson D, Katon W et al (2013) Improving confidence for self-care in patients with depression and chronic illnesses. Behav Med 39:1–6. [PubMed: 23398269]

Macartney S, Bishaw A, Fontenot K (2013) Poverty rates for selected detailed race and Hispanic groups by state and place: 2007–2011. American Community Survey Briefs. Available at: http://www.census.gov/prod/2013pubs/acsbr11-17.pdf 2014

McAllister M, Dunn G, Payne K et al (2012) Patient empowerment: the need to consider it as a measurable patient-reported outcome for chronic conditions. BMC Health Serv Res 12:157. PMID: 22694747

McFarland MR, Wehbe-Alamah HB (2015) Leininger's culture care diversity and universality: a worldwide nursing theory. Jones and Bartlett, Burlington

Mola E (2013) Patient empowerment, an additional characteristic of the European definitions of general practice/family medicine. Eur J Gen Pract 19(2):128–131. https://doi.org/10.3109/13814788.2012.756866

Muenchberger H, Kendall E (2010) Predictors of preventable hospitalization in chronic disease: priorities for change. J Public Health Policy 31(2):150–163. https://doi.org/10.1057/jphp.2010.3

Murgic L, Hebert PC, Sovic S et al (2015) Patient autonomy: views of patients and providers in transitional (post-communist) country. BMC Med Ethics 16:65. https://doi.org/10.1186/12910-015-0059-z

Negarandeh R, Oskouie F, Ahmadi F et al (2006) Patient advocacy: barriers and facilitators. BMC Nurs 5:3. https://doi.org/10.1186/1472-6955-53

Noddings N (1984) Caring: a feminine approach to ethics and moral education. UC Berkeley, Berkeley

Nutbeam D (1998) Health promotion glossary. Health Promot Int 13(4):349–364

Nygardh A, Malm D, Wikby K et al (2012) The experience of empowerment in the patient-staff encounter: the patient's perspective. J Clin Nurs 21:897–904. [PubMed: 22081948]

O'Connor AM, Bennett CL, Stacey D et al (2009) Decision aids for people facing health treatment or screening decisions. Cochrane Database Syst Rev (3):CD001431

O'Flynn N, Britten N (2006) Does the achievement of medical identity limit the ability of primary care practitioners to be patient-centred? A qualitative study. Patient Educ Couns 60(1):49–56

Oxford Dictionary (2017) Advocate. Available at https://en.oxforddictionaries.com/definition/advocacy

Peytremann-Bridevaux I, Arditi C, Gex G et al (2015) Chronic disease management programmes for adults with asthma. Cochrane Database Syst Rev. https://doi.org/10.1002/14651858.CD007988.pub2

Rappaport J (1981) In praise of paradox: a social policy of empowerment over prevention. Am J Commun Psychol 4:1–25

Rappaport J (1984) Studies in empowerment: Introduction to the issue. Prev Hum Serv 3:1–7

Rawls J (1971) A theory of justice. Harvard University Press, Boston

Rees S (1991) Achieving power: practice and policy in social welfare. Allen & Unwin, St. Leonards

Renders CM, Valk GD, Griffin S et al (2001) Interventions to improve the management of diabetes mellitus in primary care, outpatient and community settings. Cochrane Database Syst Rev (1):CD001481. PMID: 11279717

Roosevelt E (1958) Excerpt of speech at the UN, NYC in your hands: a guide for community action for the tenth anniversary of the Universal Declaration of Human Rights March 27. Available at http://www.eduplace.com/kids/socsci/nyc/books/bke/sources/bkd_template.jsp?name=roosevelte&bk=bkd&state=ny

Rose SM (1990) Advocacy/empowerment: an approach to clinical practice for social work. J Sociol Soc Welf 17(2):Article 5. Available at: http://scholarworks.wmich.edu/jssw/vol17/iss2/5. Accessed 28 March 2017

Rose SM, Black BL (1985) Advocacy and empowerment: mental health care in the community. Routledge & Kegan Paul, London

Salmon P, Hall GM (2004) Patient empowerment or the emperor's new clothes. J R Soc Med 97:53–56

Sandman L, Granger BB, Ekman I et al (2012) Adherence, shared decision-making and patient autonomy. Med Health Care Philos 15:115–127

Seedhouse D (2004) Health promotion: philosophy, prejudice and practice. Wiley, Chichester

Selanders LC, Crane PC (2012) The voice of Florence Nightingale on advocacy. Online J Issue Nursing 17. Available at http://www.nursingworld.org/MainMenuCategories/ANAMarketplace/ANAPeriodicals/OJIN/TableofContents/Vol-17-2012/No1-Jan-2012/Florence-Nightingale-on-Advocacy.html

Shaw BA, Krause N (2001) Exploring race variations in aging and personal control. J Gerontol B Psychol Sci Soc Sci 56:S119–S124

Shor I, Freire P (1987) A pedagogy for liberation: dialogues in transforming education. Bergin and Garvey, South Hadley

Souliotis K, Agapidaki E, Evangelia L et al (2016) Assessing patient participation in health policy decision making in Cyprus. Int J Health Policy Manag 5(8):461–466

Thompson AGH (2006) The meaning of patient involvement and participation in health care consultations: a taxonomy. Soc Sci Med 64:1297–1310

Tomajan K (2012) Advocating for nurses and nursing. Online J Issue Nurs 17. Available at http://www.nursingworld.org/MainMenuCategories/ANAMarketplace/ANAPeriodicals/OJIN/TableofContents/Vol-17-2012/No1-Jan-2012/Advocating-for-Nurses.html

Tronto JC (2012) Partiality based on relational responsibilities: another approach to global ethics. Eth Soc Welf special issue: gender justice. Taylor & Francis 6(3):303–316. https://doi.org/10.1080/17496535.2012.704058. Accessed 29 March 2017

UNHRC (1948) Universal declaration of human rights. Available at http://www.ohchr.org/EN/UDHR/Pages/Language.aspx?LangID=eng

Vahdat S, Hamzehgardeshi L, Hessam S et al (2014) Patient involvement in health care decision making: a review. Iran Red Cres Med J 16(1):e12454. https://doi.org/10.5812/ircmj.12454

Vargas-Bustamante A, Chen J (2011) Physicians cite hurdles ranging from lack of coverage to poor communication in providing high quality care to Latino patients. Health Affairs 30:1921–1929. [PubMed: 21976336]

Velasquez M, Andre C, Shanks T et al (1990) Justice and fairness. Available at https://www.scu.edu/ethics/ethics-resources/ethical-decision-making/justice-and-fairness/

Wallerstein N (2006) What is the evidence on effectiveness of empowerment to improve health? WHO Regional Office for Europe. Health Evidence Network report, Copenhagen. Available at: http://www.euro.who.int/Document/E88086.pdf

Wallerstein N, Bernstein E (1994) Community empowerment as a basis for healthcare reform. Health Educ Q 21(2):141–148

Wang NE, Gisondi MA, Golzari M et al (2003) Socioeconomic disparities are negatively associated with pediatric emergency department aftercare compliance. Acad Emerg Med 10:1278–1284. [PubMed: 14597505]

Weingart SN, Zhu J, Chiappetta L et al (2011) Hospitalized patients' participation and its impact on quality of care and patient safety. International J Qual Health Care 22(3):269–277

Weingarten SR, Henning JM, Badamgarav E et al (2002) Interventions used in disease management programmes for patients with chronic illness—which ones' work? Meta-analysis of published reports. BMJ 325(7370):925

WHO (1986) The Ottawa charter for health promotion. Available at http://www.who.int/healthpromotion/conferences/previous/ottawa/en/index4.html

WHO (1995) The world health report 1995-bridging the gaps. Available at http://www.who.int/whr/1995/en/

WHO (2009) WHO guidelines on hand hygiene in health care: first global patient safety challenge clean care is safer care. Available at https://www.ncbi.nlm.nih.gov/books/NBK144022/

Wilkinson RG (1996) Unhealthy societies: the afflictions of inequality. Routledge, New York

Williams DR, Kontos EZ, Viswanath K et al (2012) Integrating multiple social statuses in health disparities research: the case of lung cancer. Health Serv Res 47:1255–1277. [PubMed: 22568674]

Winland-Brown J, Lachman VD, O'Connor Swanson E (2015) The new 'code of ethics for nurses with interpretive statements' (2015): practical clinical application part I. Medsurg Nurs 24(4):268–271

Case Study: Zapotec Woman with HIV in Oaxaca, Mexico

28

Carol Sue Holtz

Sofia is a 35-year-old, married Zapotec Indian woman living in a remote small mountainous village, approximately 8 hours away from the capital city of Oaxaca in Mexico. Sofia lives with her 43-year-old husband, Jose, and four children, ages 5, 6, 10, and 12. She had two other children who died prior to their first birthday. She finished the third grade but is unable to read very well in Zapoteca or in Spanish and has minimum writing skills. Unable to find employment at home, Jose worked as a farm laborer in the United States for the past 4.5 years to support his family. Separated from his family for a long time, Jose dealt with his loneliness by socializing at the local bar near his work where other Mexicans congregated. He often engaged in casual sexual relations with some of the prostitutes who frequented this bar. Five months ago Jose returned home and Sofia became pregnant again. After visiting the local health department clinic, Sofia became aware that she was not only pregnant but also HIV positive. Before her diagnosis, Sofia and her husband did not know much about HIV and how a person can contract the disease. (Note: the name and location of this woman and her family are fictitious.)

According to Holtz and Sowell (2012), the Oaxaca Health Department now requires HIV testing for all pregnant women receiving prenatal care and encourages women's sex partners to be tested as well. Because Sofia tested positive for HIV, the public health nurse requested that she bring Jose to the clinic for testing; he was found to be HIV positive.

The couple is shocked, frightened, and concerned for themselves and their children. In their small community, they are concerned about the stigma and fear that they and their children will be ostracized in the community if others learn about their diagnosis. They know very little about the disease, the available treatments, and their costs. Sofia is angry and feels hurt by her husband's infidelity and blames him for bringing the disease to her and her pregnancy. She is worried about the future of their young children if she and her husband die from HIV.

28.1 Cultural Issues

Compared to other states in Mexico, the state of Oaxaca in the southern part of the country is home to a greater number of indigenous Indians, including Zapotecs. The majority of Zapotecs are Catholic, with some Protestants. Roman Catholicism was introduced by the Spaniards, but many remain resentful of the Spaniards' destruction of their original places of worship and continue to distrust outsiders. Zapotec families live mostly in small isolated areas with village

C. S. Holtz, Ph.D., R.N.
School of Nursing, Kennesaw State University, Kennesaw, GA, USA
e-mail: choltz@kennesaw.edu

© Springer International Publishing AG, part of Springer Nature 2018
M. Douglas et al. (eds.), *Global Applications of Culturally Competent Health Care: Guidelines for Practice*, https://doi.org/10.1007/978-3-319-69332-3_28

members acting as extended family with very strong traditional family and friendship ties. Zapotec women live within a male-dominant society with specific gender roles. The traditional roles of women include childbearing and child-rearing, homemaking, and assisting in farming and craft making that are considered primary male roles. Women are expected to exhibit deference to males including the father, husband, and/or older brother in decision-making as well as demonstrate respect for all family and community elders. All family members are expected to contribute to household chores and income (Central Intelligence Agency 2013; Joyce 2010; Stephen 2005).

Women, although often knowing what their husbands are actually doing, frequently do not have the traditional role of questioning their husband's infidelity or demanding the use of condoms during sexual relations; women cannot challenge their husbands about their outside sexual activities nor can they force them to get tested or treated for HIV (Joyce 2010; Sowell et al. 2013; Murphy and Stepick 1991; Stephen 2005).

28.2 Social Structural Issues

The Zapotecs live mainly in an agrarian society with lower levels of technology, and common occupations which include farming, manual labor, and labor-intensive craft making. Some community members refuse to work with the local, state, and/or the federal government because of their perceived lack of recognition and acceptance of their specific cultural lifeways and needs. Many demonstrate against the local government in hopes of receiving greater respect, tolerance, and assistance (Central Intelligence Agency 2013; Joyce 2010).

Because of low educational achievement, the Zapotecs are often employed in subsistence farming with minimal wages. Most have extremely low incomes, necessitating all family members to assist in pooling resources to generate an adequate family income. Most households have very low income with a minimal health literacy level and many also have malnutrition. Their diets

consist mainly of tortillas, beans, and corn with little fruits and vegetables. Some rural areas have up to a 75% infant mortality rate. In fact, Zapotec women believe that they must have large numbers of children in order to have a few survive to adulthood (Joyce 2010; Servicios de Salud 2007; Stephen 2005).

The majority of women have less than a third grade education, speaking mainly a non-Spanish indigenous language. Zapotec women in particular are often educated informally in only their traditional Zapoteca language and have minimal or no Spanish language skills. Language barriers pose a challenge in obtaining healthcare for Zapotec people (Joyce 2010; Sowell et al. 2013; Murphy and Stepick 1991; Stephen 2005).

Because Zapotec men lack employment opportunities in their areas of residence, they often leave their families behind for extended periods of time and go to other parts of Mexico or the United States for a period of 6 months to 5 years, working in agriculture, construction, restaurants, or factories. They send money back to their families. While working far away from their families, they encounter women in bars and frequently engage in unprotected sex with them. The men have little or no background on sex education, sexually transmitted infections, and HIV. They frequently bring home sexually transmitted infections and give them to their wives, who often have these infections during their subsequent pregnancies (Hirsch et al. 2007; Holtz and Sowell 2012; Sowell et al. 2013).

Residents within their small villages (*pueblos*) do not fully understand the nature and transmission of HIV and refuse to have anything to do with a diagnosed person once the disease is publicly known. Hence, it is imperative that the diagnosis is kept confidential or they risk being ostracized by their community. Being ostracized means exclusion from other family members or friends, not being able to be employed, and not being accepted into any community gatherings. HIV-infected individuals need to take a 3- to 16-hour bus ride from their local village to the main HIV clinic (COESIDA) in the metropolitan capital city of Oaxaca. In order to maintain their privacy, they inform their families and friends that they are going to seek treatment for TB or other infections which are more socially acceptable. The state of Oaxaca charges patients on a sliding scale for all public health clinic visits, but those who have no ability to pay receive free care (Holtz and Sowell 2012; Sowell et al. 2013).

28.3 Culturally Competent Strategies Recommended

The following assessment, intervention, and evaluation strategies are recommended in advocacy and empowerment of the Zapotec individual, family, and/or community. Healthcare providers need to have knowledge of the Zapotec culture including gender roles, geographical and societal factors that impact the population's health, the culture of the Zapotec people in Oaxaca, and the role of women within the culture.

28.3.1 Individual-/Family-Level Interventions

- Advocate for maintaining privacy and confidentiality of records and interactions with patients.
- During the initial clinic visit, perform a complete health and cultural assessment, obtaining information regarding sociodemographic data, health history, cultural background, vocation, individual/family income, language skills, highest level of completed education, knowledge about HIV, and a self-evaluation of their own healthcare situation and needs, including stigma of the HIV illness.
- Use culturally and linguistically appropriate communication. If the patient speaks a Zapotec dialect that the healthcare provider cannot understand and speak, obtain a professional interpreter.
- Advocate for gender-congruent care.
- Encourage the wife's participation in decisions while accommodating the traditional role of the husband as the family decision-maker.

- Promote women's empowerment by showing respect and empathy and encouraging their participation in their care.
- Facilitate women's ability to seek adequate healthcare, food, and shelter for themselves and their children as needed.
- Promote health literacy by using pictures/posters for health education and disease management.
- Obtain support from social services for appropriate financial, housing, job, and community services.

28.3.2 Organizational-Level Interventions

- Establish policies and structures to promote healthcare access by the population.
- Allocate funding for affordable and comprehensive HIV health services, including disease management, health education, social services, and mental health support/counseling services.
- Secure funding for transportation of individuals and families to and from the special HIV clinic (COESIDA).
- Implement training of health providers on cultural and social issues that influence care of HIV-affected individuals and families. Emphasize the need for privacy and confidentiality.
- Collaborate with other community stakeholders and leaders to implement a culturally appropriate education for school children and adults on HIV disease prevention and treatment and ways to combat stigma.

28.3.3 Community-/Societal-Level Interventions

- Use the leadership role of the State of Oaxaca Health Department and its branch of the COESIDA clinic (HIV care) in promoting culturally appropriate, accessible, and affordable HIV care services. Priority consideration should be given to the financial and geographic limitations to accessing these services.

- Promote community-wide awareness of HIV disease diagnosis, prevention, treatment, and supportive services (Hirsch et al. 2007; Holtz and Sowell 2012; Murphy and Stepick 1991; Servicios de Salud 2007; Smallman 2007; Sowell et al. 2013).
- Integrate the unique cultural, environmental, and socioeconomic history and conditions of the people in combating stigma and prevention of HIV. Incorporate the impact of gender-differentiated roles in HIV prevention, stigma, and care.
- Collaborate with local communities and their leaders to assess and plan prevention strategies in schools, health clinics, places of worship, and other public venues within the community.
- Utilize community leaders and healthcare providers to promote widespread "buy in" of initiative planning and implementation.
- Engage in a community-wide effort to promote education of girls and women and increasing local employment opportunities.

Conclusion

Advocacy and empowerment strategies must be included in the social and cultural context of the Zapotec Indians. Being a female, Zapotec Indian with HIV/AIDS heightens the vulnerability of women within a male-dominated society. The stigma of HIV is compounded by the difficulty of keeping the diagnosis a secret from extended close-knit relationships in small villages. Zapotec women are often proud and strong, who strive to live each day caring for themselves and their families. Their culture provides a vibrant work ethic and strong religious background, and many are talented in wood carving, weaving, sewing, and ceramic making. However, once they are affected by HIV, they face the added challenges from their geographic isolation, lack of education, poor nutrition, and poverty. Advocacy and empowerment of the

Zapotec women should include assuring their participation in decisions about their health, facilitating appropriate access to resources and services, and providing financial support.

- Zapotec society's gender-defined roles and social infrastructure create the necessity for men to leave their communities and families to seek employment in distant places for long periods of time. Prolonged separation from their loved ones and lack of awareness of HIV predispose these men to engage in unprotected casual sex. Often, HIV is undiagnosed until their wives back home get pregnant and acquire the infection from their husbands when they return home. Because of their traditional subservience to the male, compounded by low literacy and lack of knowledge of HIV, women are unable to question their men on their sexual activities or demand that they use condoms; they expose themselves and their fetus to HIV. HIV is preventable, but initiatives should be planned and implemented within the cultural and social structural realities of the population. The task of promoting widespread community awareness of the infection, its diagnosis, prevention, and management requires culturally competent strategies targeting individuals, families, and communities by individual healthcare providers, organizations, and society in general (Hirsch et al. 2007; Holtz and Sowell 2012; Murphy and Stepick 1991; Servicios de Salud 2007; Smallman 2007; Sowell et al. 2013). The state of Oaxaca Department of Health, particularly COESIDA, needs to take the leadership in transforming HIV care and prevention at the micro and macro levels of their society. Advocacy and empowerment of Zapotec women affected with HIV require not only individual-level strategies but, more significantly, institutional and community leadership in eradicating the stigma associated with HIV, educating men on the disease and its transmission, and strengthening protection of women from unprotected sex.

References

Central Intelligence Agency (CIA) (2013) Adult HIV/ AIDS prevalence in Mexico. Available at: http://www. indexmundi.com/mexico/hiv_aids_adult_prevalence_ rate.html

Hirsch J, Meneses S, Thompson B et al (2007) The inevitability of infidelity: sexual reputation, social geographies, and marital HIV risk in rural Mexico. Am J Public Health 9(6):986–996. https://doi.org/10.2105/ AJPH.2006.088492

Holtz C, Sowell RL (2012) Oaxacan women with HIV/ AIDS: resiliency in the face of poverty, stigma, and social isolation. Women Health 52(6):517–535. https://doi.org/10.1080/03630242.2012.690839

Joyce A (2010) Mixtecs, Zapotecs, and Chatinos. Wiley-Blackwell, West Sussex, pp 1–42

Murphy A, Stepick A (1991) Social inequality in Oaxaca. Temple University Press, Philadelphia

Servicios de Salud (2007) Health prevention and promotion: panoramic epidemiology of HIV/AIDS in the State of Oaxaca 1986-2007. Department of Epidemiology of the Centro de Salud de Oaxaca

Smallman S (2007) The AIDS epidemic in Latin America. The University of North Carolina Press, Chapel Hill

Sowell RL, Holtz C, VanBrackle L et al (2013) Depression in HIV-infected women: implications for mental health services. Online J Med Med Sci Res 2(1):6–12

Stephen L (2005) Zapotec women: gender, class and ethnicity in globalized Oaxaca, 2nd edn. Duke University Press, Durham

Case Study: Maternal and Child Health Promotion Issues for a Poor, Migrant Haitian Mother

29

Twenty-five-year-old Nathaly migrated to the United States from Haiti 5 months ago. She is 38 weeks pregnant and experiencing labor pains. She is brought to the labor and delivery department of a large urban hospital by her cousin. She had one prenatal visit with a midwife in Haiti about 6 months ago but did not seek healthcare since she arrived in the United States. Nathaly was examined and found to be in labor. Her cousin speaks English fluently but was unable to stay with Nathaly throughout labor and childbirth because she needed to pick up her 9-year-old daughter from school and stay with her at home after. An interpreter from the language line service was engaged to speak to Nathaly about her medical history and to obtain her consent for admission and treatment.

Nathaly completed high school and worked as a waitress in Port-Au-Prince until the city was devastated by an earthquake in 2010. She moved back home to be with her mother in rural Haiti when her father, a carpenter, died in 2012. She was planning to go to college in Haiti but became pregnant; she left her 3-year-old son with her mother in Haiti. Her mother sells housewares and farm products in the local market to support Nathaly's two younger sisters who are still in school. Nathaly's husband, a teacher in Haiti,

objected to her migrating and has not been involved with her current pregnancy. Nathaly was hoping to find a job in the United States and help her family in Haiti, but she has been unsuccessful. She speaks French and Creole and only speaks limited English.

Nathaly, her cousin, and her cousin's 9-year-old daughter live in a two-bedroom apartment in a predominantly Caribbean/Haitian community in Northeastern United States, approximately 3 miles from the hospital. There is a West Indian store that sells Haitian food about half a mile away and a supermarket about ten blocks from their residence. She describes her neighborhood as "relatively safe with occasional gun violence."

Nathaly is in the United States on a temporary visa and is unsure if she will go back to Haiti after the birth of her baby. She admits that she is not adequately prepared for childbirth and has no income nor health insurance. She only has minimal amount of cash for some baby supplies and depends on her cousin for support (food and shelter). Her cousin is employed as a certified nursing assistant (CNA) earning less than $28,000.00 per year. Her cousin admits that it has been difficult to manage financially with the high cost of living in the United States. One in five (20%) Haitians in the United States lives in poverty as compared to 1 in 7 (14%) in the total US population (U.S. Central Intelligence Agency 2017). Nathaly's cousin is her only family member in the United States. Her cousin moved to

J. Hyatt, Ph.D., D.N.P., C.N.M.
Nurse Midwifery Program, School of Nursing,
Rutgers University, Newark, NJ, USA
e-mail: hyattjs@sn.rutgers.edu

© Springer International Publishing AG, part of Springer Nature 2018
M. Douglas et al. (eds.), *Global Applications of Culturally Competent Health Care: Guidelines for Practice*, https://doi.org/10.1007/978-3-319-69332-3_29

this community 10 months ago and is not familiar with the resources available for pregnancy and childbirth in the area.

29.1 Cultural Issues

In Haitian culture, pregnancy is considered normal; hence, many women do not seek prenatal care. Women living in the rural areas of Haiti are more likely to be delivered by untrained midwives at home (Colin and Paperwalla 2013). Like most cultures, Haitians tend to maintain traditional beliefs and practices pertaining to labor and childbirth. According to Colin and Paperwalla, the women can be very expressive when having pain by being loud; others may groan or become quiet and passive. They are also known for rubbing their abdomens, walking, squatting, or sitting when in pain.

Because of the language barrier, a face pain scale was used to ascertain Nathaly's level of pain. Initially, her pain level was at six out of ten, but she refused pain medication because she had her first baby without medicine. She opted to walk around her room, groaning loudly and sometimes squatting when in pain. After she was determined to be 6 cm dilated with a pain level of eight out of ten, Nathaly decided to take the pain medication after being assured that the medicine would not affect the baby. She agreed to take the intravenous medication but refused epidural analgesia.

During the health assessment, Nathaly is comfortable sharing her belief with another nurse who speaks French. She relates her fear that her mother-in-law (who apparently dislikes her) is trying to put "a voodoo/bad spell" on her baby. Her cousin urged her to come to the United States to prevent the spell on the baby. In Haiti, it is a common belief that if a pregnant woman has an enemy, her enemy can cast a bad spell or voodoo on the baby resulting in harm to the pregnancy (Colin and Paperwalla 2013). Nathaly admits that she feels safer in the United States and does not want to go back to the rural area in Haiti after having the baby. She is concerned about not working, being uninsured, not speaking English

well, and being dependent on her cousin who has to support her and her own daughter.

Nathaly's fear of spell on her baby is not uncommon in the Haitian culture. Although the majority of Haitians practice Catholicism, some have strong beliefs in the voodoo religion (Alvarado 2011). Understanding and respecting Nathaly's beliefs and values are essential to caring for her and her baby and creating a trusting patient/provider relationship. Respecting her culture without marginalizing her beliefs promotes trust in the healthcare provider (Colin and Paperwalla 2013). Health providers need to have specific knowledge about Haitian cultural practices regarding health and illnesses to facilitate communication and foster culturally competent assessment and care (Douglas et al. 2014).

Migrants experience the stressors stemming from loss of familiar culture and way of life when exposed to different social milieu, values, and norms. Adult migrants may experience "child-like dependence" because of the need to cope with a new way of life, new language, and new behaviors. Nathaly is faced with a new culture, language barriers, and financial dependence on her cousin. She is referred to a social worker to assist her in securing health insurance and other available social programs including women, infant, and children (WIC). She is also referred to a Haitian church that has been providing support and food supplies to underserved women and children in the community.

29.2 Social Structural Factors

Haiti is considered the poorest country in the western hemisphere (U.S. Central Intelligence Agency 2017). In 2012, 58.5% of Haitians were living below or at the poverty level (World Bank 2016). Lack of adequate infrastructure and resources for healthcare in particular has contributed to poor healthcare and subsequent high infant and maternal mortality. According to the US Central Intelligence Agency (2017), Haiti's maternal mortality rate was estimated at 359 deaths/100,000 live births in 2015. In 2016 Haiti's infant mortality rate was 48.2 deaths/1000 live births. These are alarmingly high rates when compared to their neighbors, the Dominican Republic and Jamaica, with 2016 infant mortality rates of 18.1 deaths/1000 and 13.1 deaths/1000 births, respectively. In 2016, about 52.4% of rural Haiti had inadequate drinking water, while 80.8% had unimproved or poor sanitation facilities (U.S. Central Intelligence Agency 2017).

Prior to her migration to the United States, Nathaly lived and experienced the environmental disadvantages of living in rural Haiti which can impact her pregnancy outcome. Fortunately for Nathaly, the neighborhood in which she now lives, is considered fairly safe with adequate access to transportation and healthy food. Because she is unemployed and dependent on her cousin's income, she has limited ability to purchase healthy food. Lack of health insurance, language difficulty, and unfamiliarity with, or lack of awareness of community resources are significant factors that can negatively influence her access to health services and quality care for herself and her baby. It could not be ascertained how much weight Nathaly gained during her pregnancy, blood type, HIV status, or blood glucose level. Laboratory and other diagnostic assessments are usually done during prenatal care, providing significant information about the mother and baby's health status. In Nathaly's case, these were not available until admission. Lack of baseline and prenatal care puts Nathaly and her baby at risk for labor and birth complications. After 7 h, Nathaly gave birth to a 6-pound baby boy who appeared to be grossly normal.

29.3 Culturally Competent Strategies Recommended

Advocacy and empowerment for Nathaly and her family must be informed by the social structural and cultural factors in Haiti and in their new environment. In the United States, Haitians are considered one of the most at-risk populations (U.S. Central Intelligence Agency 2017). Based on the problems identified for Nathaly, the following are the recommended culturally competent advocacy and empowerment (Douglas et al. 2014).

29.3.1 Individual-/Family-Level Interventions

- Empower clients by integrating socioeconomic, linguistic, and literacy factors during interactions, including:
  - Promoting awareness of the importance of prenatal care, postpartum follow-up, and growth and developmental assessment of the baby
  - Selecting interpreters and health education approaches
  - Obtaining comprehensive health history and providing health education and counseling
  - Providing postpartum education on immediate and long-term needs including breastfeeding and importance of follow-up care for mother and baby
- Respect and accommodate client's preferences and unique cultural beliefs and practices while promoting safe and supportive care by:
  - Developing awareness of Haitian cultural beliefs and practices relevant to pregnancy, birthing, and child care
  - Ensuring confidentiality of information shared by clients to prevent marginalization of their traditional beliefs and practices
  - Ensuring privacy while conducting examinations and honoring the cultural value of modesty and preference for gender congruent practitioner
- Advocate for client's access to appropriate social services and culturally congruent community resources by:
  - Facilitating referral to appropriate social services to assist with application for health insurance and nutritional programs for mother and baby
  - Providing information on English classes for immigrants offered in the local community
  - Providing information on available programs for job training and occupational mentorship in the community
  - Linking client with Haitian churches and community support networks
  - Connecting the client with legal advocates to assist legalization of her immigration status in the United States

29.3.2 Organizational-Level Interventions

- Advocate for organizational responsiveness to healthcare for vulnerable Haitian population by:
  - Assessing adequacy of organizational infrastructure of services and care delivery
  - Training of staff and administrators in culturally competent care
  - Ensuring presence of interpretation and translation services (language line, certified interpreters) for prominent languages of the populations being served
  - Ensuring adequate certified interpreters (in person) when the patient speaks a language that is different from the healthcare providers
  - Ensuring availability of printed material and signage with low literacy level and in the major languages of the population served
- Recruit and maintain a culturally diverse workforce by:
  - Determining presence of culturally congruent staff that Haitian patients can communicate and identify with
  - Integrating cultural competence in staff hiring, job descriptions, and promotion requirements
- Promote engagement of the organization with vulnerable communities by:
  - Conducting free health fairs in the community (such as in public housing, local parks, and churches)
  - Establishing partnership with local Haitian community centers and coalitions, churches, and radio and television stations to provide information on pregnancy and childbirth in English, French, and Haitian Creole
  - Encouraging staff participation in research on the Haitian population to identify significant health challenges including demographic, socioeconomic, and epidemiological data

29.3.3 Community-/Societal-Level Interventions

- Empower the Haitian community by:
  - Inviting community participation in planning of social and health programs that will benefit the community
  - Establishing collaborative partnership with the Haitian church and the Haitian Community Coalition to assist with health education and communication with the Haitian population
  - Collaborating with community leaders and organizations to conduct health fairs providing free health assessment, counseling, and treatment referrals
  - Collaborating with Haitian community leaders and organizations to seek participation in local and statewide policies and programs that impact their community

Conclusion

Nathaly is typical of Haitian immigrants who are confronted by sociocultural factors that can significantly impact their lives. Although she has a high school education, she is unemployed, and her capacity for employment is limited because of her temporary visa, lack of English proficiency, and caretaking responsibilities for her baby. Her lack of prenatal care and exposure to the limitations of her previous rural residence and her current situation will impact the present and future health of her baby as well as her own.

Nathaly needs culturally competent advocacy and empowerment to navigate the challenges of a new environment and social vulnerability. These strategies should not only focus on her current state of being but should include strategies that will improve her capacity to maintain a healthy life for her and her baby. Advocacy and empowerment for vulnerable individuals and families necessitate multisectoral approaches addressing individual and family needs as well as transformation of services and supports offered by organizations and present in the community. The current political climate in the United States severely limits the future of Nathaly and her baby because of her lack of permanent legal status as immigrant. Advocacy and empowerment strategies must address this issue and not just limited to maternal and child health. Legal status is prerequisite to their survival.

References

Alvarado D (2011) The voodoo hoodoo spellbook. Weiser Books, San Francisco. ISBN 1-57863-513-6

Colin J, Paperwalla G (2013) People of Haitian heritage. In: Purnell L (ed) Transcultural health care: a culturally competent approach, 4th edn. F. A. Davis, Philadelphia, pp 269–287

Douglas M, Rosenkoetter M, Pacquiao D et al (2014) Guidelines for implementing cultural competent nursing care. J Transcult Nurs 25(2):109–121

U.S. Central Intelligence Agency (2017) The world factbook. Central America and Haiti 2017. Available at: https://www.cia.gov/library/publications/the-world-factbook/geos/ha.html

World Bank (2016) World development indicators. Available at: http://data.worldbank.org/country/haiti#cp_wdi

Case Study: Caring for a Pakistani Male Who Has Sex with Other Men

Rubab I. Qureshi

Fifty-year-old Mr. M, of Pakistani descent, came in for a consultation at a local urgent care center. He states that he is married with no children and that his wife lives in Pakistan. He has no immediate family members in the United States. He immigrated to the United States 20 years ago and drives a taxicab for a living. He is bilingual in his native language, *Pashto* that is spoken in the Khyber Pakhtunkhwa province of Pakistan and fluent in English. Mr. M completed high school before migrating to the United States. He has no health insurance. He provides financial support for his wife and parents in Pakistan. He tries to visit Pakistan every year and had recently returned from a 6-week visit a month ago. He smokes occasionally but does not drink alcohol.

Mr. M complains of urethral discharge with some dysuria for a week. He had similar episodes in the past, but he took some antibiotics he had brought back from Pakistan and got better. However, he forgot to bring back some antibiotics from his last trip. He is reluctant to talk about his sex life. After some probing questions, he admits that he is uncomfortable because he has never discussed "this" with anyone. He identifies as heterosexual but has sex with other men (MSM) occasionally. He describes his wife as a simple woman from a farming family and does not want to migrate to the United States. Many men from his village have migrated to Middle Eastern countries like Saudi Arabia, Dubai, and Kuwait, leaving their families in Pakistan and visiting them regularly. He feels lonely and likes company. He does not like going to other women, because it would be cheating on his wife.

As he becomes more comfortable with the health provider, Mr. M says that he had been living with a male Caucasian friend until a year ago. They had sex occasionally but were not exclusive of other relationships. He says that sex with other men is different. He does not use a condom all the time. Over the years he had multiple sexual partners but was never in a long-term one-on-one relationship. He just "hooks up with a friend when he wants to." He has a circle of nine to ten friends who call on each other when they want to. He had a casual sex encounter with a couple of men while in Pakistan. He met them in Karachi, a large bustling metropolis, before catching a connecting flight to his village. He admits doing "all kinds of things" without specifying oral or anal sex; no condoms were used.

When asked about his wife, Mr. M says that "she is fine and would never discuss female problems with me [him]." He had not heard from her. His wife wanted a family, but Allah had not blessed them with children. His family had suggested that he marry a second time, but he is "fine with things the way they are." He laughs and says, "one woman is enough."

R. I. Qureshi, M.D., Ph.D.
School of Nursing, Rutgers University,
Newark, NJ, USA
e-mail: rubab.qureshi@rutgers.edu

M. Douglas et al. (eds.), *Global Applications of Culturally Competent Health Care: Guidelines for Practice*, https://doi.org/10.1007/978-3-319-69332-3_30

Mr. M is told that he might have a sexually transmitted infection and needs some tests to confirm the diagnosis. If confirmed, he is advised to inform his sexual partners of his diagnosis, so they can get tested and treated if necessary. Mr. M admits that he may only tell the friends he had sex with but would not share this with his wife—"she does not have to know."

30.1 Social Structural Issues

Pakistan is a predominantly Muslim country comprised of 192 million people (PBS 2016). It is bordered by Afghanistan, Iran, China, and India. Pakistan is a developing country with high rates of poverty and unemployment. This has encouraged a steady stream of emigres with large diasporas of Pakistanis in neighboring Gulf States, the United Kingdom, Canada, and the United States.

Social hierarchy and opportunities are generally structured by male dominance infusing gender-based sociocultural dichotomy in all spheres of life. Gender roles and expectations define masculine roles. Males act as the family link to the external world (providing for the family, shopping, outside interactions, etc.). In contrast, females' lives are circumspect and limited to the management of domestic activities (Hussain et al. 2015). Males are valued and socialized in an environment emphasizing their superiority over females. It starts at birth when the birth of a male child is celebrated with pomp and the female child is met with apprehension (Qureshi 2010). Gender roles are inculcated early when boys and girls play different games and boys are encouraged to be tough and chastised if they show weakness (Hussain et al. 2015). Girls are socialized to be weak, delicate, sensitive, emotional, and dependent, while boys are raised to be strong, aggressive, brave, and the protectors of the family honor (*izzat* in Urdu and *namus* in Pashto) (Hussain et al. 2015; Qureshi 2010).

It is not uncommon for women to be excluded from property and land inheritance, but are given dowries at the time of marriage. Men make key decisions for the women in their families including marriages and even contraception. In Pakhtun culture it is a rarity for a woman to seek divorce from her husband. More family resources are allocated to raising boys, getting them educated and employed. Very few women are educated and even fewer participate in the work force (Qureshi 2010). Traditional gendered roles are encouraged, and contemporary social roles are discouraged, especially for females (Hussain et al. 2015). Internalized gendered behaviors are reflected at the institutional level in gender segregation in most social spheres.

30.2 Cultural Issues

Pakistan is comprised of five major distinct ethnic groups based on culture and language. These include Pashtuns/Pakhtuns in Khyber Pakhtunkhwa, Punjabis in Punjab, Sindhis in Sindh, Baluch and Barhui in Baluchistan (Zaman 2014). Pakistani culture is a conglomeration of shared cultures bound by a common national and religious identity. Historically these geographical neighbors share a rich history and identities. Pakistan and India were part of the Indian subcontinent ruled by the British until 1947. The Pakhtuns are ethnically close to Afghanistan and share a similar culture, while the Punjabis have cultural similarities with the Indian Punjab. Pakhtuns adhere to a tribal culture, *Pashtunwali* (tribal code) and considered the most patriarchal and most traditional adherents of Islam than other ethnic groups.

The family is the cornerstone of ethnic societies in Pakistan (Zaman 2014). It is not uncommon for extended families to live together and decision-making is shared with deference to the older members of the family (Nath 2005; Zaman 2014). Most marriages are arranged and considered a family duty. Family loyalty and honor (*izzat* in Urdu) are inculcated in child-rearing (Nath 2005; Zaman 2014). Whereas men enjoy greater autonomy, women are held to a stricter code and closely guarded (Zaman 2014).

Men and women have very few opportunities to socialize. Any romantic dalliance is often clandestine because of fear of damaging the family honor (*izzat/namus*) if discovered. Such relationships can have terrible consequences such as honor killing by the women's family. Single men socialize freely and with greater freedom, but societal structures and lifestyles are not conducive to developing or maintaining a gay identity. Homosexuality is illegal and considered a crime in Pakistan. Although Islam condemns homosexuality as a sin, in some parts of the country homosexual relationships are not uncommon (Jaspal and Siraj 2011; Nath 2005).

Among the Pashtuns, variant patterns of sexual identity go against the tenets of Islam and violators may be severely punished (Nath 2005). Sexuality cannot interfere with tradition, and as long as the institution of marriage is not threatened, what men do in their private lives is tolerated. There is no acceptance of a gay identity or "coming out," and gay men may be pressured into marriage to lead "normal" lives (Nath 2005). There are no "gay" rights, and gay men have to be covert and keep their relationships secret (Nath 2005). Oftentimes erotic love between two males is reduced to anal penetration and is subject to ridicule in public spheres. In this context, some men who prefer to have sex with men exclusively reported feelings of shame, dissonance, guilt, and fear of persecution (Jaspal 2012).

Within a close-knit family structure, sexuality, sex education, and preventive care are rarely discussed. Consequently overall knowledge about sexual health is low (Rehan 2002). In addition, there are no reliable data on the prevalence of sexually transmitted infections (STIs), and not surprisingly the official rates of STIs are grossly underestimated (Maan et al. 2011; Nath 2005). Pakistani immigrant gay men who have strong transnational ties and second generation gay men are likely to behave like their counterparts in Pakistan because their cultural context remains the same (Jaspal 2012).

30.3 Culturally Competent Strategies

Advocacy and empowerment of Pakistani immigrant MSM need to be informed by their cultural and religious traditions and degree of connected-ness with families back in Pakistan. Sexual and gender minorities may feel uncomfortable disclosing their identities orally or in writing in healthcare settings. For Pakistani MSM, disclosure to family members and co-ethnics is difficult because of entrenched gendered roles including sexual roles of males. Failure to disclose adds to their invisibility and isolation from social resources and support.

30.3.1 Individual Level Interventions

1. Advocate for using appropriate literacy level in oral and written communication, signage, and teaching materials for foreign-born migrants even if they speak English well.
2. Obtain comprehensive health and sociocultural assessment including migration history, socioeconomic status, religious beliefs, cultural traditions, and practices including sexual practices, social support and transnational ties, literacy level, language preference, need for interpreter, etc.
3. Promote privacy and confidentiality of interactions to allow the client to open up and discuss his problem freely. Privacy and confidentiality should be assured when using medical interpreters.
4. Advocate for gender-congruent provider if preferred by the client.
5. Facilitate client referral to social services to apply for health insurance and other social resources. Many immigrants who are self-employed or non-naturalized citizens may not have health insurance.
6. Promote client empowerment by enhancing his understanding of his condition, diagnosis, treatment, and prevention and follow up by:
   • Providing explanations on the following: (a) need for a battery of tests for STIs including HIV, (b) types of specimens to be collected including urethral discharge, (c) adherence to prescribed treatment regimen and follow-up to prevent or treat microbial resistance, (d) avoidance of all sexual contact during treatment and for 7 days after treatment, (e) prevention of self-exposure to STIs and transmission of STIs to others,

(f) need to inform all his sexual partners about his condition and how to seek help, and (g) some states may require the provider to report his case to the health authority.

- Allowing the client time to ask questions, clarify ambiguities and express his feelings.
- Offering additional support for the client to reach out for further questions or concerns.

7. Being aware that MSM may not consider themselves as gay or bisexual. This is especially significant for Mr. M who was socialized in an environment where private sexual practices are tolerated for as long as these do not interfere with his role as a married man and family provider.

30.3.2 Organizational Level Interventions

1. Ensure language interpretation assistance for clients with less English proficiency.
2. Employ navigators to assist clients in using the various services of the organization as well as resources in the community.
3. Foster a sexual and gender minority (SGM) friendly environment by:
   (a) Participating in the Human Rights Campaign's Health Equality Index, an annual survey that examines hospital policies toward SGM patients.
   (b) Implementing regulations and standards for visitation and nondiscrimination from the Department of Health and Human Services and Joint Commission.
   (c) Providing SGM health competency/sensitivity training to staff and administrators.
   (d) Revising forms used to elicit information appropriate for SGM clients.
   (e) Advertising inclusive philosophy of the organization.
4. Recruit and maintain a culturally diverse staff representing the population groups in the community.

30.3.3 Community Level Interventions

1. Advocate for research on sexual minority immigrants from South Asian countries including Pakistan and inclusion of these groups in national databases, e.g., Behavioral Risk Factor Surveillance System, Centers for Medicare and Medicaid Services, etc.
2. Disseminate information on organizations providing care specific for sexual and gender minorities.
3. Facilitate development of social networks and community outreach to SGM members particularly from South Asian countries using multiple formats.

Conclusion

Sexual minorities have a long, almost universal history of persecution and discrimination which makes disclosure difficult. Stigma attached to SGM is widespread in many countries, and some religions consider variant sexuality as sinful and a cultural taboo. These cultural norms contribute to the invisibility of this group which contribute further to their health vulnerability. Members of the SGM community also experience overt discrimination and bias from healthcare providers which deter them from seeking care services. Advocacy and empowerment of SGM clients must occur at the individual, institutional, and societal levels. Improving their health is difficult when they need to hide their sexual identity and sexual practices. Social and cultural transformation requires legal protection of SGM individuals. Macrosocial changes are needed to combat marginalization and stigmatization of SGM individuals. Such changes begin at the level of the individual but are not sustainable unless organizational support and community reform occur. Culturally competent advocacy and empowerment of SGM groups need to negotiate with the realities of the social and cultural contexts of stigma and discrimination.

References

Hussain M, Naz A, Khan W et al (2015) Gender stereotyping in family: an institutionalized and normative mechanism in Pakhtun society of Pakistan. SAGE Open 5(3):2158244015595258

Jaspal R (2012) 'I never faced up to being gay': sexual, religious and ethnic identities among British Indian and British Pakistani gay men. Cult Health Sex 14(7):767–780

Jaspal R, Siraj A (2011) Perceptions of 'coming out' among British Muslim gay men. Psychol Sex 2(3):183–197

Maan MA, Hussain F, Iqbal J et al (2011) Sexually transmitted infections in Pakistan. Ann Saudi Med 31(3):263–269. https://doi.org/10.4103/0256-4947.81541

Nath S (2005) Pakistani families. In: Ethnicity and family therapy. Guilford, New York, pp 407–420

PBS (2016) Population Census. Available at: http://www.pbs.gov.pk/content/population-census

Qureshi RI (2010) Experiences of pregnancy, childbirth and post-partum period in urban and suburban immigrant Pakistani women. New Jersey Institute of Technology. Available at: http://archives.njit.edu/vol01/etd/2010s/2010/njit-etd2010-102/njit-etd2010-102.pdf

Rehan N (2002) Profile of men suffering from sexually transmitted infections in Pakistan. J Ayub Med Coll Abbottabad 15(2):15–19

Zaman RM (2014) Parenting in Pakistan: an overview. In: Selin H (ed) Parenting across cultures. science across cultures: the history of non-western science, vol 7. Springer, Dordrecht, pp 91–104

Part VIII
Guideline: Multicultural Workforce

Culturally Competent Multicultural Workforce

31

Dula Pacquiao

Guideline: Nurses shall actively engage in the effort to ensure a multicultural workforce in health care settings. One measure to achieve a multicultural workforce is through strengthening of recruitment and retention efforts in the hospitals, clinics, and academic settings.

Douglas et al. (2014: 110)

31.1 Introduction

The trend toward increasing diversity in world populations has been associated with globalization supported by advances in technology and internationalization of economy. Technology has allowed easier world travel and movement of people, reducing physical distances and heightening awareness of cultural diversity. As part of the global economy, people are now living and working in environments exposed to diversity, requiring more interactions with people from diverse backgrounds. The global economy has intensified competition for resources worldwide, moving human and material capital across regions and nations to maximize productivity and profitability. Organizations are becoming more diversified to remain competitive.

Today's world gradually is becoming more global in its outlook, and as the marketplace becomes increasingly global in nature, the need for multiculturalism in the workplace will continue to grow. For many people, encounters with people from different racial and ethnic backgrounds as well as national origins occur most frequently in the workplace (Martin and Nakayama 2010). Workplaces are places where individuals from diverse cultures convene and collaborate. Recent immigrants comprise more than half of the total workforce in the USA (Okoro 2012). Diversity challenges are not limited to businesses and healthcare organizations but also involve academic institutions.

31.2 Definition of Multicultural Workforce

Understanding a multicultural workforce requires an expanded definition of cultural diversity to encompass differences between people in an organization including age, generation, national origin, race, ethnicity, class, gender, sexual orientation, religion, education, disability, language and communication, and life experience (Okoro 2012). Workforce diversity also includes differences in personality, cognitive style, tenure in the organization, organizational role, and work preferences. Diversity requires acknowledging, understanding, accepting, and valuing differences among people; it involves how people perceive themselves and how they perceive others, which affect their interactions (Mayhew 2017).

D. Pacquiao, Ed.D., R.N., C.T.N.-A., T.N.S.
School of Nursing, Rutgers University, Newark, NJ, USA

School of Nursing, University of Hawaii, Hilo, Hilo, HI, USA

© Springer International Publishing AG, part of Springer Nature 2018
M. Douglas et al. (eds.), *Global Applications of Culturally Competent Health Care: Guidelines for Practice*, https://doi.org/10.1007/978-3-319-69332-3_31

31.3 Drivers of Workforce Diversity in Healthcare

31.3.1 Global Healthcare Workforce Shortage

The World Health Organization estimated that the worldwide shortage of healthcare workers including doctors, midwives, nurses, and other healthcare workers rose from 4.3 million to 7.2 million in 2013. This shortage is predicted to increase to 12.9 million by 2035 (WHO 2013). The number of countries with health workforces well below the basic threshold of 23 skilled health professionals/10,000 people increased from 75 in 2006 to 83 in 2013. While the largest shortages are predicted in parts of Asia, sub-Saharan Africa will be most severely affected. Internal and international migration of health workers exacerbates regional and global shortages. The pattern of internal migration flows from rural to urban areas, while international migration flows from low- and mid-income countries to high-income countries in North America and Western Europe (Allutis et al. 2014). International migration may occur among neighboring countries in the same region or continent. This is motivated by several factors, including better wages and more opportunities for employment, educational advancement, and career mobility. Some health workers migrate to escape poverty, violence, and disease epidemics in their home country (Allutis et al. 2014; Kingma 2007).

Many countries in North America, Europe, the Middle East, and Oceania actively import health service labor to sustain their own healthcare system, while African countries (Zimbabwe, Nigeria, Ghana, Zambia, and South Africa) experience a net outflow of health workers. Seventy percent of health workers from African countries (approximately 65,000 physicians and 70,000 nurses) have migrated to high-income countries (Clemens and Petersen 2008). Nearly all European members of the Organization for Economic Cooperation and Development (OECD) increasingly rely on recruiting health workers from abroad to fill their shortages. In contrast to Estonia, Slovakia, and Poland that have little reliance on foreign medical doctors, Switzerland, Slovenia, Ireland, and the UK have very high reliance on foreign health workers especially medical doctors. A study of ten countries in the European Union (EU) found that one third of migrant doctors came from outside EU: 60% in France and Italy and 80% in Ireland and the UK (Dussault et al. 2009).

Worldwide, nurses comprise the largest group of healthcare workers as well as the largest migrant group among all categories of healthcare workers. In the USA, the number of companies engaged in international nurse recruitment rose from about 40 in 1990 to 270 in 2009 (Eckenwiler 2009). About 8% of US Registered Nurses (RNs) are foreign-educated with the Philippines as the major source country accounting for more than 30% of US foreign-educated nurses. Nurse immigration to the USA has tripled since 1994 to about 15,000 annually (Aiken 2007). The USA employs the most international nurses, but foreign-educated nurses comprise only 4% of its nursing workforce, compared to the UK and Ireland (8%) and Canada (6%). The top six countries that export nurses are the Philippines, Canada, India, Nigeria, Russia, and Ukraine (Walker 2010).

High-income countries have resorted to foreign recruitment to address their workforce shortages instead of developing an adequate plan for sustainable workforce development within their own countries. International recruitment has created the phenomenon of "brain drain," a shortage of highly educated and skilled health workers within the source countries, which has catastrophic effects on the quality of care, disease burden, and mortality in these countries (Allutis et al. 2014; Kingma 2007). The "brain drain" has worsened conditions in source countries that are likely to be low-income, resource poor, and plagued by shortages of manpower particularly highly skilled professionals and well-qualified educators; shortages are worse in rural areas.

31.3.2 Government Policies

The pattern of migration of Filipino internationally educated nurses (IENs) illustrates how the drivers of migration work. Filipino IENs comprise the largest group of migrants with the USA as the favored destination country. Filipino nurses emigrate because of high unemployment at home despite a glut of nurses because the local economy could not absorb the large numbers of graduates, creating tight competition and less opportunity for advancement. Low wages have prompted Filipino physicians to retrain as nurses for employment abroad.

According to Jurado (2013), both the US and Philippine governments have played a major role in creating the "push" and "pull" for nurse migration. The Philippines was colonized by the Americans in 1898 after the Spanish-American War that ended centuries of Spanish rule since 1521. Except for a brief period of Japanese occupation during World War II, the American occupation finally ended in 1946 when the Philippines gained its independence. During the occupation, Americans were confronted with health issues in the Philippines from epidemics of typhoid, cholera, smallpox, and tuberculosis. In addition to introducing mass public education, the Americans were instrumental in developing hospitals, public health programs, and training of doctors and nurses in the Philippines. The Americanization of Philippine nursing was paved by American teachers and textbooks and further training of nurses in the USA; these nurses subsequently assumed leadership positions in nursing education and service. The American influence in the country's professional nursing and healthcare has remained strong with English as the medium of collegiate instruction (Pacquiao 2003). According to Masselink (2009) countries that were colonized may have been introduced to the colonizer's language and educational systems, facilitating ease of migration to the colonizing country. Consequently, Filipino nurse graduates are preferred targets of foreign nurse recruitment. In fact, nursing shortages with corresponding opening of visa entry to the USA are the major influence in local nursing enrollment in the Philippines (Jurado and Pacquiao 2015). US immigration policies since after World War II have paved the way for thousands of Filipino IENs to enter the country legally by creating different entry visa categories (temporary and permanent status), extending their legal residence in the USA after expiration of their temporary work visas and allowing adjustment of their temporary status to permanent residents (Jurado 2013).

The Philippine government has encouraged labor emigration because Filipinos working in other countries send significant remittances that bolster the dollar revenues of the country critical to the payment of its foreign debt. Since the time of President Marcos, the government has encouraged overproduction of nurses for export. Large numbers of nurses are unemployed due to limited employment opportunities in healthcare. Healthcare jobs offer low wages, so many nurses seek employment outside of healthcare (Jurado 2013).

31.3.3 Increased Global Demand for Healthcare Services

Healthcare workforce shortages have been attributed to high demand for healthcare services because of the increasingly aging population, population growth, higher prevalence of chronic and noncommunicable diseases, and expansion of primary care services (WHO 2013). The UN's Millennium Development Goals and Alma-Ata's declaration of "healthcare for all" have given impetus to the global agenda to provide universal access to healthcare. Increased recognition of the social determinants of health has pushed the need for primary care services that promote health beyond disease-based care (ICN 2006). The shortage is also attributed to lack of workforce planning, inadequate funding for students entering the professions, inadequate numbers of faculty constraining enrollments, and growth of alternative work opportunities for women (AACN 2014; ICN 2006).

In the USA, there are 6804 geographical areas, populations, and facilities with a shortage of primary medical practitioners, 5598 with a shortage of dental professionals, and 4730 with shortage of mental health professionals (HRSA 2017a). In addition, 4221 areas are designated as medically underserved areas or populations that have too few primary care providers, high infant mortality, high poverty, or high elderly population (HRSA 2017b). It is predicted that by 2025, there will be a shortage of 23,640 primary care physicians (general, family, and internal medicine) (HRSA 2016). Buerhaus et al. (2009) have predicted that the imbalance in the supply and demand for nurses will be worsened by the mass retirement of aging American nurses. The RN workforce is expected to grow from 2.71 million in 2012 to 3.24 million in 2022, representing an increase of 19%. In 2022, 525,000 nurses will be needed to replace those who will retire, bringing a total of 1.05 million job openings to meet the increased demand and replacement (AACN 2015).

Several studies have indicated that the insufficient nurse staffing contributes to higher stress levels among nurses, which has a negative impact on their job satisfaction and retention, as well as patient safety and survival (AACN 2015). Adequate nursing staffing was associated with decreased patient hospital stay, rehospitalization, infections, and mortality. Studies in 12 countries in Europe, USA, and Canada found fewer patient deaths in intensive care units that were staffed with higher percentages of nurses with baccalaureate degrees (Aiken et al. 2014). A consensus exists among consumers, nurses, physicians, and healthcare administrators regarding the significant impact of nurse staffing ratios on quality of care and patient outcomes (Aiken et al. 2012). The Institute of Medicine (2010) has called for increasing the numbers of baccalaureate and doctorally-prepared nurses to meet this need.

31.3.4 Population Diversity

The growing population diversity has highlighted the need for greater representation of racial and ethnic minorities among healthcare professionals.

By mid-twenty-first century, it is predicted that the USA will cease to have a majority race. Ethnic and racial minorities will increase from 37% to nearly 50% of the total population as compared to white Americans who will decrease from 69.4% to 50.1%. Hispanics will experience 187% growth and African Americans 71%; Hispanics and African Americans will comprise 24.4% and 14.6% of the population in 2050, respectively (Colby and Ortman 2015; Okoro 2012).

Currently, over 33 million people speak Spanish in the USA, more than 10 million speak another European language, and more than 8 million speak an Asian language (Okoro 2012). However, today's health professional workforce does not proportionally reflect all racial and ethnic groups; whites comprise more than 80% of the health professional workforce. While Asian Americans are well represented in health careers, the representation of African Americans, Hispanics, and Native Americans is much lower. When combined, these groups represent over 30% of the US population, yet these minorities are underrepresented among physicians, registered nurses, dentists, pharmacists, and allied health professionals (Valentine et al. 2016).

31.3.5 Existence of Health Inequities

There is mounting evidence of health disparities in access to health services and health outcomes across population groups within the same region and across different nations. Worldwide, there is overwhelming evidence demonstrating poorer health among those with lower socioeconomic status and groups who experience a history of systemic discrimination, marginalization, and disempowerment. These groups are likely to live in neighborhoods with meager resources and higher health risks as well as encounter prejudice and discrimination when accessing health services (see Chap. 1).

In the USA, racial and ethnic minorities comprise the majority of people living in areas designated as health professional shortage areas (Mitchell and Lassiter 2006). According to the

American College of Physicians (2010), minorities have less access to healthcare than whites and receive poorer quality of care even when access-related factors such as insurance status and income are controlled. For example, 34% of Hispanics are uninsured as compared to 13% among whites, more minority women avoid doctors' visits because of cost, and racial and ethnic minority Medicare beneficiaries with dementia are 30% less likely than whites to use anti-dementia medication. Compared to white Americans, African Americans are less likely to receive certain treatments, wait longer for kidney transplants, are more likely to die from cancer from all causes, and have higher infant mortality rates. Hispanic and African Americans are more likely to die from diabetes complications than white Americans (AACN 2014).

Countries with universal access to health services have focused on social determinants and social inequalities to address health inequity, defining the latter as avoidable and unfair differences (see Chap. 1). By contrast, the USA lacks a universal program for accessing healthcare services. Hence, efforts have focused on increasing representation of racial and ethnic minorities in health professions, training, and development of health practitioners and students in culturally competent care and changes in organizational infrastructure and health delivery. It should be noted that development of all healthcare practitioners and students in culturally competent care has been recommended by international and national stakeholders alike.

31.4 Advantages of a Multicultural Workforce

Multiculturalism in the workplace can create a sense of cultural awareness among workers as employees are exposed to different ideas and perspectives. Encounters with diverse perspectives can stimulate reflection on one's own ways of thinking and doing. Diverse viewpoints can generate new and innovative solutions (Lewis 2017). As a result of exposure to cultural differences, curiosity can be stimulated and employees are motivated to learn more about other cultures. Knowledge of cultural differences can promote tolerance in the workplace and implementation of work approaches that are informed by this knowledge (Green et al. 2015). Exposure to different viewpoints and cultures can build tolerance of different perspectives, which in turn can foster improved collaboration and cooperation. Employees from diverse backgrounds thrive in an organizational climate of inclusion and openness (Mayhew 2017). The effectiveness of a diverse workforce depends on a climate of multiculturalism that permeates every aspect of the organization (Greenberg 2004).

Organizations can draw from a greater variety of abilities offered by diverse employees, such as, multilingual proficiencies, and work-related expertise and life experiences in other cultures. Companies may benefit from a workforce with a larger social network than just one ethnic group that can generate an interest in providing products and services in many ethnic communities. An organization providing goods and services that appeal to several ethnic groups is more likely to be successful with workers who can communicate with these groups.

Employees with diverse backgrounds can also improve global competitiveness of their organizations because they are familiar with their own country—the customs, traditions, and language of the people. They can act as cultural brokers and facilitate bridging with global customers (Bovee and Thill 2008). Workforce diversity has become a powerful tool for recruitment and retention of the best employees in order to sustain an organization's competitive edge (Cadrain 2008). An effective multicultural workforce can increase an organization's success, competitiveness, and adaptability in a global marketplace. A multicultural workforce offers a greater pool of talents, ideas, and work ethic that can enhance organizational effectiveness.

Healthcare organizations gain these same benefits from a diverse workforce. A review of studies in healthcare by the US Health Resources and Services Administration (HRSA 2006) revealed that patients are more likely to receive quality preventive care and treatment when they share race, ethnicity, language, and/or religious experiences with their providers. A diverse workforce and the diverse perspective it provides contribute many benefits, including enhanced communication, increased healthcare access, greater patient satisfaction, decreased health disparities, and improved problem-solving for complex problems and innovation. Given a choice, racial and ethnic minority patients are more likely to select health professionals of the same racial and ethnic background as themselves. Patients are more likely to report greater satisfaction with care and higher quality of care received when they share a common racial and ethnic background as well as language with their providers. Minority providers improve access to care in underserved areas more than nonminority providers; they are more likely to practice in underserved communities and care for large numbers of minority patients (HRSA 2006).

Diversity in health professional educational environments improves the quality of education and ability to treat patients from different sociocultural backgrounds by broadening students' perspectives. Diversity improves learning outcomes, thinking and intellectual engagement, motivation, social and civic skills, and empathy and understanding of racial and cultural differences (AACN 2015).

31.5 Challenges of a Multicultural Workforce

As the workforce becomes increasingly global and culturally diverse, organizations are challenged to communicate more effectively interpersonally, interculturally, and in groups (Lauring 2011). Internal and external communication is essential for an organization to maintain its competitive edge and sustainable growth in a global market. Perceptual, cultural, and language barriers need to be overcome for diversity to succeed. Communication affects productivity and overall business performance, individually and in groups (Gupta 2008). Ineffective communication results in confusion, lack of teamwork, and low morale.

Performance and productivity of human capital in the global market depends largely on the effectiveness of business communication and employees' competence in interpersonal communication, intercultural sensitivity, and nonverbal communication (Nagourney 2008). By expanding avenues for communication and providing ongoing feedback, organizations can establish a culture that values diversity in their employees (Hannay and Fretwell 2011).

Another challenge is resistance from employees to accept and accommodate differences. Productive diverse teams require a robust organizational leadership commitment to allocate resources and create the infrastructure and management systems supportive of active participation and success of diverse employees (Kokemuller 2017). Organizational leaders have the daunting challenge of motivating and promoting harmony among diverse employees while facing challenges from the community and business competitors.

There are costs involved in cultivating an effective multicultural workforce. Ongoing development of managers and future leaders among the diverse pool of employees can facilitate organizational adaptability to internal and external challenges. There are associated costs to global recruitment, training, and development of diverse employees. There are costs associated with litigation involving internal workforce diversity and community diversity. Managers need to adapt to changing responsibilities and social norms by ensuring that practices are aligned with regulatory and legal provisions, e.g., protection against sexual discrimination and harassment, Equal Employment Opportunity, etc. (Greenberg 2004).

A diverse workforce poses increased potential for discrimination because when people with obvious distinguishing traits are placed together, employees with prejudices could use them against others. Diversity management is so critical to preventing such risks. Organizations need to provide cultural awareness and sensitivity training to help create a culture of tolerance and acceptance of differences (Kokemuller 2017).

31.6 Strategies for Building Effective Multicultural Healthcare Workforce

31.6.1 Workforce Planning and Development

Public and private stakeholders worldwide have called for the need for all nations to develop a sustainable workforce. Measures are needed through global and multilateral agreement among countries to prevent unethical manpower outflows that endanger any country's health. Multilateral agreements among governments should address ways to compensate for the loss of financial investment in the education of healthcare professionals and the negative consequences on population health and healthcare services in source countries. While migration of health professionals has benefited their families and countries through their remittances, these gains are hardly used for improviwng overall population health, healthcare infrastructure, and educational systems. Source countries are also accountable for their lack of policies promoting retention and engagement of health professionals in their own healthcare systems.

A significant strategy recommended is improving the supply of sufficient numbers of students entering and graduating from health professions schools, particularly for racial and ethnic minority students. Attracting racial and ethnic minorities should begin early by increasing awareness of communities of healthcare professions and by engaging minority healthcare professionals in recruiting potential students. Healthcare organizations, including professional associations and schools, should develop long-standing partnerships with primary and secondary schools, the media, and communities to promote interest in healthcare professions. Partnerships among stakeholders in the public and private sectors with health professionals can create sustainable programs and policies on recruitment and workforce development, such as the partnerships between the Institute of Medicine and Robert Wood Johnson Foundation and between Johnson and Johnson and nursing

professional stakeholders (IOM 2010; Johnson and Johnson 2016).

To enhance admission of racial and ethnic minorities in medicine, the Sullivan Commission (2004), which is comprised of multiple healthcare stakeholders, recommended using quantitative and qualitative criteria for admission to medical schools to enhance the competitive edge of racial and minority students who may not do as well in traditional measures for admission. To improve the quality of pipeline schools in minority neighborhoods, several initiatives have evolved such as summer enrichment programs to improve students' proficiency in science, math, communication, and critical thinking as well as awareness of college-level expectations. Cooperative after-school and summer internship programs between high schools and local organizations connect students with mentors in health professions and expose them to different healthcare settings. Professional schools have created an infrastructure to provide academic, financial, and psychological support for disadvantaged students.

31.6.2 Training and Development

Various chapters of this book (Chaps. 1–11) are focused in more detail on development of cultural competence among healthcare workers. This section highlights the process of fostering global citizenship outlook and skills critical to culturally competent practices of healthcare workers. Developing cultural knowledge and awareness must emphasize empathic understanding of the social and cultural contexts of people's lives. Fostering the development of cultural curiosity in learners by communicating enthusiasm about knowing other cultures should be developed early in education. Much influence is exerted by teachers and mentors who are keenly interested in cultural phenomena and diversity. Curricular integration and selection of learning experiences should be carefully planned to prevent marginalization of certain groups by building unquestioned superiority of others. Empathic and compassionate understanding is enhanced by using different methods of learning using videos, case studies, home visits, travel-learn, etc. Listening to actual narratives by the people provokes empathy and compassion among listeners.

The method of instruction must move away from a listing of descriptions of people's characteristics and ways of life toward an understanding of how social, environmental, and historical circumstances have shaped people's life chances and current life situations. Stereotypes and monolithic generalizations of cultures should be avoided. Actual encounters, observations, and experiences in different social contexts are superior in promoting appreciation of the holistic context of people's lives. Exposure of learners to diversity, disadvantaged communities, and diverse groups should be aimed at developing comparative knowledge of cultures and compassionate understanding of how and why certain people live differently. Teachers and mentors should facilitate discovery of hidden forces that contribute to how people behave and live. For example, learning health disparities must not be limited to morbidity and mortality but should promote understanding of why certain groups have fewer resources and have greater health liabilities than others; learners must be made aware that poor health is not merely caused by poor genes or unhealthy life choices.

Critical reflection can be facilitated by open and respectful dialogue focusing on critiquing and challenging individual opinions. This is built upon the foundation that each one has value and a positive contribution to the collective wisdom and decision. Honest and genuine dialogue should be facilitated in order to challenge individual opinions and come up with equitable solutions. The potential impact of recommended solutions must be examined thoroughly to develop a full understanding of the consequences of each solution on individuals, families, organizations, and communities.

Teachers and mentors must model the learner's role and the value of humility to facilitate growth and mutual respect among learners. This approach builds trust essential for openness and acceptance of differences. While standards for practice are essential to follow, these should not blindly dictate actions and decisions. Rather, the personal, social, environmental, and historical factors must be considered in determining the proper course of action. Peer mentors should be trained and made available to facilitate individual level and unit level cultural competence.

Development of intercultural communication is critical. Health workers deal with different levels and types of diversity in healthcare. Flexibility and adaptability are extremely important in interactions. The ability to understand others, work with human and material communication aids, and reach diverse groups hinges upon one's knowledge of cultural differences, commitment to diversity and equity and available resources. Conflict management skills are essential in intercultural communication as most conflicts are associated with cultural differences. Training and actual practice in advocacy skills to identify, question, and challenge injustices in the workplace should be provided. Promoting trust and cooperation requires the ability to create bonds and attachments emphasizing similarities with others, recognizing and bridging differences, and building mutual capacity by linking with appropriate social networks. Conflict management is a significant skill to develop as many conflicts arise from sociocultural differences. Training should be provided in negotiation, cultural brokering, and helping others navigate the healthcare system. Multilevel and interprofessional communication skills should emphasize the skills of collaboration, role clarification, and leadership to resolve conflicts and enhance patient/family-centered communication (Arain et al. 2017).

31.6.3 Global Citizenship Values

A critical foundation of culturally competent practice is the development of a global outlook and global citizenship skills. Reysen and Katzarska-Miller (2013) define global citizenship as "awareness, caring, and embracing cultural diversity while promoting social justice and sustainability, coupled with a sense of responsibility to act" (p. 858). As global citizens, individuals have a keen awareness of global trends and issues, appreciate the interconnectedness among people, and position themselves within a larger global context (Cesario 2016). Global citizens are self-actualized in inherently synergistic values such as the desire for relatedness and compassion for others (Cooper 2016). Relatedness allows for the flourishing of the values of mutuality and care for others and rejection of oppressive or exploitative relationships.

31.6.4 Valuing Diversity

Global citizens have an empathic understanding of the feelings and experiences of others, including both people who experience oppression and the oppressors (Lemberger and Lemberger-Truelove 2016). Empathy and compassion draw humans together, building meaningful and transformative connections and social capital. Global citizens have actualized their "wants" that may be dysergistic in nature such as the quest for individual competence, success, and uniqueness toward more prosocial values of mutual trust and reciprocity. Dysergistic wants can be tempered by the principle of *equifinality* that accepts the multiple ways by which problems can be solved and the myriad ways by which individuals can achieve (Cooper 2016). Cultural heterogeneity provides a means whereby each person can actualize their authentic being as a unique and distinctive person by tapping into their unique traditions and wisdom to build on the wisdom of others. Cultural heterogeneity allows people to actualize their desires for competence and significance without undermining these in others.

31.6.5 Commitment to Social Justice

Social justice is grounded in the principles of human rights and equality, consistent with societal efforts to provide equitable treatment and a fair allocation of health resources to all citizens (Matwick and Woodgate 2017). Understanding, respecting, and valuing of existing diversity is the foundation that enables global citizens to challenge injustice and take action in personally meaningful ways (Jones 2016). True justice must

activate the human potentialities in both the advocates and those who are advocated for (Freire 2000). Empathy allows a deeper appreciation of experiences and feelings of others, including both people who experience oppression and the oppressors. Compassion allows the practitioner to accept another person's humanity, even when their position as an oppressor or oppressed person is not understandable. Empathy and compassion draw humans together. By helping people trust, recognize, and articulate their true feelings and experiences along with developing skills for dialogue and negotiation (Cooper et al. 2012), advocacy for social justice can be informed by the context in which injustice occurs and allow best practices for advocacy and empowerment to occur (Ratts et al. 2016).

31.6.6 Recruitment and Retention

The best recruitment strategy is generated from the positive testimonial from employees and consumers of care. Racial and ethnic groups tend to gravitate toward members of their own group and seek care from organizations that value their culture and understand their language and communication. Job promotion and recognition of minority employees are positive advertisements for recruitment of diverse workforce and consumers. As organizational leaders, they can serve as mentors and role models for their group. Capitalizing on the cultural identity and community affiliation of diverse employees can establish the link between the community and the organization. By engaging diverse staff, consumers, and communities, the organization can benefit from their input in recruiting potential employees, develop interest in health professions in their community, and improve its services. Partnering with local schools (secondary and collegiate) by offering cooperative work experiences, internships, and clinical affiliations can generate long-term interest and commitment in students to work in the organization.

A diverse workforce flourishes in an organizational climate that values expressions of diversity and using diversity to develop innovative practices that others can support. Organizational leaders should develop the structure and management systems supportive of diversity. Further discussion of leadership strategies to promote this organizational climate is presented in Chap. 10.

Organizational investment in continuing education of employees for advanced degrees nurtures loyalty and commitment of employees to stay in the organization. Management systems built on fairness, respect, and appreciation of diversity contribute to a sense of value and belonging among diverse staff. Organizational leaders, mentors, and preceptors should have training in advocacy for these values. Orientation of new staff should include not only the technical aspects of their work but also the culture of the organization and the community in which it is nested. Concrete explanations with demonstrations of policies and protocols of care will minimize confusion and misinterpretation for multicultural staff. Soliciting feedback of diverse employees in a non-threatening way will enhance their security and sense of belonging as well as increase their participation in unit decisions.

Staff retention is enhanced by how employees fit within the organization. Organizational norms and cultural nuances are best learned through bicultural mentors who can nurture multicultural perspectives within the context of the organization and the community. Training and modeling of professional behaviors (communication, conflict management, decision-making, etc.) for diverse employees require a concerted effort by all staff. This is particularly important for nurses who were socialized in a hierarchical culture and gender-differentiated behaviors. Training should include both oral and written expression particularly for those who are nonnative speakers of the mainstream language of the culture.

Advocacy for diverse staff with aggressive patients and abusive co-workers should be fostered as well as assist their development of self-advocacy skills. Many cultures across the globe do not value assertiveness and confrontation; hence healthcare professionals from these cultures need to learn the cognitive, expressive, and emotional components of this interactive style. Effective communication enhances achievement of desired outcomes and ability to influence others. Understanding cultural differences among all staff and administrators promotes development of empathy and compassion for others. In this environment, mutual trust, reciprocity, and engagement with others thrive.

Conclusion

The value of workforce diversity has been documented in studies in businesses, healthcare, and education. In healthcare, language and racial/ethnic concordance between health providers and patients have positive impact on patient's health behaviors, satisfaction with care, and access to care. However, the approach to increase the proportional representation of diverse patients among healthcare professionals is challenged by market forces, globalization, and increasing movement of populations across the world. Therefore, training and development of all health professionals and students in culturally competent care must be instituted while continuing efforts to recruit and graduate large numbers of diverse health professionals.

Culturally competent practice in a diverse world with long-standing disparities in healthcare access and outcomes that impact more negatively the disadvantaged and diverse minorities should be grounded in the values of global citizenship. The model presented in Chap. 1 emphasizes the need for healthcare professionals grounded with a compassionate understanding of social inequities that impact health. It requires commitment to the principles of social justice, equity, and human rights protection. Cultural competence can assist in transforming vulnerable groups when it is grounded in these principles. Culturally competent healthcare professionals have a common grounding in a global citizenry emphasizing a collective outlook that respects and treats others as part of oneself and a common humanity. Global citizenship is built on empathy and compassion for others that can foster common bonds and social connectedness for a common good—promote well-being and health of everyone. Cultural competence development must be centered on building inherent prosocial tendencies to be connected with others in a climate of mutual trust and respect that transcends cultural differences.

References

AACN (2014) Fact sheet. The need for diversity in healthcare workforce. http://www.aapcho.org/wp/wp-content/uploads/2012/11/Need ForDiversityHealthCareWorkforce.pdf. Accessed 31 May 2017

AACN (2015) Talking points: HRSA report on nursing workforce projections through 2025. http://www.aacn.nche.edu/media-relations/HRSA-Nursing-Workforce-Projections.pdf

Aiken LH (2007). U.S. nurse labor market dynamics are key to global nurse sufficiency. Health Serv Res. 42(3 Pt 2): 1299–1320. https://doi.org/10.1111/j.1475-6773.2007.00714.x

Aiken LH, Sermeus W, Van den Heede K et al (2012) Patient safety, satisfaction, and quality of hospital care: cross sectional surveys of nurses and patients in 12 countries in Europe and the United States. BMJ 344:e1717. https://doi.org/10.1136/bmj.e1717

Aiken LH, Sloane DM, Bryneel L et al (2014) Nurse staffing and education and hospital mortality in nine European countries: a retrospective observational study. Lancet 383(9931):1824–1830

Allutis C, Bishaw T, Frank MW (2014) The workforce for health in a globalized context—global shortages and international migration. Global Health Action 7:23611. https://doi.org/10.3402/gha.v7.23611

American College of Physicians (2010) Racial and ethnic disparities in health care. Author, Philadelphia, PA. http://www.acponline.org/advocacy/where_we_stand/access/racial_disparities.pdf

Arain M, Suter E, Mallinson S et al (2017) Interprofessional education for internationally educated health professionals: an environmental scan. J Multidiscip Healthc 10:87–83

Bovee CL, Thill JV (2008) Business communication today, 9th edn. Prentice Hall, Boston

Buerhaus PI, Auerbach DI, Staiger DO (2009) The recent surge in nurse employment: causes and implications. Health Aff 28(4):w657–w668. https://doi.org/10.1377/hlthaff.28.4.w657

Cadrain D (2008) Sexual equity in the workplace. HR Magazine 53(9):44–48,50

Cesario S (2016) Sustainable development goals for monitoring action to improve global health. Nurs Women's Health 20(4):427–431. https://doi.org/10.1016/j.nwh.2016.06.001

Clemens MA, Petersen G (2008) New data on African health professionals abroad. Human Resour Health 6:1. https://doi.org/10.1186/1478-4491-6-1

Colby SL, Ortman JM (2015) Projections of the size and composition of the US population: 2014–2060. Current population reports. https://www.census.gov/content/dam/Census/library/publications/2015/demo/p25-1143.pdf

Cooper M (2016) The fully functioning society: a humanistic-existential visions of an actualizing, socially just future. J Humanistic Psychol 56(6):581–594. https://doi.org/10.1177/0022167816659755

Cooper M, Chak A, Cornish F et al (2012) Dialogue: bridging personal, community and social transformation. J Humanistic Psychol 55:70–93. https://doi.org/10.1177/0022167812447298

Douglas M, Rosenketter M, Pacquiao D, Clark Callister L, Hattar-Pollara M, Lauderdale L, Milsted J, Nardi D, Purnell L (2014) Guidelines for implementing culturally competent nursing care. J Transcult Nurs 25(2):109–221

Dussault G, Fronteira J, Cabral J (2009) Migration of health personnel in the WHO European region. WHO Regional Office, Copenhagen

Eckenwiler LA (2009) Care worker migration and transnational justice. Public Health Ethics 2:171–183

Freire P (2000) Pedagogy of the oppressed. Bloomsbury Academic, New York

Green K, Lopez M, Wysocki A, et al (2015) Diversity in the workplace: benefits, challenges and the required managerial tools. https://edis.ifas.ufl.edu/pdffiles/HR/HR02200.pdf

Greenberg J (2004) Diversity in the workplace: benefits, challenges and solutions. http://www.multiculturaladvantage.com/recruit/diversity/diversity-in-the-workplace-benefits-challenges-solutions.asp

Gupta S (2008) Mine the potential of multicultural teams. HR Magazine 53(10):79–80

Hannay M, Fretwell C (2011) The higher education workplace: meeting the needs of multiple generations. Res Higher Educ J 10:1–12

HRSA (2006) The rationale for diversity in the health professions: a review of evidence. http://www.readbag.com/bhpr-hrsa-healthworkforce-reports-diversityreviewevidence.

HRSA (2016) National and regional projections of supply and demand for primary care practitioners: 2013–2025. USDHHS, Rockville, MD

HRSA (2017a) Designated health professional shortage areas. https://ersrs.hrsa.gov/ReportServer?/HGDW_Reports/BCD_HPSA/BCD_HPSA_SCR50_Smry_HTML&rc:Toolbar=false

HRSA (2017b) Data warehouse: medically underserved areas /populations. https://ersrs.hrsa.gov/ReportServer?/HGDW_Reports/BCD_MUA/BCD_MUA_State_Statistics_HTML&rc:Toolbar=false

ICN (2006) The global nursing shortage: priority areas for intervention. Author, Geneva, Switzerland

IOM (2010) The future of nursing: leading change, advancing health. National Academies Press, Washington, DC

Johnson and Johnson (2016) Campaign for nursing's future. https://www.discovernursing.com/sites/default/files/media/press1796178328/Campaign%20for%20Nursing%27s%20Future_Overview_5%203%2016.pdf

Jones S (2016) Global citizenship. Aust Nurs Midwifery J 23(10):48

Jurado LF(2013).Social construction of Filipino foreign-educated nurses in the US. PhD dissertation. Rutgers University, Newark, NJ

Jurado LF, Pacquiao DF (2015) Historical analysis of Filipino nurse migration to the US. J Nurs Pract

Appl Rev Res 5(1):4–18. https://doi.org/10.13178/jnparr.2015.0501.1303

Kingma M (2007) Nurses on the move: a global overview. Health Res Educ Trust 42(3):1281–1298. https://doi.org/10.1111/j.1475-6773.2007.00711.x

Kokemuller N (2017) Advantages and disadvantages of multicultural workforce. http://smallbusiness.chron.com/advantages-disadvantages-multicultural-workforce-18903.html

Lauring J (2011) The social order of interaction in international encounters. J Bus Commun 48:231–255

Lemberger ME, Lemberger-Truelove TL (2016) Bases for a more socially just humanistic praxis. J Humanistic Psychol 56(6):571–580. https://doi.org/10.1177/0022167816652750

Lewis J (2017) The advantages of multiculturalism in the workplace. http://smallbusiness.chron.com/advantages-multiculturalism-workplace-15239.html

Martin J, Nakayama T (2010) Intercultural communication in contexts, 4th edn. McGraw-Hill, New York

Masselink LE (2009) Health professions education as a national industry: framing of controversies in nursing education and migration in the Philippines. PhD Dissertation, University of North Carolina at Chapel Hill

Matwick A, Woodgate R (2017) Social justice: a concept analysis. Public Health Nurs 34(2):176–184. https://doi.org/10.1111/phn.12288

Mayhew R (2017) How to manage and motivate a multicultural workforce. http://smallbusiness.chron.com/manage-motivate-multicultural-workforce-10985.html

Mitchell DA, Lassiter SL (2006) Addressing health care disparities and increasing workforce diversity: the next step for the dental, medical and public health professions. AJPH 96:2093–2097

Nagourney E (2008) East and West part ways in test of facial expression. NY Times. http://www.nytimes.com/2008/03/18/health/18face.html. Accessed on 13 May 2017

Okoro EA (2012) Workforce diversity and organizational communication: analysis of human capital performance and productivity. J Diver Manag 7(1):57–62

Pacquiao DF (2003) People of Filipino heritage. In: Purnell LD, Paulanka B (eds) Transcultural health care: a culturally competent approach. F. A. Davis Company, Philadelphia, pp 138–159

Ratts M, Singh J, Nassar-McMillan AA, et al. (2016) Multicultural and social justice counseling competencies: guidelines for the counseling profession. J Multicult Couns Dev 44: 28–48.

Reysen S, Katzarska-Miller I (2013) A model of global citizenship: antecedents and outcomes. Int J Psychol 48(5):858–870. https://doi.org/10.1080/00207594.2012.701749

Sullivan Commission (2004) Missing persons: minorities in the health profession. http://www.aacn.nche.edu/media-relations/SullivanReport.pdf

Valentine P, Wynn J, McLean D (2016) Improving diversity in the health professions. NCMJ 77(2):137–140

Walker J (2010) The global nursing shortage. Migration, brain drain and going forward. Johns Hopkins Nursing. http://magazine.nursing.jhu.edu/2010/08/the-global-nursing-shortage/

WHO (2013) Global health workforce shortage to reach 12.9 million in coming decades. http://www.who.int/mediacentre/news/releases/2013/health-workforce-shortage/en/

Case Study: Internationally Educated Nurses Working in a Canadian Healthcare Setting

32

Louise Racine

Anita is a 21-year-old nurse who recently completed her baccalaureate in nursing from a nursing school in Manila. Anita has aspired to pursue a nursing career abroad to avail of better working conditions, better pay, and a chance to pursue higher nursing education. She decided to immigrate to Canada and settle in a western Canadian province. She needed to have her credentials reviewed and approved by a provincial regulatory body to determine her eligibility to take the Canadian licensure exam (NCLEX) for entry to practice as a registered nurse/RN in Canada. Anita passed her NCLEX exam. She benefitted from the financial support of her Canadian employer. The employer paid Anita's fees to write her NCLEX as it did for all recently hired internationally educated nurses. The employer provided a 6-month allowance to pay Anita's rent. Anita stays in a rented apartment with other Filipino nurses. Anita has very few Canadian friends outside work. Anita is fluent in English, and she does not have problems communicating with her patients in English.

Anita was hired in an urban hospital to work on a surgical care unit of 40 beds. Her employer provided her with 1-week orientation training where she and other internationally educated nurses learned policies, protocols, equipment, and technology. Following this orientation, Anita was matched with a Canadian nurse mentor for 2 full weeks. Nurses in this tertiary care hospital perform 12-h shifts. Anita completed the training, and the mentor informed the head nurse (nurse manager) that Anita was secure enough to practice without direct supervision by a colleague.

Anita seems to perform quite well but has frequently been observed by the head nurse to talk in her native language, *Tagalog*, with her Filipino colleagues on the unit. Her co-workers and other nurses have been irritated by this behavior and complained to the nurse in charge of the unit. Anita and her colleagues were reminded to speak in English during working hours to prevent conflicts with other nurses. More recently, Anita encountered a problem with a patient. She needed to draw a blood sample from a central intravenous port line. After the nurse manager received a complaint from the patient, she asked Anita and her mentor to come to her office. The nurse manager stated:

> For instance, let's say they [Filipino nurses] are asked to take a sample from a port line. They say, Yes. Yes. I know. I know. Yes. Yes. Then the patient comes to my office and tells me, I do not think Anita knows how to access the port line. Other nurses do it another way. They [Filipino nurses] will not admit to not knowing how to do the procedure. Instead, the patient comes to tell me. Why have you not told me that you were uncomfortable performing that technique?

L. Racine, Ph.D.,C.N.M.,F.A.C.N.M., FAAN
College of Nursing, University of Saskatchewan, Saskatoon, SK, Canada
e-mail: louise.racine@usask.ca

© Springer International Publishing AG, part of Springer Nature 2018
M. Douglas et al. (eds.), *Global Applications of Culturally Competent Health Care: Guidelines for Practice*, https://doi.org/10.1007/978-3-319-69332-3_32

The nurse manager has assumed that internationally educated nurses will not disclose practice skills deficit reflecting their lack of professional accountability. This behavior has been attributed by the nurse manager and other nurses to the internationally educated nurses' fear of losing their jobs and being forced to return to their country. If procedures and techniques are not adequately followed, this creates risks to patient safety and quality of care. While failure to disclose lack of practice skills also arises among domestic trained nurses, the attribution is only applied to internationally educated nurses, creating a major risk of *othering* internationally educated nurses based on an ethnocentric bias. Othering is a process of social stratification by which the color of the skin (race) or other attributes (speaking English with a foreign accent) are used to marginalize culturally different peoples (Racine 2003). Canales (2010) argues that othering is both exclusionary and inclusionary "often using the power within relationships for domination and subordination with the potential consequences of alienation, marginalization, decreased opportunities, internalized oppression, and exclusion" (p. 5).

The case study reveals how important it is for nurses to understand the interplay of race, gender, and social class within health workplaces in general and nursing workplaces in particular. O'Brien-Pallas et al. (2007) suggest that internationally educated nurses experience more physical and emotional abuse in the workplace than Canadian nurses. Issues of "everyday racism" (Essed 1991) have been documented within Canadian nursing workplaces (Beaton and Walsh 2010; Calliste 1993; Das Gupta 2009; Newton et al. 2013; Racine 2009; Reimer Kirkham 2003; Ronquillo et al. 2011; Salami and Nelson 2014). Also, instances of racism and ethnocentrism have been reported within international nursing work contexts (Bae 2011; Huria et al. 2014; Mapedzahama et al. 2012; McKillop et al. 2013; Puzan 2003; Schroeder and DiAngelo 2010). Racism in nursing does not represent a new phenomenon per se, yet little progress has been made in eliminating problems of cultural incompetency within health organizations and nursing workplaces (Douglas et al. 2014; Racine 2014).

32.1 Social Structural Factors

Nurse migration is a trend not likely to decrease in the coming years as migration is a human right. Furthermore, some supplying countries train their nurses for export to high-income countries for economic purpose. Workplace diversity is becoming increasingly important in healthcare settings in the United States, Canada, and other Western nations. As the nursing workforce and demographic patterns change, it is important for nurses to understand cultural diversity in nursing and health workplaces. The Sullivan Commission on Diversity in the Healthcare Workforce report (2004) underlines three principles for increasing diversity within health and nursing workforce in the United States. These principles are designed to: (1) increase ethnocultural diversity in the health workforce through hiring and retention of minority peoples, (2) facilitate and implement changes within health organizations to support ethnocultural diversity, and (3) promote openness to explore new and nontraditional paths to nursing and allied health professions.

Globalization brings increased ethnic and cultural diversity within healthcare organizations that affects the way nurses deliver care and how they interact with nurses coming from other countries. More than ever, nurses must be culturally competent and safe in their everyday practice regardless of the health settings in which they work. Cultural competency and cultural safety are key skills for nurses to acquire and sustain. The International Council of Nurses (2013), Canadian Nurses Association (2015), Canadian Association of Schools of Nursing (2014), American Nurses Association (1998), American Organization of Nurses Executives (2015), and the US Department of Health and Human Services (2017) are among the major regulatory nursing bodies and health organizations that recognize the moral and ethical duty of nurses to advocate and provide culturally competent care.

Cultural diversity implies the notion of cultural differences which means how individuals and groups vary based on some ethnic, racial, and cultural attributes. Andrews and Boyle (2012) define diversity as "differences in race, ethnicity, national origins, religion, gender, sexual orientation, ability or disability, social and economic status or class, education, and related attributes of groups of people in society" (p. 5). The notion of diversity creates the need for nurses to become culturally knowledgeable and conscious of their attitudes toward people from other ethnocultural groups. The concepts of race and ethnicity are often conflated and emerge as problematic issues arising from cultural conflicts or misunderstandings between individuals and groups. It is therefore, important to understand the differences between ethnicity and race.

Ethnicity and race constitute different concepts, although they may overlap. Eriksen (2010) defines ethnicity as "the relationships between groups whose members consider themselves distinctive" (p. 10). Belonging to an ethnic group may be used to categorize individuals and groups based on some norms or values that can cause prejudice. This phenomenon is called ethnocentrism. Ethnocentrism refers to a "universal tendency of human beings to think that their ways of thinking, acting, and believing are the only right and proper ways" (Purnell 2013: 7).

Race refers to "a group of human beings socially defined by physical characteristics. Determining which characteristics constitute a particular race, the selection of markers and, therefore, the construction of the racial category itself, is a choice human beings make" (Cornell and Hartmann 2007: 25). Purnell (2013) argues that "race as a social meaning, assigns status, limits or increases opportunities, and influences interactions between patients and clinicians" (p. 8). Race can be used as a means of stratification through social and cultural othering where discrimination arises from the "visibility of one's Otherness" (Canales 2010: 5).

32.2 Cultural Competency

Cultural competency is a concept that arises from the seminal work of Madeleine Leininger who trained as a nurse and an anthropologist (McFarland and Wehbe-Alamah 2017). Leininger (2002) postulates that "culture is an integral and essential aspect of being human, and the culture care aspects cannot be overlooked or neglected" (p. 4). Campinha-Bacote (2002) defines cultural competency as an "ongoing process in which the health care provider continuously strive to achieve the ability to effectively work within the cultural context of the client [individual, family, and community]" (p. 181). Campinha-Bacote (2002) builds on the assumption that cultural competency is an ongoing process of being and becoming. She describes five interrelated concepts: (1) cultural awareness, (2) cultural knowledge, (3) cultural skill, (4) cultural encounters, and (5) cultural desire. Campinha-Bacote (2002) underlines that to be effective, this model "requires health care providers to see themselves as becoming culturally competent rather than already being culturally competent" (p. 181).

On top of being culturally competent with their practice with individuals and groups, nurses must also become aware of power relations within their workplaces. Becoming aware of power differentials associated with race, gender, and social class represents the first step toward becoming culturally safe. Cultural safety originates from the groundbreaking work of Irihapeti Ramsden, a Maori nurse who described the persistent inequities affecting indigenous peoples of New Zealand (Nursing Council of New Zealand 2011; Ramsden 1993). Cultural safety is defined as "nursing or midwifery action to protect from danger and/or reduce risk to patient/client/community from hazards to health and well-being" (Papps and Ramsden 1996: 493). While cultural competency helps us to understand other people's attitudes and behaviors, nurses also need to understand the limitations of systemic barriers in maintaining health and social inequities. Cultural safety requires nurses to be aware of power relations in their interactions with individuals, groups, communities, or colleagues at work.

The delivery of culturally competent care is a fundamental standard of ethical practice set by international and national nursing regulatory bodies. The International Council of Nursing (2013) mentions that "in providing care, the nurse promotes an environment in which the human rights, values, customs and spiritual beliefs of the individual, family, and community are respected" (p. 2). In a position statement on discrimination and racism in health care, the American Nurses Association (1998) underlines that nurses must strive to eradicate discrimination within health workplaces and guide practice from a social justice perspective. Similarly, an expert panel for Global Nursing and Health established by the American Academy of Nursing and members of the Transcultural Nursing Society (2010) report the need to apply universal standards of practice for culturally competent nursing care in the world. Arising from that report, Douglas et al. (2014) underline the need for nurses to apply Guideline 8 to support a multicultural workforce. The ongoing issue of nurse migration illustrates the need for health agencies to develop strategies to address cultural conflicts and support internationally educated nurses in their adaptation to their new working environment (Douglas et al. 2014).

32.3 Culturally Competent Strategies Recommended

Internationally educated nurses from middle- and low-income countries need to be mentored and supported in the receiving countries. Based on Anita's case study, the following recommendations are likely to facilitate the creation of a multicultural workforce and strengthen the recruitment and retention of a culturally diverse nursing labor force.

32.3.1 Individual Interventions

- Be aware that international nurses may have been educated in different healthcare settings where technology may be limited as compared to that of Western countries.
- Document the practice skills and ensure that international nurses disclose lack of knowledge or skills to create a culture of patient safety.
- Domestic-educated nurses need to receive cultural competency training to prevent the harmful effects of racism and ethnocentrism in stereotyping ethnocultural groups based on one individual's actions.
- International nurses need to know the healthcare system, the official language, and the cultural norms of the receiving countries.
- Provide international nurses the opportunity to speak their languages while ensuring that it does not create conflicts at the workplace or interfere with patient care.
- Pair up international nurses with another international nurse of the same ethnocultural group who has successfully integrated in the unit and the healthcare organization.

32.3.2 Organization Level Interventions

- Develop programs of mentoring for internationally educated nurses to support their social, cultural, and professional integration.
- Develop a policy of zero tolerance of racism and other forms of discrimination based on gender, social, class, sexual orientation, disability, religion, language, or ethnicity at work.
- Develop a charter of rights that apply to all levels of the organization and staff.
- Make cultural competency a shared value of the organization.
- Create activities to support the celebration of cultural diversity.
- Implement professional development activities geared toward developing cultural competency and cultural safety skills within the organization.
- Facilitate the reporting of discrimination at work and support initiatives to prevent and address discrimination in the workplace.

- Create a positive work environment to avoid discrimination and bullying that can affect international nurses' job satisfaction and work relations.
- Acknowledge that race relations must be managed to avoid disrupting the mission of the organization.
- Equip nurses, healthcare practitioners, and staff with conflict management training.
- Support policy development and interventions to increase cultural competency and safety in health care.
- Develop collaboration between ethnic communities, professional organizations, and healthcare regulatory bodies to formulate culturally competent care delivery through multicultural workforce.
- Organize coalitions to promote recruitment, graduation, and hiring of multicultural workforce in health care.

Conclusion

The twenty-first-century context of globalization, massive displacements of refugees from low-income to high-income countries, and nurse migration compels nurses to apply cultural competency knowledge and cultural safety attitudes within health workplaces. Although many efforts to achieve culturally competent and safe practices (Racine 2014) have been defined, much actions need to be done as internationally educated nurses still face discrimination within Western countries' healthcare systems (Mortell 2013). Nurses have an ethical duty to respect other persons' and groups' cultural beliefs related to health and illness. Respect of otherness intersects with culture and cultural competency to move beyond the boundaries of race and ethnicity to the culturally different other in a humanistic and caring way (Andrews and Boyle 2012).

References

American Academy of Nursing & the Transcultural Nursing Society (2010) Standards of practice for cultural competent nursing care. Executive summary. http://www.tcns.org/files/Standards_of_Practice_for_Culturally_Compt_Nsg_Care-Revised_.pdf

American Nurses' Association (1998) Discrimination and racism in health care. Position statement. http://www.nursingworld.org/MainMenuCategories/Policy-Advocacy/Positions-and-Resolutions/ANAPosition Statements/Position-Statements-Alphabetically/Copy-of-prcidisrac11118.html

American Organization of Nurse Executives (2015) AONE Nurse manager competencies. Author, Chicago, IL

Andrews MM, Boyle JS (2012) Transcultural concepts in nursing care, 6th edn. Wolters Kluwer, Lippincott, Williams & Wilkins, Philadelphia, PA

Bae SH (2011) Organizational socialization of international nurses in the New York metropolitan area. Int Nurs Rev 59:81–87

Beaton M, Walsh J (2010) Overseas recruitment: experiences of nurses immigrating to Newfoundland and Labrador. Nurs Inq 17(2):173–183

Calliste A (1993) Women of exceptional merits: immigration of Caribbean nurses to Canada. Can J Women Law 6:85–102

Campinha-Bacote J (2002) The process of cultural competence in the delivery of healthcare services: a model of care. J Transcult Nurs 13(3):181–184.

Canadian Association of Schools of Nursing (2014) Position statement: education of registered nurses in Canada. Author, Ottawa, ON

Canadian Nurses Association (2015) Promoting cultural competency in nursing. Position statement. Author, Ottawa, ON

Canales MK (2010) Othering: difference understood? A 10-year analysis and critique of the nursing literature. Adv Nurs Res 33(1):15–34

Cornell S, Hartmann D (2007) Ethnicity and race. Making identities in a changing world, 2nd edn. Pine Forge Press, Thousand Oaks, CA

Das Gupta T (2009) Real nurses and others. Racism in nursing. Fernwood, Halifax, NS

Douglas MK, Rosenkoetter M, Pacquiao DF, et al (2014) Guidelines for implementing culturally competent nursing care. J Transcult Nurs 25(109). https://doi.org/10.1177/1043659614520998

Eriksen TH (2010) Ethnicity and nationalism. Anthropological perspectives, 3rd edn. Pluto Press, London

Essed P (1991) Understanding everyday racism. An interdisciplinary theory. Sage, Newbury Park, CA

Huria T, Cuddy J, Lacey C et al (2014) Working with racism: a qualitative study of the perspectives of Maori (Indigenous Peoples of Aotearoa New Zealand) registered nurses on a global phenomenon. J Transcult Nurs 25(4):364–372

International Council of Nurses (2013) Position statement of cultural and linguistic competence. http://www.icn.ch/images/stories/documents/publications/position_statements/B03_Cultural_Linguistic_Competence.pdf

Leininger M (2002) Culture care theory: a major contribution to advance transcultural nursing knowledge and practices. J Transcult Nurs 13(1):189–192

Mapedzahama V, Rudge T, West S, et al. (2012) Black nurses in white space? Rethinking the in/visibility of race within Australian nursing workplace. Nurs Inq, 19(2): 153–164.

McFarland MR, Wehbe-Alamah HB (2017) The theory of cultural care diversity and universality. In: McFarland MR, Wehbe-Alamah HB (eds) Leininger's transcultural nursing: concepts, theories, research and practice, 4th edn. McGraw-Hill, New York, pp 1–35

McKillop A, Sheridan N, Rowe D (2013) New light through old windows: nurses, colonists, and indigenous survival. Nurs Inq 20(3):265–276

Mortell S (2013) Delving into diversity-related conflict. Nurs Manag 44(4):28–33

Newton S, Pillay J, Higginbottom G (2013) The migration and transitioning experiences of internationally educated nurses: a global perspective. J Nurs Manag 20(4):534–550

Nursing Council of New Zealand (2011) Guidelines for cultural safety, the Treaty of Waitangi and Maori health in nursing education and practice. Author, Wellington, NZ

O'Brien-Pallas L, Tomblin Murphy G, Birch S et al (2007) Health human resources modelling: challenging the past, creating the future. Canadian Health Services Research Foundation, Ottawa, ON

Papps E, Ramsden I (1996) Cultural safety in nursing: the New Zealand experience. Int J Qual Health Care 8(5):491–497

Purnell LD (2013) Transcultural health care. A culturally competent approach. F.A. Davis, Philadelphia, PA

Puzan E (2003) The unbearable whiteness of being in nursing. Nurs Inq 10(3):193–200

Racine L (2003) Implementing a postcolonial feminist perspective in nursing research related to non-Western populations. Nurs Inq 10(2):91–102

Racine L (2009) Haitian-Canadians' experiences of racism in Quebec; a postcolonial feminist perspective. In: Agnew V (ed) Racialized migrant women in Canada. Essays on health, violence, and equity. University of Toronto Press, Toronto, ON, pp 265–274

Racine L (2014) The enduring challenge of cultural safety in nursing. Can J Nurs Res 46(2):6–9

Ramsden I (1993) Cultural safety in nursing education in Aotearoa (New Zealand). Nurs Prax N Z 8(3):4–10

Reimer Kirkham S (2003) The politics of belonging and intercultural health care. West J Nurs Res 25(7):762–780

Ronquillo C, Boschma G, Wong ST et al (2011) Beyond greener pastures: exploring contexts surrounding Filipino nurse migration in Canada through oral history. Nurs Inq 18(3):262–275

Salami B, Nelson S (2014) The downward occupational mobility of internationally educated nurses to domestic workers. Nurs Inq 21(2):153–161

Schroeder C, DiAngelo R (2010) Addressing whiteness in nursing education. The sociopolitical climate project at the University of Washington school of nursing. Adv Nurs Sci 33(3):244–255

Sullivan Commission on Diversity in the Healthcare Workforce (2004) Missing persons: minorities in the health professions. The Sullivan Alliance to Transform the Health Professions, Alexandria, VA

U.S. Department of Health and Human Services (2017) The National CLAS Standards. The Office of Minority Health. https://minorityhealth.hhs.gov/omh/

Case Study: Recruitment of Philippine-Educated Nurses to the United States

Leo Felix Jurado

Twelve nurses from the Philippines were recruited by an agency for a long-term care facility at a suburban area in the southern region of Midwestern United States. The nurses signed a contract with the agency in the Philippines stipulating the following: (a) a minimum of 2-year employment at the facility, (b) advanced payment by the agency for their airfare with the amount to be deducted from their salary over a period of 1 year, (c) free accommodation in a furnished apartment and transportation to and from work for the first 3 months of employment, (d) agency will facilitate processing of necessary papers for employment (social security cards and RN license), and (e) differential pay for working during evenings and night shifts and weekends.

The nurses arrived during the winter month of February and were housed in a two-bedroom unfurnished apartment two miles away from the facility. None of them confronted the recruiting agency about their housing. They all started working a month upon arrival after obtaining their social security cards and RN licenses except for five nurses who agreed to work as nursing assistants while waiting for their RN licenses that took 6–8 weeks. Because they were not provided assistance with transportation, the nurses used a taxicab or walked in bitter cold to work and for grocery shopping. This experience was stressful as it entailed much expense and the winter weather was particularly difficult for newcomers from a tropical country. Some Filipino nurses in the facility offered them a ride when they worked the same schedule. When they inquired from the recruitment agency about the free transportation, they were informed that the contract they signed was recently revised.

Upon receipt of their first paycheck, the nurses discovered that their hourly rate was five dollars less than what was written in their contract in addition to the automatic deduction for their airfare. They were not paid differentials for working off shifts and weekends. Half of them worked on evenings, and the other half worked on night shifts. The nurses also found out that they have to pay about 200 dollars from each paycheck for health coverage.

The nurses realized that the recruitment agency reneged on the terms of the contract they signed in the Philippines. They requested to meet with the agency administrator but were denied each time they called the agency. When the nurses threatened to resign en masse, the administrator sent them a letter stating that they will have to pay $30,000.00 each to breach the contract. The nurses were also concerned that their immigration papers (green cards) were kept by the agency as they used the agency's address to apply for immigration. They had legal documentation to enter and work in the United States.

L. F. Jurado, Ph.D., R.N., APN, FAAN
Department of Nursing, William Paterson University, Wayne, NJ, USA
e-mail: juradol@wpunj.edu

© Springer International Publishing AG, part of Springer Nature 2018
M. Douglas et al. (eds.), *Global Applications of Culturally Competent Health Care: Guidelines for Practice*, https://doi.org/10.1007/978-3-319-69332-3_33

The nurses also experienced challenges at work. Oftentimes, the staffing was so inadequate increasing their workload from 15–20 residents to 30 residents per nurse. Some of the nurses found some of the nursing assistants to be uncooperative and argumentative. When asked for assistance, some nursing assistants refused because they were busy or were missing from the unit for long periods of time. To avoid conflict, the nurses did not report them to the nurse managers or supervisors. Often, the nurses did not finish their tasks at the end of the shift and were told that they will not be paid overtime. Nevertheless, they continued working beyond their shift until the tasks were completed.

The hardships at work and in their living conditions took a toll on the nurses. Four of them left their employment after only 6 months and lived with their relatives in other states without ever receiving their green cards from the agency. Two nurses reached out to the local chapter of the national organization of Filipino nurses (Philippine Nurses Association of America) for help. The national organization investigated their complaint and referred them to a law firm. After legal pursuit, all the nurses were able to get out of their contract without paying any fees for breach of contract and received restitution from the recruitment agency.

33.1 Social Structural Factors

Internationally educated nurses (IENs) will continue to contribute to the multicultural workforce in the United States and globally. They bring diversity in the workplace because of their variant knowledge, skills, and caring approaches. According to NCSBN (2017), the Philippines tops the list, followed by India, among IENs that sit for the licensing exams during the past 5 years. Other countries supplying IENs to the United States include Puerto Rico, South Korea, Jamaica, and Canada.

Filipino nurses comprise the largest group of emigres to the United States and other developed countries including the Middle East, the United

Kingdom, Australia, New Zealand, and other Asian countries (Singapore and Japan) (Brush and Sochalski 2007; Choy 2003; Jurado and Pacquiao 2015). Emigration is motivated by economic, social, and political factors. Governmental and private institutions in the Philippines and the United States have facilitated the emigration of Filipino nurses. Immigration policies have helped ease the nursing shortages in the United States. The Philippine government has pushed emigration by production of nurses primarily for export because of very limited employment opportunities in the local market; dollar remittances from overseas workers significantly contribute to the nation's ability to pay for its foreign debt (Jurado 2013).

33.2 Cultural Factors

The family-centered social structure of Filipinos plays a major role in the emigration of nurses to developed countries. The family is a major influence in the career choice of their children and in propagating the idea that working abroad is a pathway to help the entire family back home. Filipinos view education as key to economic success. The educational achievement of children enhances the family's well-being and reputation in the community. Success of the children in finding lucrative employments abroad means support for the family through remittances sent back home to assist siblings in pursuing their education and the family's economic well-being (Jurado 2013).

At least 81% of Filipinos are Catholics (Pew Research Center 2015) who believe in the power of God to resolve problems (Fuchs 1967). The Filipino value of *bahala na* (*bathala* or God in Tagalog) is attributed to their strong religious belief manifested in the common philosophical expression used when confronted with problems (Morgan 2013), "come what may; whatever will be, will be; or leave it to God." Filipinos tend to accept what comes their way, appreciate what they have, and leave the rest to God, believing that God is on their side if they give their all. This belief may be viewed negatively because of the tendency to avoid conflict, accept status quo, or rely on others to solve their problems. On the other hand, it can be positive because it gives them strength and confidence to endure and be buoyed by the hope that everything will turn out for the best if God wills it.

Filipino culture emphasizes *utang na loob* (debt of gratitude), a debt of gratitude for those who have sacrificed or performed deeds on ones' behalf. A son or daughter has *utang na loob* to their parents, and it is the child's obligation to return the favor as the parents grow older. *Utang na loob* has a deeper meaning as it reflects sharing of one's *kapwa* (personhood) with others. Failure to reciprocate the kindness and good deeds of others is tantamount to losing face or *hiya*, which can bring shame to oneself, one's family, or community (Flores 2012; Hays 2015).

Collectivistic societies like the Philippines often use high-context communication. Filipinos have a particular way of behaving in different situations. Among insiders (fellow Filipinos or in-group), the expectation is to speak in a common language familiar to the group; communication tends to be implicit and indirect without having to elaborate. Nonverbal communication speaks louder than words. In contrast, individualistic cultures like the Western world, low-context communication is predominant. Direct, explicit, and more elaborate communication is common. The goal of high-context cultures is to maintain harmony, while the goal of low-context cultures is the giving and getting of information (Storti and Bennhold-Samaan 1997).

Filipinos avoid direct confrontation by keeping calm and controlling emotions until a crisis develops and the situation becomes intolerable. This is demonstrated in the case study by the Filipino nurses' behavior toward the recruitment agency and nursing assistants they worked with. They prefer harmony and conflict avoidance and rely upon others such as the Philippine Nurses Association of America to intervene on their behalf. Maintaining "face" and upholding an individual's reputation is a significant cultural trait among Filipinos. To disagree with someone

in public or to have an outburst is considered disgraceful and can result to "loss of face." In general, the emphasis of communication is on maintaining smooth personal relationships (Jurado 2013; Pacquiao 2003).

33.3 Culturally Competent Strategies Recommended

IENs have been a part of the US multicultural healthcare workforce since the exchange visa program was initiated in 1948 (Choy 2003). Organizations that embrace diversity find that there are several benefits of a multicultural workforce. Employees from different backgrounds bring a rich array of skills, experiences, and different cultural viewpoints that can be advantageous to an increasingly diverse population of consumers. Business companies with a more diverse workforce have noted that when diverse employees are more inspired to perform in their highest potential, there is greater productivity and return of investment (Greenberg 2004).

33.3.1 Individual-Level Interventions

- Support initial adaptation of IENs to the new environment (e.g., the University of Pennsylvania Model Transition Program for IENs (Adeniran et al. 2008). The transition program should include:
  - Providing support for relocation (initial housing, heating, telephone, transportation, appropriate clothing for winter, etc.)
  - Ensuring safety of IENs who are more likely to work on off shifts and walking to work or home
  - Designating a responsible person with whom IENs can seek help during emergencies
  - Connecting IENs with support groups at work and in the community (churches, ethnic grocery stores, Filipino workers and organizations, etc.)

- Implement comprehensive and adequate orientation for IENs to develop their understanding of:
  - Own cultural values and those of co-workers
  - American dominant and variant cultural values and organizational values/expectations
  - Differences in communication styles, conflict management, and professional communication
  - Differences in care modalities (technology, nutrition, drugs, diagnostics, etc.)
  - Caring approaches to multicultural patients
  - Ways of negotiating with patient and organizational hierarchy
  - Legal and ethical aspects of professional nursing in the state and country (regulatory and accreditation requirements)
  - Individual professional accountability and leadership role expectations
- Implement bicultural mentorship program for IENs for an extended time period beyond the initial orientation in order to:
  - Promote advocacy and empowerment of IENs at work to build teamwork, confront discrimination, and ensure equitable workload
  - Foster cross-cultural communication, communicating with people perceived to be in higher status and authority, conflict management, decision making, and care approaches
  - Help identify lingering issues and measures for addressing them
  - Promote further understanding of organizational values and expectations including evaluations by peers, administrators, and patients
- Encourage dialogue between IENs and administrators to determine relocation needs, job-related issues, and other challenges by:
  - Visiting their residence
  - Connecting them with Filipino workers and community
  - Facilitating their access to religious, food, and other venues.

33.3.2 Organizational-Level Interventions

- Develop a job orientation curriculum with input from other Filipino IENs, organizations, and multidisciplinary staff, and use evidence from relevant research including regulatory and accreditation requirements, organizational policies and procedures, professional and variant communication patterns (slang, common idiomatic expressions, jargon, and colloquial terms), care technology, nutrition, pharmacology, managing psychiatric patients, health insurance and payment for care services, delegation, performance evaluation, employment benefits and salaries, etc.).
- Implement a bicultural program for multidisciplinary staff, unit staff, educators, and administrators including:
  - Need for IEN recruitment and their potential contribution to the organization
  - Awareness of cultural differences between IENs and themselves
  - Advocacy for IENs against bias and discrimination from staff and patients
  - Work and social engagement of staff with IENs
  - Role modeling for IENs
- Develop an organizational climate of multiculturalism and cultural competence by:
  - Integrating multiculturalism and cultural competence in organizational policies, hiring and staffing, staff education, leadership training, staff and leadership performance evaluation, patient surveys, language services, social services, etc.
  - Celebrating workforce diversity through publications, websites, and organizational events
  - Creating a formal structure dedicated to promote workforce diversity and organizational teamwork
  - Engaging IENs in establishing policies and procedures promoting equity, accessibility, and affordability of patient care services to diverse patients
  - Creating an office with dedicated personnel to ensure that the above goals are met

- Consulting with diversity experts in promoting continued development of staff and administrators
- Engaging diverse communities in organizational policy development and care improvement
- Developing unit champions who can facilitate valuing diversity at the grassroots level
- Promoting continuing education and leadership development of staff and IENs

33.3.3 Community/Societal-Level Interventions

- Develop social network of support for IENs through collaboration with ethnic professional nursing associations such as the Philippine Nurses Association of America, Asian American Pacific Islander Nursing Association, National Indian Nurses Association, Hispanic Nurses Association, etc. They can provide educational programs, consultation, and mentorship to organizational leaders and staff including IENs.
- Engage in ethical recruitment of IENs.
    - Develop partnership with reputable recruitment agencies.
    - Collaborate with the Philippine Nurses Association of America and its state chapter. PNAA works with the Philippine Commission of Filipinos Overseas (CFO), the Migrant Heritage Commission, and the Philippine consular offices in the United States to (1) ensure protection of Filipino IENs, (2) provide comprehensive predeparture orientation, (3) maintain statistics of Filipino IENs in different countries, and (d) track and follow up on reported violations of contract violations and related abuses.
    - Develop thorough knowledge of immigration, recruitment, and relocation policies in both the United States and countries supplying IENs.
    - Scrutinize and preapprove all work contracts offered to IENs by recruitment agencies.

- Distinguish actual employment offers by the organization and other specifications by the recruitment agency.
    - Maintain open dialogue with IENs to identify issues.
- Facilitate reporting of unscrupulous practices to appropriate agencies by:
    - Familiarizing with the Voluntary Code of Ethical Conduct for Recruitment of Foreign-Educated Health Professionals to the United States published by the Alliance for Ethical International Recruitment Practices (2011) which includes legal adherence, communication, contract, immigration and labor practices, transition support, working with local authorities, respecting prior agreements, and selecting recruitment countries
    - Partnering with ethnic professional organizations and consular offices
- Engage diverse communities in supporting adaptation of IENs.
    - Identify ethnic community leaders and stakeholders interested in workforce diversity. For example, Filipino church groups and physicians have been supportive of initiatives for Filipino IENs.
    - Invite participation of ethnic communities in organizational events and develop policy initiatives for the community as well as IENs.

Conclusion

IENs particularly Filipino nurses have contributed to increasing the multicultural workforce in the United States and other developed countries for more than half of a century. Culturally competent strategies at the individual, organizational, and community levels are recommended to promote ethical recruitment, smoother transition, and effective integration of IENs in their social and work environments. Comprehensive transitional programs were found to promote increased job satisfaction and retention of IENs (Adeniran et al. 2008). In return, IENs contribute to the provision of quality care, patient safety, and positive patient outcomes (Jurado 2013).

References

Adeniran RK, Rich VL, Gonzalez E, et al (2008) Transitioning internationally educated nurses for success: a model program. Online J Issues Nurs 13(2). http://www.nursingworld.org/MainMenuCategories/ANAMarketplace/ANAPeriodicals/OJIN/TableofContents/vol132008/No2May08/TIENS.html

Alliance for Ethical International Recruitment Practices (2011) Voluntary Code of Ethical Conduct for the recruitment of foreign educated health professionals to the United States. http://www.cgfnsalliance.org/wp-content/uploads/2014/11/THE-CODE11.pdf

Brush BL, Sochalski J (2007) International nurse migration: lessons from the Philippines. Policy Polit Nurs Pract 8(1):37–46. https://doi.org/10.1177/1527154407301393

Choy CC (2003) Empire of care: nursing and migration in Filipino American History. Duke University Press, Durham, NC

Flores R (2012) The typical Filipino family. http://www.filipino-heritage.com/filipino-family.html

Fuchs L (1967) Those peculiar Americans. Meredith Press, New York

Greenberg J (2004) Diversity in the workplace: benefits, challenges, and solutions. The multicultural advantage. http://www.multiculturaladvantage.com/recruit/diversity/diversity-in-the-workplace-benefits-challenges-solutions.asp

Hays J (2015) Social relations in the Philippines: utang na loob, bayanihan and pakikisama. Facts and Details. http://factsanddetails.com/southeast-asia/Philippines/sub5_6c/entry-3868.html#chapter-5

Jurado L (2013) Social construction of Filipino nurses in the Philippines and as foreign-educated nurses in the United States. PhD Dissertation, Rutgers, The State University of New Jersey

Jurado L, Pacquiao DF (2015) Historical analysis of Filipino nurse migration to the US. J Nurs Pract Appl Rev Res 5(1):4–18. https://doi.org/10.13178/jnparr.2015.0501.1303

Morgan R (2013) What is the meaning of BAHALA NA? https://rosalindarmorgan.com/

NCSBN (2017) NCLEX fact sheet. https://www.ncsbn.org/search.htm?q=NCLEX+Fact+Sheet

Pacquiao DF (2003) People of Filipino heritage. In: Purnell LD (ed) Transcultural health care: a culturally competent approach. F. A. Davis Company, Philadelphia, pp 138–159

Pew Research Center (2015) Facts about Catholicism in the Philippines. http://www.pewresearch.org/fact-tank/2015/01/09/5-facts-about-catholicism-in-the-philippines/

Storti C, Bennhold-Samaan L (1997) Culture matters: the Peace Corps—cultural workbook. Government Printing Office, Washington, DC

Case Study: Health Care for the Poor and Underserved Populations in India

34

Joanna Basuray Maxwell

Ramesh, a 12-year-old male, is brought to a low-cost clinic by his parents in the city of Kochi, in the state of Kerala in South India. Ramesh has been suffering from severe asthma for several years. He appears younger and underdeveloped for his age. Ramesh's parents had previously sought several doctors who repeatedly informed them that Ramesh has asthma. Ramesh's parents had sold all their belongings to pay for his health care prior to this last visit. The family lives in a thatched-roof hut. His parents are in their early 30s; his father is the sole family breadwinner working as a day laborer.

Ramesh's history indicates that he had been a normal boy until the age of 10 months when he started waking up during the night with respiratory wheezing that has worsened over time. Auscultation of his lungs reveals clear breath sounds, but severe wheezing is heard over his right lower lobe. The physician suspected foreign body aspiration and referred the family for follow-up at a nearby medical university hospital. At the medical center, a plastic bead was removed from Ramesh's lung, immediately relieving his wheezing. While Ramesh's condition was resolved, it took much from his family's meager income to reach a physician who was able to correctly diagnose and treat his problem. The chronic need for medical services for Ramesh to treat a correctable condition has further devastated the family's already meager resources.

34.1 Cultural and Social Factors

Gender is a social determinant of health in India (see Chap. 1) placing females in all age groups at a higher health risk than males. Being a male son, Ramesh's health is a priority in the traditional Indian culture. An increasing aging population includes women who are living longer than men in worse health than elder men. Indian cities are overpopulated as 40% of the population has migrated into major cities to improve their economic conditions and access to basic services, such as health care. The urban poor suffer many hardships including vulnerability to respiratory illnesses such as asthma, cardiovascular disease, and diabetes.

Poverty has been defined by the Indian Government as a "multidimensional problem that includes low access to opportunities for developing human capital and to education, health, family planning, and nutrition" (Nolan et al. 2014: 2). Urbanization is seen as a structural determinant of health due to the ill effects of "rapid and unplanned" urbanization leading to slums and exposing urbanites to undesirable living conditions and sanitation. Children under 5 years of

J. B. Maxwell, Ph.D., R.N.
Department of Nursing, Towson University,
8000 York Road, Towson, MD 21252, USA
e-mail: jmaxwell@towson.edu

© Springer International Publishing AG, part of Springer Nature 2018
M. Douglas et al. (eds.), *Global Applications of Culturally Competent Health Care: Guidelines for Practice*, https://doi.org/10.1007/978-3-319-69332-3_34

age experience higher incidence of developmental delays and stunting as well as higher mortality rates than their nonpoor and non-slum counterparts.

My interviews of two Indian health service providers (a social worker and a physician) who have worked in India and in the United States offered a multiple-layered perspective on the social and cultural factors in India. According to K. Cunningham (social worker) and D. Suskind, MD (personal communication, August 25, 2017), physicians in India are confronted by large numbers of patients who generally come to the clinic or hospital with severe life-threatening conditions. Because of these long lines of patients to be seen, it is rare to see a physician take the time to do a physical examination, such as assessing lung sounds or evaluating findings followed by a plan of treatment. Poor and illiterate patients are verbally intimidated and sent home with a prescription. For example, parents accompanying a child, like Ramesh are scolded for not responsibly taking care of the child to prevent the asthma attack. A physician's diagnosis assumes a culturally biased lens that results in further neglect, oppression, and alienation of people of lower socioeconomic status (K. Cunningham and D. Suskind, personal communication, August 25, 2017).

Physicians are not compensated adequately for an exhausting workday dealing with a heavy workload. In order to support their middle-class and upper middle-class lifestyle, many physicians work in private practice where they are paid per-patient visit generated from self-paying patients (Basuray 2002; Sharma 2015). Doctors attempt to exercise control of their work environment by displaying arrogance, rudeness, and abuse toward other health providers such as nurses. Nurses' work is largely subsumed under the physician's plan of treatment. Majority of nurses are educated in a 3-year diploma program at a teaching hospital setting. Few programs offer a master's degree in nursing with specific clinical concentrations (Indian Nursing Council 2017).

The structure and management of clinics and hospitals in large cities of India are based on a Western healthcare delivery system that was originally introduced by the British in the eighteenth century. The educational preparation and professional practice of Indian physicians and nurses in India are influenced by the British medical model. Although the government acknowledges Indian indigenous health systems based on generic healthcare practices such as Ayurveda, Unani, and Siddha, professional education and training of healthcare practitioners has been consistently based on the Western biomedical model (Basuray 2002).

As the population growth increases, millions of people will never receive health care as most Indians cannot afford health insurance to cover hospitalization cost. Many poor people are uninformed about health insurance plans (Basuray 2002). According to the World Bank report (2012), about 25% (approximately 300 million) of India's population had access to either private insurers or insurance providers through the government. However, health insurance in India only covers inpatient hospitalization and hospital-based treatment but not outpatient visits. As a result, 70% of the population have to pay out of pocket for these services, increasing the financial burden on individuals and families (World Bank 2012).

India is experiencing a major workforce crisis through a shortage of practicing physicians. In 2016, the Medical Council of India reported the doctor/patient ratio of 1:1681 (Chatterjeel 2016). Despite large enrollment and graduation rates in medicine and nursing, India lacks qualified professional practitioners to provide preventive and primary care to its people (Nolan et al. 2014). According to Sharma (2015), 8% of the 25,300 primary centers nationwide had no doctor on the premises; 38% lacked lab technicians, and 22% lacked pharmacists. Vacancies among healthcare assistants included 50% females and 61% males. The shortage of medical specialists included 83% surgeons, 83% pediatricians, and 76% obstetricians and gynecologists. There is also a shortage of healthcare assistants. Sharma also highlighted high absenteeism among physicians compounding the shortage. Physician shortage is critical in remote rural areas as many physicians are unwilling to work in these areas because of poor infrastructure (e.g., unpaved roads), limited medical resources, and lack of opportunity for professional development that is only accessible in large city hospitals (Sharma 2015).

34.2 Culturally Competent Strategies

34.2.1 Individual/Family-Level Interventions

- Recognize human potential of every citizen to achieve optimum health.
  - Seek health provider volunteers to assist with managing patient admission and assessment.
  - Promote integrity of the family by accommodating traditional family roles in care of family members.
  - Observe and listen to patients with respect and genuine attentiveness.
  - Maintain patients' dignity and their right to health care.
  - Create an environment that encourages open and trusting interaction between patients and health providers.
- Promote health provider awareness of the impact of social determinants on health outcomes.
  - Increase awareness of the impact of poverty, class/caste, illiteracy, gender, religion, and language proficiency on physical and mental health and access, utilization, and adherence with health care.
  - Promote self-reflection on the impact of workload and work environment on one's own behavior toward vulnerable patients.
  - Promote critical reflection on the influence of personal and cultural bias on one's behavior toward vulnerable patients.

34.2.2 Organizational-Level Interventions (Clinic and City Hospitals)

- Develop systems for addressing multifaceted problems of the poor and underserved.

  - Build a strong social service component to health services.
  - Use appropriate interpreters to assist in communicating with illiterate and poor patients.
  - Use gender-congruent community advocates to assist patients.
- Restructure workplace services and resource utilization.
  - Evaluate workload of staff and streamline their roles and responsibilities.
  - Utilize auxiliary personnel to assist with nonprofessional tasks and responsibilities.
  - Develop team approach to healthcare services by delegating expanded professional responsibilities to nurses and other health professionals.
  - Provide training for volunteers or "paraprofessionals" to manage patient traffic and some administrative tasks.
- Design educational programs and ongoing training of interprofessional staff in the following areas:
  - Impact of social determinants on population health, health behaviors, and access, utilization, and adherence with health services.
  - Culturally competent care that is respectful of gender, age, religious, language, and social class differences. Use creative teaching methods such as simulation and modeling. Reward culturally competent outcomes.
  - Indigenous health practices, practitioners, values, and beliefs of individuals and communities.
- Collaborate with private, business, faith-based organizations and the community to promote access by underserved populations to preventive and primary healthcare services.
  - Seek funding and participation in community-based initiatives for the underserved.
  - Promote community empowerment by opening health education classes for patients, families, and communities on preventive measures for healthy living, health promotion, and illness prevention

(including pregnancy, child-rearing, and adult health behaviors). Offer information on health promotion and illness prevention.

– Collaborate with indigenous health practitioners in the community in promoting access to primary healthcare services.

34.2.2.1 Community/Societal-Level Interventions

- Collaborate with schools of nursing and medical colleges to integrate social determinants of health in the curriculum.
  – Increase emphasis on managing the care of patients and communities from lower socioeconomic levels and culturally diverse populations.
  – Increase the focus on health promotion and prevention of illness.
  – Strengthen educational training of nurses for leadership roles in health promotion and illness prevention.
- Promote partnerships among academic institutions, businesses, health organizations, and local communities to improve the living conditions of the people by expanding access to health screening especially for children, females, and the elderly.
- Develop multisectoral collaboration among public and private entities, professionals, and academicians to improve living conditions of slum dwellers and those living in poverty to promote their access to potable water and sanitation, enhance safety inside and outside their homes, and control environmental pollution.
- Develop sustainable partnerships and multisectoral collaboration to influence public policies impacting health such as retention of healthcare professionals, universal access to quality health care, and combating unequal treatment of the poor, women and children, the elderly, and other disadvantaged groups.
  – Explore indigenous health systems in the community as a point of referral when appropriate and in agreement with patients' health beliefs.

Conclusion

Ramesh and his parents provide a classic profile of a family in India that is from a lower socioeconomic level with a male child who is ill. This family reflects the interplay between gender, socioeconomic status, and healthcare infrastructural variables that influence healthcare decisions, access, and utilization of services and health outcomes of the Indian population. The cultural factors compounded by lack of access to health care are based on the parents' level of income and a healthcare system that is inadequate for the underserved population.

Healthcare professional shortage particularly of physicians has reached a crisis level. Reorganization of the public healthcare system is critical to promote access of populations to primary care services and improve their living conditions. The role of professional nurses should be expanded to increase their leadership and participation in health promotion and disease prevention. Changes in the educational preparation of healthcare professionals are imperative to emphasize population health promotion by addressing social determinants of health vulnerability. Genuine collaboration between indigenous and allopathic health practitioners can help address the multiple and complex health needs of the population.

References

Basuray J (1997) Nurse Miss Sahib: colonial culture-bound education in India and transcultural nursing. J Transcult Nurs 9(1):14–19

Basuray J (2002) India: transcultural nursing and healthcare. In: Leininger MM, McFarland MR (eds) Transcultural nursing: concepts, theories, research and practice, 3rd edn. McGraw-Hill, New York, pp 477–491

Chatterjeel S (2016) India has just 1 doctor for every 1,681 persons: MCI. http://timesofindia.indiatimes.com/life-style/health-fitness/health-news/India-has-just-1-doctor-for-every-1681-persons-MCI/articleshow/52102964.cms

Dixit U (2011) Development of nursing education in India: post-independence. http://hinsar.hitkarini.com/wp/?p=479

Indian Nursing Council (2017) Nursing programs. http://www.indiannursingcouncil.org/nursing-programs

Nolan LB, Balasubramaniam P, Muralidharan A (2014) Urban poverty and health inequality in India. http://paa2014.princeton.edu/papers/140103

Sharma DC (2015) India still struggles with rural doctor shortages. Lancet 386(10011):2381–2382. https://doi.org/10.1016/S0140-6736(15)01231-3

The World Bank (2012) Government-sponsored health insurance in India: are you covered? http://documents.worldbank.org/curated/en/644241468042840697/pdf/722380PUB0EPI008029020120Box367926B.pdf

Part IX

Guideline: Cross Cultural Leadership

Attributes of Cross-Cultural Leadership

35

Dula Pacquiao

Guideline: *Nurses shall have the ability to influence individuals, groups, and systems to achieve outcomes of culturally competent care for diverse populations. Nurses shall have the knowledge and skills to work with public and private organizations, professional associations, and communities to establish policies and guidelines for comprehensive implementation and evaluation of culturally competent care.*

Douglas et al. (2014: 110)

35.1 Global Context for Leadership

According to Friedman (2007), international systems have arisen from dramatic changes in the global economy and global landscape making historical and geographic divisions increasingly irrelevant. Markets, technology, information systems, and telecommunication systems are interweaving globally, thus shrinking the world and enabling humans to connect farther, faster, deeper, and cheaper. On the other hand, globalization and modernization have created a new world order—a "runaway world" that is out of control and filled with risks and cultural complexity (Giddens 2003). Modern society is becoming a risk society that is increasingly preoccupied with its future and safety and in controlling the risks associated with modernization and human activity. According to Giddens, risk needs to be controlled, but active risk-taking is central to a dynamic economy and an innovative society.

Globalization is associated with major trends that place businesses, politics, popular culture, and health on the world stage. It is a process resulting from a combination of forces that is increasing the flow of information, goods, capital, and people across political and geographic boundaries. It has its own rules, logic, pressures, and incentives that can affect directly or indirectly countries, businesses, and communities, worldwide (Cohen 2010). An overarching feature of globalization is integration as threats and opportunities flow among those who are interconnected. Centers of economic activity are shifting profoundly regionally and globally. A demographic trend pushing this macroeconomic shift is the aging population particularly in the developed world with profound impact on the growth of the workforce, economic productivity, and innovations in technology and services. Mass retirement and aging of the nursing workforce in the United States is predicted to create acute nursing shortages and increased burden and demands on healthcare and social services (see Chap. 31). The demands of an aging population will need realignment of economic activity and priority in both private and public sectors.

Geographic and social environments have been transformed by technology and enhanced connectivity, changing the way people and organizations interact, operate, and thrive (Aggarwa 2011). Growth of foreign-owned and affiliated companies has become a worldwide trend as local markets open to meet growing local demand

D. Pacquiao, Ed.D., R.N., C.T.N.-A., T.N.S.
School of Nursing, Rutgers University, Newark, NJ, USA

School of Nursing, University of Hawaii, Hilo, Hilo, HI, USA

© Springer International Publishing AG, part of Springer Nature 2018
M. Douglas et al. (eds.), *Global Applications of Culturally Competent Health Care: Guidelines for Practice*, https://doi.org/10.1007/978-3-319-69332-3_35

for economic growth and survival. Ongoing shifts in labor and talent are prompted by migration of jobs to low-wage countries. Demand for well-trained workers in knowledge-intensive industries has precipitated a global search for talented workers (Cohen 2010). Nontraditional business models and blurring of corporate borders have prompted the growth of large, complex organizations that require innovative decision techniques and management strategies to compete in a highly complex and unpredictable market. An international labor market is facilitated by shifting population demographics, technological connectivity, global migration, international sourcing of labor, and local workforce shortages.

Indeed, globalization, technological innovation, and demographic changes have transformed human life. Technology has a significant role in shaping global policies, economies, culture, and systems (Fritsch 2011). Globalization also creates problems with distance and disconnection on human relations and leadership. The trend toward globalized communities is accompanied by dissolution of local identity and cultural distinctiveness. In fact, this transformative aspect of globalization has fueled the movement toward national entrenchment (Giddens 2003). The rise of nationalistic populism in the United States and Europe is evidence of the counterreaction to globalization. Hofstede and Hofstede (2005) believe that a new world order is inevitable necessitating attention to national identities in cross-cultural interactions.

While globalization is generally considered in economic terms, it has broader effects in other areas such as health and social structures. Globalization has changed the dynamics of health across populations. International trade of goods and services can negatively impact social determinants of health such as access to employment, education, and social support as well as increase health risks. By contrast, sharing of knowledge and resources through enhanced technology can have positive effects (Canadian Nurses Association 2009). Inequities in health and environmental degradation result from social norms, policies, and practices that promote economic exploitation and unfair distribution of power, wealth, and social resources (WHO 2008). For example, polluting industries are usually sited in poorer countries and in underprivileged neighborhoods. Globalization initiatives must be examined along with other issues as social and economic development of global populations, health equity, and environmental justice (WHO 2006).

35.2 Global Leadership

Leadership is the process of influencing, facilitating, and organizing a group with an aim of accomplishing a vision, purpose, or significant goal (Pierce and Newstrom 2011). Leadership is substantially distinct in global and domestic or local leadership. The global context significantly increases the valence, intensity, and complexity of the structure and processes involved (Lokkesmoe 2009). Global leaders inspire a group of people to willingly pursue a positive vision in an effectively organized fashion while fostering individual and collective growth in a context characterized by significant levels of complexity and relationships across different spatiotemporal dimensions (Mendenhall et al. 2012).

Global leaders face higher degrees of complexity and uncertainty as there is need for adapting to different cultures and leadership style preferences based on different cultural norms and values. They need to simultaneously create global integration and local responsiveness and balance commercial and cultural concerns (Cohen 2010). Uncertainty is a consequence of lack of uniformity in customer preferences, competitive circumstances, economic conditions, employee relations, or governmental regulations across the various countries and cultures. Although the world is increasingly becoming borderless, there are linguistic, cultural, political, temporal, economic, and social boundaries that exist (Bingham, Felin, and Black 2000).

Global leaders face greater complexity inherent in the multiplicity of stakeholders, competitors, cultures, and governments involved. The rapid movement of capital, information, and people necessitates complex and interdependent arrangements across different units and sites of operations. Complexity results from ambiguity presented by massive information, lack of certainty, nonlinear and equivocal events, and outcomes. Lack of certainty from rapidly changing systems creates a state of flux and complexity (Lane et al. 2006).

In healthcare, globalization has resulted in increased cultural diversity in both workforce and clientele posing a challenge for leaders while addressing global trends and domestic realities. Organizations need to be concerned with the dominant social and cultural norms of society in which they are nested (Hofstede and Hofstede 2005). Organizations are comprised of multicultural groups including racial, ethnic, gender, sexual identity, language, religious, generational, work roles, education, immigration status, socioeconomic and educational status, physical and mental health status, etc. Healthcare leaders also deal with different governmental and regulatory bodies and private entities, different cultures of affiliate organizations, and different geographic communities. While technology has produced great innovations in healthcare, it has posed issues regarding unequal access to technology, privacy, and quality of life. Technology and growth of large healthcare organizations have shaped the way people work and interact within and across organizations.

The changing context of society significantly impacts leadership. Leaders need to adapt to the evolving social and cultural milieu of the environments outside and within the organization. Leaders need to grasp the interconnectivity between local events and global trends. Aging of the local population promotes outsourcing and importation of goods, services, and workers. Catastrophic events in other countries can lead to mass migration of refugees and vulnerable populations to the country and local community with intense need for access to comprehensive services. Leaders need to recognize the impact of local and national policies and initiatives on both local and global populations. Preferential immigration policies of one country can deplete resources in another. Mass migration of internationally educated healthcare professionals to wealthier (receiving) countries has depleted available manpower in poorer (sending) countries impacting their population morbidity and mortality. Conversely, the mass influx of internationally educated workers in organizations has consequent changes in interpersonal relationships, communication, role performance, leadership behaviors, and systems.

35.3 Attributes of Cross-Cultural Leadership

35.3.1 Global/World Citizenship

A global citizen is someone who identifies with being part of an emerging world community and whose actions contribute to building this community's values and practices (Israel 2017). Gillis Jr (2011) contends that there is a shortage of developed and prepared leaders with global leadership competency that includes a body of knowledge, skill, or ability to motivate, influence, and enable individuals across national boundaries and cultural diversity to contribute to the accomplishment of an organization's goal. Nussbaum (2013) identifies a global crisis because we have become "nations of technically trained people who are useful profit makers" but lack the ability to challenge authority, think in terms of the good of the world, and concern for the lives of others. Nussbaum proposes development of world citizenship that allows one not only to view oneself within one's own customs and beliefs but as someone belonging to the world—citizens in an interlocking world (Gorman and Womack 2017; Teshima 2010).

According to Nussbaum (2003), world citizens have three abilities: (1) to criticize one's own traditions and engage in discourse based on mutual respect for reason; (2) think as a citizen of the whole world, not just some local region or group; and (3) imagine what it would be like to be in the position of someone very different from oneself. Education for world citizenship needs to be multicultural emphasizing awareness, knowledge, and respect of cultural differences.

Education for world citizenship is grounded in the humanities and liberal education as the foundation for fostering compassionate understanding of others, developing habits of critical thinking and reflection and the value of social justice.

35.3.2 Cultural Intelligence

A significant attribute of cultural competence is critical reflection. Cultural intelligence is a system of cognitive structures and processes and multiple types of cultural knowledge and skills linked by cultural metacognition that promote effective patterns of intercultural interactions and behaviors (Thomas et al. 2012). Cultural knowledge is the foundation for comprehending and decoding one's behavior and those of others. It includes content knowledge (culture, social interactions, and history), procedural knowledge (effect of cultural knowledge on one's nature), and knowledge of cross-cultural encounters (reflective learning of culture-specific and culture-general aspects). Knowledge allows one to grasp the internal logic and model behavior of another culture and negotiate between similarities and differences across cultures (Lane et al. 2000).

Cultural skills in a variety of domains include information gathering or perceptual, interpersonal, action, and analytical skills. Cultural skills are related to emotional intelligence that includes important traits as world mindedness and openness (Caligiuri 2000). Cultural metacognition is the knowledge of and control over one's thinking and learning activities in the cultural domain involving core mental processes that transcend environmental context. Metacognition allows the ability to consciously and deliberately monitor, regulate, and orchestrate one's knowledge processes and cognitive and affective states to accomplish cognitive tasks or goal (Thomas et al. 2012).

What constitutes intelligent behavior may differ from one cultural environment to another (Johnson et al. 2006). The GLOBE study of foreign business executives and managers working in different countries worldwide revealed the need for adaptation of leadership style to the dominant national culture. Values, ideas, and beliefs of a culture or culture clusters determine its conception of effective leadership. History and culture shape leadership practices and follower expectations (House and Javidan 2004; Dorfman et al. 2004).

35.3.3 Compassion and Empathy

Nussbaum (1997) identifies compassion as a psychological link between our own self-interest and the reality of another person's good or ill. Compassion however is purely emotional and without thought. She emphasizes development of empathy—an imaginative and emotional understanding of what it might be like to be in the shoes of a person different from oneself (Nussbaum 1997; Teshima 2010). Empathy is a deep understanding of another's point of view and experiences that may be different from their own. Empathy and compassion foster values of mutuality, interconnections and reciprocal social obligation (Story 2011).

35.3.4 Social Justice Identity

Social justice identity is the attainment of pervasive internalization of the values of social justice in one's life as demonstrated by a consistent and profound commitment to foster social equity (Singh et al. 2010). The goals of social justice are beneficence, justice, and respect for people's rights and dignity (APA 2010). Social justice requires multicultural competence (Kaplan et al. 2014). Leadership practices that reflect social justice promote the agency and empowerment of individuals and groups and systemic change in order to promote equity and fairness for the oppressed and marginalized members of society (Ratts 2009). Leaders engage in ongoing self-examination, sharing power, giving voice to the weak, facilitating consciousness raising, building strengths, and leaving others with the tools for social change (Dollarhide et al. 2016).

Leaders engage in advocacy to empower individuals, groups, and organizations to promote social and systemic change. Leaders interact with structures, organizations, or institutions that are perceived as oppressive by marginalized groups (Constantino et al. 2007) Leaders initiate interventions at both individual and societal levels to promote greater levels of social justice and respond to institutional, systemic, and cultural barriers impeding well-being (Crethar et al. 2008). Promoting social justice and sustainability along with a responsibility to act on behalf of others is inherent in global citizenship (Reysen and Katzarska-Miller 2013). Becoming aware of the larger global context, understanding one's interconnectedness with the world and valuing existing diversity are the foundation for challenging injustice and taking action in personally meaningful ways (Jones 2016) based on the principle of human rights and equality (Cesario 2017).

35.3.5 Capacity for Self-Transformation

Engagement in personal transformation requires motivation to learn and commitment to ongoing development of personal knowledge and skills (Caligiuri and Tarique 2009). Personal transformation requires critical reflection – a meaning-making process that helps one set goals, use what was learned to inform future action, and consider the real-life implications of one's thinking. It is the link between thinking and doing and can be transformative (Rodgers 2002). Engaging in critical reflection helps articulate questions, confront bias, examine causality, contrast theory with practice, and identify systemic issues which help foster critical evaluation and knowledge transfer (Ash and Clayton 2009: 27). Critical reflection is learned through practice and feedback (Rodgers 2002).

Personal transformation is built on developing social judgment skills built on a big picture and long-term orientation (cause-effect, interdependencies, consequences) considering multiple constituents' perspectives. It also involves

self-awareness that in turn develops the ability to have self-confidence, self-reliance, and self-insight, as well as social and cultural awareness. Cultural self-awareness and self-reliance promote the courage to take a stand, openness, self-confidence and self-insight, and valuing diversity (Peterson 2004). It involves self-regulation and the ability to control impulses, maintain integrity, and remain flexible as one adapts to new situations. In other words, self-regulation is thinking before acting and capacity for behavioral flexibility and adaptability (Mumford et al. 2000). Self-transformed leaders are excellent coaches and mentors to others.

35.3.6 Community Engagement

Leaders with social justice orientation have the right and responsibility to recognize and raise awareness of the root causes of inequity in global health and participate in finding solutions. They are aware that individuals and communities have a right to be informed of their rights as citizens of a particular state and participate fully in defining their healthcare needs and deciding on approaches to address those needs (Dollarhide et al. 2016).

Leaders in healthcare should engage in addressing social determinants of health in vulnerable populations. Social determinants are best addressed at the community level to create broader impact on populations through systemic change. Leaders can promote engagement of their organizations in building social capital for health in vulnerable communities. Social capital are resources that become available for use or exchange based on social connections, mutual acquaintance, and/or social recognition gained through associations in a stable network of mutually established relationships. Resources may be actual or potential in the form of material, information, psychological support, and/or social relationships (Eriksson 2011; Walther 2014).

Culturally competent leaders can foster trust between communities and their organization and among other communities and organizations. Leaders can determine informal and formal social groups in the communities where people are engaged on a steady basis. Fostering trust and social cohesion can be enhanced by promoting the structure and process for people to engage with each other. Trust is the foundation for building mutual respect, reciprocity, and social norms. Trust among close-knit groups that regularly meet each other such as families, local churches, and social groups has the structure and process for developing bonding capital. Bonded groups can develop networks with outside groups (Bridging capital) to gain greater potential for sharing information and resources through horizontal collaboration and cooperation. Connections among various church groups and social groups in different communities demonstrate bridging capital. Linking capital involves vertical ties between people in different formal or institutional groups (Eriksson 2011). Engagement of healthcare organizations and public schools with the community to decrease obesity in young children is an example of linking capital.

Leaders need to have strong networking skills for establishing and maintaining relationships within an organization and across a range of stakeholder groups to build social networks and mutual capacity. Networking should involve domestic and global connections that can be called upon to facilitate changes. Leaders should maintain a high degree of engagement with their professional, work, and community organizations. They can model volunteerism and community engagement for others. Involvement in policy making is valuable in developing multiple perspectives on issues and in critically reflecting on the best course of action. Leaders should design systems within their organizations to facilitate active participation of communities and stakeholders in decision making. They should strengthen participation of management and staff in policy and program development and evaluation. High impact assessment of policies and programs on the population particularly the vulnerable groups should be standard practice.

Conclusion

The capacity for cross-cultural leadership can be learned (Northouse 2004). Training and development should focus on the attributes that are presented through formal training, developmental activities, and self-help activities (Yukl 2002). High-contact training activities are more likely to change behaviors of trainees (Caligiuru and Tarique 2009; Gillis Jr 2011). High-contact activities include experience working in other countries, global teams, experiential learning, and coaching. By contrast, low-contact activities include intercultural training, assessment, and reflection exercises. Direct experience with diversity can be facilitated within an organization and through engagement with diverse teams, patients, and communities. It is extremely important to promote encounters with diversity in different contexts to gain multiple perspectives, compassionate empathy, and reflexivity. Coaching and feedback are important to promote cultural metacognition and critical reflection.

Bonding, bridging, and linking strategies should be modeled and fostered to expose prospective leaders to diversity. Incentives and recognition of community engagement by workers can promote transformation of individuals and communities. Leaders must mentor advocacy and empowerment of disadvantaged individuals and communities to help develop social justice identity in others. Compassion, empathy, critical reflexivity, social justice, and global mind-set are best developed through direct experience and exposure to diversity and vulnerability. Innovative training must incorporate direct experiences with diverse patients and peers and community engagement with ample feedback and coaching provided. Leaders as mentors and coaches can facilitate opportunities for others to observe demonstration of desired leadership attributes.

Effective leadership is evident in how organizations and groups are influenced to achieve personal transformation of individuals and social change for vulnerable communities. Cross-cultural leadership aims to create high impact solutions to population health through organizational initiatives. Cross-cultural leaders are effective because they maintain active engagement with a vast network of diverse groups and resources that can be relied upon to promote goal achievement.

References

Aggarwa R (2011) Developing a global mindset: integrating demographics, sustainability, technology, and globalization. J Teach Int Bus 22(1):51–69

APA (2010) Ethical principles of psychologists and code of conduct. http://www.apa.org.ethics/code/principles.pdf. Accessed 2 Dec 2017

Ash SL, Clayton PH (2009) Generating, deepening, and documenting learning: the power of critical reflection in applied learning. J Appl Learn High Educ 1(1):25–48

Bingham CB, Felin T and Black JS (2000). An intreview with John Pepper: What it takes to be a global leader. Human Resource Management 39(2-3):287–291

Caligiuri PM (2000) The big five personality characteristics as predictors of expatriate's desire to terminate the assignment and supervisor-rated performance. Pers Psychol 53:67–88

Caligiuru P, Tarique I (2009) Predicting effectiveness in global leadership activities. J World Bus 44:316–346

Canadian Nurses Association (2009) Position statement on global health and equity. https://www.cna-aiic.ca/~/media/cna/page-content/pdf-en/ps106_global_health_equity_aug_2009_e.pdf?la=enwww.cna-aiic.ca. Accessed 1 Dec 2017

Cesario SK (2017) What does it mean to be a global citizen? Beyond Borders. http://nwhjournal.org/article/S1751-4851(16)30340-3/pdf. Accessed 2 Dec 2017

Cohen SL (2010) Effective global leadership requires a global mindset. Ind Commer Train 42(1):3–10

Constantine MG, Hage SM, Kindaichi MM et al (2007) Social justice and multicultural issues: implications for the practice and training of counselors and counseling psychologists. J Couns Dev 85:24–29

Crethar HC, Rivera ET, Nash S (2008) In search of common threads: linking multicultural, feminist, and social justice paradigms. J Couns Dev 86:269–278

Dollarhide CT, Clevenger SD, Edwards K (2016) Social justice identity: a phenomenological study. J Humanist Psychol 56(6):624–645

Dorfman PW, Hanges PJ, Brodbeck FC (2004) Leadership and cultural variation: identification of culturally endorsed leadership profiles. In: House RJ, Hanges PJ, Javidan M et al (eds) Culture, leadership and organizations: the GLOBE study of 62 societies. Sage, Thousand Oaks, CA, pp 669–719

Eriksson M (2011) Social capital and health implications for health promotion. Glob Health Action 4:5611. https://doi.org/10.3402/gha.v4i0.5611

Friedman T (2007) The world is flat. Farrar, Straus and Giroux, New York. ISBN 0-374-29278-7

Fritsch S (2011) Technology and global affairs. Int Stud Perspect 12(1):27–45

Giddens A (2003) Runaway world: how globalization is reshaping our lives. Routledge, New York

Gillis J Jr (2011) Global leadership development: an analysis of talent management, company types and job functions, personality traits and competencies, and learning and development methods. Doctoral dissertation, University of Pennsylvania. http://repositoryupenn.edu/edissertations/1177

Gorman D, Womack K (2017) Cultivating humanity with Martha Nussbaum. Interdiscip Lit Stud 19:145–148

Hofstede G, Hofstede GJ (2005) Cultures and organizations. Software of the mind. McGraw-Hill, New York

House RJ, Javidan M (2004) Overview of GLOBE. In: House RJ, Hanges PJ, Javidan M et al (eds) Culture, leadership and organizations: the GLOBE study of 62 societies. Sage, Thousand Oaks, CA, pp 9–28

Israel RC (2017) What does it mean to be a global citizen? Kosmos J Glob Transf. http://www.kosmosjournal.org/article/what-does-it-mean-to-be-a-global-citizen. Accessed 2 Dec 2017

Johnson JP, Lenartowicz T, Apud S (2006) Cross-cultural competence in international business: toward a definition and a model. J Int Bus Stud 37:525–543

Jones S (2016) Global citizenship. Aust Nurs Midwifery J 23(10), 48

Kaplan DM, Tarvydas VM, Gladding ST (2014) 20/20: a vision for the futures of counseling: the new consensus definition of counseling. J Couns Dev 92:366–372

Lane HW, DiStefano JJ, Maznevski ML (2000) International management behavior: text, readings and cases. Blackwell, Malden, MA

Lane HW, Maznevski ML, Mendenhall ME (2006) Globalization: Hercules meets Buddha. In: Scholz G (ed) Global talent: an anthology of human capital strategies for today's borderless enterprise. Human Capital Institute, Washington, DC, pp 3–32

Lokkesmoe KJ (2009) Grounded theory study of effective global leadership development strategies. Perspectives from Brazil, India and Nigeria. University of Minnesota. ProQuest, Ann Arbor, MI

Mendenhall ME, Reiche BS, Bird A et al (2012) Defining the 'global' in global leadership. http://blog.iese.edu/reiche/files/2010/08/Defining-the-global-in-global-leadership.pdf. Accessed on 2 Dec 2017

Mumford MD, Zaccaro SJ, Harding FD et al (2000) Leadership skills for a changing world: solving complex social problems. Leadersh Q 11(1):11–35

Northouse PG (2004) Leadership theory and practice. Sage, London

Nussbaum M (1997) Cultivating humanity: a classical defense of reform in liberal education. Harvard University Press, Cambridge, MA

Nussbaum M (2003) Compassionate citizenship. Humanity initiative. http://www.humanity.org/voices/commencements/martha-nussbaum-georgetown-university-speech-2003. Accessed 1 Dec 2017

Nussbaum M (2013) Liberal education and global community. Association of American Colleges and

Universities. 16 May 2013. http://uca.edu/liberalarts/files/2013/05/Liberal-Education_Nussbaum.pdf. Accessed 1 Dec 2017

Peterson B (2004) Cultural intelligence: a guide to working with people from other cultures. Intercultural Press, Yarmouth

Pierce JL, Newstrom JW (2011) Leaders and the leadership process, 6th edn. McGraw-Hill, New York

Ratts MJ (2009) Social justice counseling: toward the development of a fifth force among counseling paradigms. J Humanistic Counsel 548:160–172

Reysen S, Katzarska-Miller I (2013) A model of global citizenship: antecedents and outcomes. Int J Psychol 48(5):858–870

Rodgers C (2002) Defining reflection: another look at John Dewey and reflective thinking. Teach Coll Rec 104(4):842–866

Singh AA, Urbano A, Halston M et al (2010) School counselors' strategies for social justice change: a grounded theory of what works in the real world. Prof Sch Couns 13:135–145

Story JSP (2011) A developmental approach to global leadership. Int J Leadersh Stud 6(3):375–389

Teshima I (2010) Nussbaum discusses liberal arts education, global citizenship. http://www.wm.edu/news/stories/2010/nussbaum-discusses-liberal-arts-education,-global- citizenship-123.php. Accessed 1 Dec 2017

Thomas DC, Stahl G, Ravlin EC et al (2012) Development of cultural intelligence. In: Mobley WH, Wang Y, Li M (eds) Cultural intelligence assessment. Advances in global leadership, vol 7. Emerald Group Publishing, Bingley, pp 5–39

Walther M (2014) Bourdieu's theory of practice as theoretical framework. In: Walther M (ed) Repatriation to France and Germany. mir-Edition. Springer Gabler, Wiesbaden. https://doi.org/10.1007/978-3-658-05700-8_2

WHO (2006) Ottawa charter for health promotion. WHO/HPR/HEP/95.1. Author, Geneva

WHO (2008) Maximizing positive synergies between health systems and global health initiatives. Author, Geneva

Yukl G (2002) Leadership in organizations, 5th edn. Prentice Hall, Englewood Cliffs, NJ

Case Study: Integrating Cultural Competence and Health Equity in Nursing Education

36

Susan W. Salmond

As a nation, the United States is facing a health-care crisis; our current system of care is unsustainable. The United States' national health expenditure (i.e., the annual health spending) grew 5.8% in a single year to $3.2 trillion in 2015. This amounted to $9990 per person, and the number is projected to continue to grow 1.3% faster than gross domestic product (GDP) per year from 2015 to 2025 (Salmond and Echevarria 2017). Despite outspending all other comparable high-income nations, our health-care system ranks last or near last on measures of health, quality, access, and cost. The United States has higher infant mortality rates; higher mortality rates for deaths amenable to health care (mortality that results from medical conditions for which there are recognized health-care interventions that would be expected to prevent death); higher lower-extremity amputations due to diabetes; higher rates of medical, medication, and lab errors; and higher incidence of chronic illness and disease burden than comparable countries (Peterson-Kaiser Health Tracker System 2015).

Our country is more racially and ethnically diverse, and it is projected that by 2044, no one racial group will make up a majority of the country's population. Yet, Americans' health and access to health care is unequally influenced by ethnicity, income, education, and where they live. Despite successful national efforts to increase the number of Americans with health insurance (through the Affordable Care Act), at the end of 2015 there were still 28.5 million Americans without health insurance. People of color are at higher risk of being uninsured (Kaiser Family Foundation 2016). Although health insurance isn't the only factor in access to health care, it is an important one. In the United States, ethnic minorities including African Americans, Asian Americans, Native Americans, and Latinos experience well-known health disparities, i.e., a higher relative burden of illness, injury, disability, or mortality.

These groups have a higher prevalence of chronic conditions along with higher rates of mortality and poorer health outcomes, when compared with the white population. For example, the incident rate of cancer among African Americans is 10% higher than among whites. African Americans, Native Americans, and Latinos are also approximately twice as likely to develop diabetes as white people are, and Asians are 1.6 times as likely. We are a nation facing an epidemic of chronic disease. In fact, chronic disease accounts for three-quarters of America's direct health expenditures. As of 2012, about half of all adults—117 million people—had one or more chronic health conditions. One of four adults had two or more chronic health conditions.

S. W. Salmond, Ed.D., R.N., A.N.E.F., FAAN
School of Nursing, Rutgers University,
Newark, NJ, USA
e-mail: susan.salmond@rutgers.edu;
salmonsu@sn.rutgers.edu

Many chronic diseases can be prevented. Health risk behaviors are unhealthy behaviors which lead to chronic disease. Four of these health risk behaviors—lack of exercise or physical activity, poor nutrition, tobacco use, and drinking too much alcohol—cause much of the illness, suffering, and early death related to chronic diseases and conditions (Centers for Disease Control and Prevention 2017).

These patterns cannot be denied. Improvement of health outcomes requires greater emphasis on keeping people well and preventing and managing chronic illness. Care across the continuum must be better coordinated necessitating cross professional teams partnering not only with patients and family but with community groups contributing to improving health and well-being of its members. A culturally competent health care and health professional education system and a shift toward population health are a prerequisite to improving health outcomes and quality of care and contributing to the reduction of racial and ethnic health disparities.

36.1   Changing Nursing Education to Respond to Changing Health-Care Needs

This case study presents the journey of one School of Nursing's efforts to prepare its students to be culturally competent nursing leaders prepared to address the challenges of improving population health and quality care in tomorrow's health-care industry. The School of Nursing at the center of this case study is based in the northeastern United States; it is a well-established, sizeable School of Nursing that is part of a much larger state university. The School is grounded in an urban, economically challenged, highly diverse city and serves a diverse student body with approximately 50% of students belonging to a minority ethnic group.

The process of reenvisioning the School and curriculum to enhance cultural competence, to promote cultural diversity, and later to move toward population health has been a journey—a journey that will continue as the School is always

dealing with faculty turnover; changing demographics of faculty, staff, and students; as well as changes in the broader community and political backdrop. The leadership of the School recognized that there were deficits among faculty in cultural awareness and knowledge. Students raised concerns that the learning environment was not inclusive and that to some degree subtle discrimination was occurring. This sense of alienation was not conducive to student personal and academic development and the problem needed to be addressed. Additionally, there was little involvement of the School in the larger community. Clinical practicums were predominantly hospital-based, and the School and most of its faculty were not vested in ongoing activities to promote improvement in clinical care in the local clinical agencies or in improving the health of those in the community outside of periodic health education programs. It was a clear priority to address this issue.

36.2   Developing the Structure to Address Cultural Competence Issues

Early efforts focused on examining the School's mission and vision and commitment to diversity. At a faculty and staff retreat, the intention to address issues surrounding diversity and community involvement was raised by the Dean and actively discussed by faculty. Although not universal, most agreed with the focus and believed that student learning would be improved if the School and faculty would actively work to create an inclusive, culturally competent student and work environment. The School mission was discussed and adapted to affirm a commitment to clinical practice, scholarship, and advocacy for underserved populations and the diverse communities served by the wider university. Goals were established to look at curriculum (inclusive of clinical experiences) and the teaching-learning environment.

The Dean assumed responsibility for implementing and overseeing this process. Resources were allocated across a 5-year period. The goals were added to her own self-evaluation plan so that the larger university was aware of the School's plans and efforts and consequently would hold her accountable for achieving the goals. Additionally, these goals were reported to the School's advisory board and examined on an ongoing basis.

A diversity task force was charged with performing an overall assessment and making recommendations specific to the goal areas. This task force ultimately was voted on by faculty to become a standing committee—further attesting to our commitment to cultural competence. Members of the committee in collaboration with a faculty leader in community and cultural competence updated the School's philosophy with greater emphasis on health across the life course and in respecting and valuing cultural differences and right of choice regarding health-care issues. The philosophy and mission were discussed with all incoming students at orientation and within relevant courses. It was also discussed at faculty orientations and revisited in ongoing forums for reflection as to whether it was being actualized in our approach.

36.2.1 Assessment

A three-prong approach to assessment was taken. First, course syllabi were reviewed, examining course objectives and content, and curricular mapping was completed. Second, faculty were interviewed to understand their perceptions and to explore whether teaching within each course reflected culture or cultural competence, their perceptions on teaching diverse student groups, the overall valuing of diversity within the School, and any recommendations they had for change. The third focus was on students. Students from different levels (year group within the program) and cultures participated in focus groups to examine their experiences of inclusion, valuing diversity within the School; experiences during which they had gained insight about cultural competency and what these experiences were; and recommendations they had for change within the School.

36.2.2 Initial Findings

Cultural competence was one of eight organizing constructs for the curriculum. There was one course on health promotion and community health that had a strong focus on culture, cultural beliefs, and explanatory models for what causes illness, beliefs about approaches for curing or treating illness, and who should be involved in the process. Across the rest of the curriculum, there were course objectives highlighting cultural competence, but in discussion with faculty and students, it emerged that this content was "present but hidden" with significant variation across faculty, little incorporation of cultural competency as a main theme in case studies and simulation, and virtually no test questions specific to cultural competence other than in the one health promotion and community health course.

All identified that it was through clinical experiences that culture came alive, but in many cases, this was a "casual" learning in that students were caring for people from different cultural and socioeconomic backgrounds but sometimes with little discussion as to how this impacts assessment, planning, and delivery of care at either the individual or the population level. Almost all clinical experiences were found to be hospital-based and students had little experience with care across the continuum.

Assessment of the work environment showed a lack of diversity at the faculty level but not at the staff level, sterile hallways that did not reflect the diversity of the School, some evidence of strained relations across dominant and non-dominant groups, and a general discomfort with how to handle these situations.

36.3 The Approach

The first priority was training. Over a span of 5 years, there were multiple faculty and staff development programs to increase awareness of issues surrounding cultural competence and to build knowledge and skills—both in cultural competence itself and how to teach it. Approaches ranged from skits depicting common classroom scenarios to a series of workshops examining culture and social determinants of health. These programs often incorporated self-assessments so that each individual was forced to reflect on their own values, beliefs, implicit biases, and ways of interacting with others. Issues of power differentials between faculty and student as well as confronting issues of stereotyping and racism were included. Although this was challenging, it was felt to be fundamental to changing the culture.

Curricular changes were implemented to make the teaching of cultural competence more explicit. Case studies and simulations were developed to elicit culturally appropriate health assessment inclusive of social determinants. Teams of faculty worked on examining class-specific scenarios (i.e., the patient with heart failure or the patient with diabetes) and integrating different cultural concepts, so the case study was more about the whole person than simply the disease. A review of the revised cases showed that we had targeted the major cultural groups in our demographic region as well as common subgroups. Not only were ethnic groups examined but also diversity in religion, sexual orientation, gender identification, and generation.

As these cases were being implemented, School leadership began discussing the importance of ensuring that the curriculum truly prepared the nursing student for a future in nursing, a future very different from that faced by the nursing student just a few decades ago. We recognized that our focus on cultural competence needed to be integrated within other demands for change in nursing student preparation. We knew it was particularly important that our students be ready to contribute to the National Health and Human Services goals of improving health-care quality, emphasizing primary and preventive care, reducing the growth of health-care costs, ensuring access to culturally competent care for vulnerable populations, and improving health care and population health through meaningful use of health information technology. Resources were allocated to training for population health—understanding vulnerable and high-risk populations and the contextual conditions that increase risk exposure. Curriculum groups began to examine how to integrate upstream (e.g., social, economic, and environmental factors), midstream (e.g., working conditions and housing), and downstream (e.g., behavioral and biological determinants of disease) factors contributing to exposure within key clinical didactic courses, rather than waiting until the final community nursing clinical.

36.3.1 Diverse Faculty and Students

In addition to updating the curriculum, the School of Nursing leadership recognized that the nursing workforce of the future must reflect—in terms of ethnicity, race, and religious and cultural background—the patients they will be serving. The School of Nursing has been successful in recruiting a diverse student body to meet the needs for diversity in our field with over half of the students describing themselves as racial or ethnic minorities.

We have not been as successful in ensuring faculty diversity. Cultural competence includes ensuring that the School is a safe zone for anyone who considers themselves a minority—whether a sexual, racial, or religious minority—and actively working to create this environment. We recognized the challenge of having a diverse student body without the diversity in faculty and recognized that students looking for academic role models to encourage and enrich their learning may be frustrated in their attempts to find mentors and a community of support.

The School is implementing approaches to recruit and retain minority faculty. As part of a Robert Wood Johnson grant, we were able to support minority students in obtaining graduate degrees which had an added curricula component inclusive of the faculty role, teaching/learning, and curriculum development. Participating students had mentors to guide them through the graduate program as well as into the role of faculty and the different faculty committees, including the diversity committee. Several of these graduates continued on as full-time or adjunct faculty. To continue to support these faculty and aim for retention, resources were allocated during the first year of employment for participation in a "new faculty" development program and in the second year a scholarly writing development program.

Attempting to draw from the pipeline of diverse students, the Dean developed an aspiring faculty scholarship program for ethnic minority undergraduate students and later for doctoral students. Within these programs, students were exposed to graduate education opportunities and different faculty research and worked alongside experienced faculty in the classroom and clinical area.

Although the outcomes demonstrate that the School of Nursing has the most faculty diversity of other health professions schools and programs in the university, the reality is that that is not enough—we continue not to reflect the diversity of the students or the community we serve. We continue to actively recruit using a variety of methods including one-to-one contacts, advertising in a range of sources, and negotiating for competitive salary and development packages.

36.3.2 Curriculum Updates

We recognized the need for curricular adaptation moving from a curriculum which was strongly grounded in a systems (disease), developmental, and evidence-based practice approach to one with a greater focus on supporting clients with health promotion and prevention. We were preparing nurses with the skills to assist clients and their families with self- and disease management, coordinating care across the continuum, and working with the community to address health needs from the perspective not only of clinical care but also of the physical environment, health behaviors, and social and economic factors such as family and social support and community safety. We aimed to provide our students with a range of experiences to better understand the social, cultural, and environmental factors that can enhance wellness or increase vulnerability to illness, i.e., the social determinants of health (SDOH), and how to provide care that is culturally competent in ever-diverse settings.

The revised curriculum stresses that even when a diagnosis takes place in a health facility, getting well happens in the community, probably the same community where that individual became unwell. Didactic presentations move from the population to the individual level. First we present the epidemiology, contributing factors, and comparisons of disease statistics across geographic counties/states and across population groups; then we discuss the manifestations of illness at the individual level, contrasting that with a discussion at the group and population level for how to manage and prevent the illness across the continuum of care. More of our clinical practicums are set to be community-based, not only in primary care and post-acute care facilities but also in patients' homes and within community-based organizations where the nurse can gain a better understanding of the context in which the patient lives and the social determinants of health the patient faces.

36.3.3 Legacy Clinical Experiences

As the faculty addressed curricular change to enhance cultural competence and develop curricula to integrate population health, a supportive School goal was to "build community service capacity" by engaging in collaborative community-based service with the goal of developing community capacity for health. If we were to provide meaningful population health clinical experiences, we needed to be a partner with the community, actively addressing their priority health concerns.

One such undertaking was the development and ultimately expansion of a nursing community health center serving four public housing facilities. A lead faculty and the School Dean developed a business plan for how the School could develop and lead an interprofessional, collaborative, community-based population health initiative to improve health outcomes and well-being. We had our foot in the door as the lead faculty member had already built a connection with the communities by offering weekly health screenings and follow-ups with residents.

Demonstrating our commitment to the community, we expanded our efforts to include active partnership with the tenant association to define priority needs and allocated School resources to offer screening and health promotion programs and to have an RN hired to coordinate some of the efforts. The RN served in a dual capacity—working with the community and working with students for active participation in case finding, care coordinating and navigating, as well as designing and implementing health promotion programs. Students work alongside community members to develop culturally appropriate programs and services. They gain firsthand experience in making complex medical issues understandable for patients—being guided by community members in how to do this. They witness the reality of not being able to simply say "eat fresh fruits and vegetables" when people live in food deserts or saying "get 30 minutes of exercise a week" where people feel unsafe walking outdoors. An outcome of some of these connections has been students partnering with community agencies to start a community garden, implementation of Tai Chi programs for the elderly, using Wii fitness with pre-teens and yoga programs for youth, and parenting and child wellness programs. As a legacy partnership, these programs are ongoing, and students orient new groups of students to the community and to the specific projects so there is continuation of efforts and commitment.

In addition to the health promotion activities, the project expanded to provide primary health care "on wheels"—a mobile health van that moved from site to site. Nurse practitioner (NP) and NP students would see patients, and follow-up was done by the community registered nurse (RN) and baccalaureate students. Working with the medical school, we partnered with the community board to develop a community health worker (CHW) program. Now, CHWs, residents of the community and supervised by an RN, are part of the team for health outreach and education. Interprofessional teams of students work with a CHW, and the CHW serves a culture broker, guiding the students on culturally appropriate ways to intervene at the group and individual

level. Taking such a population-focused approach has been a win-win proposition. For the community, there is a committed school partner and improved health outcomes. For the School, we have a wealth of clinical experiences for pediatrics, maternal-child, adult health, and psych mental health that are grounded in the community demonstrating nursing's strong role in health promotion and care management within the context of real life.

Conclusion

The current state of health care in the United States is unsustainable: costs are spiraling out of control despite a health-care system that ranks last or near last on measures of health, quality, access, and cost. This cost is, in part, driven by America's epidemic of chronic disease: nearly half of American adults had one or more chronic health conditions, many of which can be prevented through lifestyle changes. The health-care system is particularly poor at meeting the needs of America's ethnic minority populations who have disproportionately borne the burden of illness and chronic disease.

The School of Nursing at the center of this case study recognized the role of nursing in leading change not only within the School institution itself but in the wider health-care system it serves. The School of Nursing recognized that it needed to make structural and curricular changes to ensure its graduates were ready to serve in the health-care system of the future. The Dean took the lead in working with faculty to address the School's mission and vision. Once the overall philosophy was agreed, she then worked with a faculty task force to establish goals to look at curriculum, the teaching-learning environment, and the work environment. Initiatives included training of faculty and updating the curriculum. Key themes woven into all initiatives were a greater emphasis on cultural competence; reorienting the curriculum to train students to provide preventive, acute, and chronic care in the community; and recruiting faculty and students that better represent the patient populations they (will) serve. Driving these changes was the Dean, who ensured that she consulted with faculty and students at every step—from development of a new framework for change to the implementation of concrete initiatives. On a big picture level, the School of Nursing is training the nurse leaders of tomorrow to drive the needed changes within our wider health-care system.

References

Centers for Disease Control and Prevention (2017) Chronic disease overview. https://www.cdc.gov/chronicdisease/overview/index.htm

Kaiser Family Foundation (2016) Analysis of the 2016 ASEC supplement to the CPS. http://www.kff.org/uninsured/report/the-uninsured-a-primer-key-facts-about-health-insurance-and-the-uninsured-in-the-wake-of-national-health-reform/view/footnotes/

Peterson Center on healthcare, Kaiser Family Foundation (2015) Health of the healthcare system: an overview. Peterson-Kaiser Health Tracker System. http://www.healthsystemtracker.org/chart-collection/health-of-the-healthcare-system-an-overview

Salmond SW, Echevarria M (2017) Healthcare transformation and changing roles for nursing. Orthop Nurs 36(1):12

Case Study: Cross-Cultural Leadership for Maternal and Child Health Promotion in Sierra Leone

Florence M. Dorwie

I was born in Sierra Leone, in Jimmi Bagbo, a headquarter of Bargo Chiefdom. Jimmi can be accessed by 36 miles of dirt road from the nearest town of Bo. I grew up in a polygamous family and my mother was the last wife of my father. My mother is a homemaker who worked as a traditional birth attendant/TBA in our village. I was delivered by a TBA. I came to the USA in 1983 after my father allowed me to leave and pursue further education despite the cultural belief that a girl's role is to bear children and prepare a home for her family. Previously, my father only sent his sons to school. I was the first of his daughters to go to school who finished high school. I was not born in wealth but was spared from poverty and risk of early marriage like many girls in my community. I emigrated alone and stayed initially with a family friend who looked after her children. Later, I worked as a nurse's aide in a long-term care facility that provided tuition support for my BSN degree. I subsequently completed my MSN and DNP and have been practicing as a primary care provider in the ambulatory clinic of a large urban hospital in a metropolitan area in the northeast.

After the brutal civil conflict in Sierra Leone (1991–2002) that devastated the healthcare infrastructure, I felt a sense of urgency and responsibility to assume a role that would be both professionally rewarding and challenging. After I completed my MSN, I established a nongovernmental organization, *Sa Leone Health Pride Inc.*, in partnership with five international colleagues. I am the Founder and Chairperson of its Board. In 2005, the NGO was registered as a tax-exempt organization in the USA and recognized as an affiliate of the UN. The goal of the organization is to reduce infant and maternal mortality in Sierra Leone primarily through education. In order to accomplish this goal, the organization conducts annual fund raising dinners, individual solicitations, grant writing, and presentations to potential donors. I developed collaboration with schools of nursing and pharmacy, hospitals, and healthcare practitioners in the USA to participate in the NGO's projects in Sierra Leone. Our initiatives and projects are published in the organization's website, www.saleonehealth.org.

Sa Leone Health Pride is registered as an NGO under the Ministry of Social Welfare and has two part-time personnel in Sierra Leone (Liaison and Coordinator). The liaison facilitates approval for project implementation and meetings between the NGO Chairperson with vital stakeholders (Ministry of Health, Chief Medical Health Officer for Clinical Services, Ministry of Education, and the Vice-Chancellor of the

F. M. Dorwie, D.N.P., R.N.C., A.P.N.-B.C.
Sa Leone Health Pride, Inc., North Bergen, NJ, USA

New York Presbyterian Columbia University Medical Center, New York, NY, USA

University of Sierra Leone). The Coordinator is in charge of all program implementations in Sierra Leone. The NGO is affiliated with the national nursing organization in Sierra Leone and collaborates with local nurses to identify needs to be addressed. Annual programs are planned based on identified needs from program participants and observations by program facilitators. Programs are jointly planned and coordinated by the Chair and in-country Liaison and Coordinator. As Chairperson, I am involved in all project implementation and evaluation that entail 1–2 visits annually in Sierra Leone.

Jimmi is comprised of about 15 villages. The nearest hospital is 36 miles away in Bo Town. It has 1 birthing clinic staffed by 5–7 maternal and child health aides (MCHAs) under the supervision of 1 registered nurse (RN). MCHAs undergo a formal training of about 6 months conducted by the RN and subsequently work as an apprentice of the RN in prenatal, birthing, postnatal, and newborn care at the clinic. They also make home visits and supervise TBAs.

The NGO has partnered with local community leaders such as the village chiefs, government and religious leaders, clinical health officials, nurses, and TBAs to build a "holding area" attached to the clinic for mothers who are sick or close to delivery as many of them live very far from the local clinic. This need was identified during our dialogue with community leaders and stakeholders in Jimmi. The leaders met with the community and asked each adult member to bring stone or sand for the building structure when they come to seek healthcare. *Sa Leone Health Pride* provided monetary assistance. Today, the clinic and its "holding area" is equipped with solar-powered electricity and running water from a well. It has expanded services for minor surgery and has hired one additional RN.

Since 2004, *Sa Leone Health Pride* has been collaborating with Sierra Leone's Ministry of Health and Sanitation in providing health education and training of women in the community, TBAs, MCHAs, and RNs on prenatal care, healthy nutrition, safe delivery, prevention of newborn and postpartal infection, umbilical care,

child development, etc. The NGO has provided kits for TBAs to prevent infection through handwashing, asepsis, and barrier techniques. It has conducted one-on-one clinical supervision of participants, providing valuable critique of their practice. It has developed a train-the-trainer curriculum to facilitate sustainable training of maternal and child health workers. In keeping with the recommendation from WHO, in 2010 the Ministry of Health has mandated that all women should be delivered in a healthcare facility and attended by trained health workers, not TBAs. TBAs have been incentivized to bring the women to the clinic or hospital for prenatal, delivery, and postnatal follow-up. MCHAs supervise the care given by TBAs at home. *Sa Leone Health Pride,* along with other NGOs, helped with the implementation of the government's mandate by helping TBAs adapt to their new role. Women who seek their care are encouraged and accompanied by TBAs to go to the clinic for delivery as well as for their scheduled prenatal, postnatal, and newborn care follow-up. *Sa Leone Health Pride* has maintained its policy to provide health education to anyone including TBAs.

In one of the annual national conferences sponsored by *Sa Leone Health Pride* in Freetown, a foreign white male presenter cited the research that "female circumcision increases susceptibility of women to HIV infection." The audience erupted and a local reporter confronted the speaker: "We don't do that in this country; men don't talk about female circumcision." The audience was offended and became disruptive, preventing the speaker from continuing his presentation. The incident required immediate intervention. I had to intervene by apologizing to the audience. The audience responded that "I did not offend them" but continued their objection to hearing the speaker further.

I met with the presenter, advising him to modify his presentation for the next round in another venue. I explained to him that this is a cultural taboo prohibiting men from openly discussing about women's sexuality, pregnancy, and female circumcision. Female circumcision is not discussed in public especially by a male to a female audience or by females to other females who are nonmembers of the Sande society. While the speaker was warned about the danger of talking about this topic the day before the conference, he was very adamant in presenting relevant research evidence.

I met with the reporters right after the incident to explain that the presenter was merely presenting a research finding which may not be specific to Sierra Leone. They informed me that they were offended by an outsider—a white male unfamiliar with their culture, telling them about something that should not be discussed in public by a male, particularly a non-native.

Cross-cultural leadership requires awareness of social and cultural issues in the context of the people and communities. Cultural awareness and sensitivity to others mandate adaptation of knowledge and decisions to prevent transgressions of taboos. Presentation of evidence-based practices and scientific facts may be offensive without thorough consideration of the sociocultural context. My role as the conference sponsor was to guide the presenter beforehand and prevent alienation of the people we were trying to reach. It was apparent that because of my long-term engagement in the community and the work that the NGO has done, mutual trust protected me from the audience's anger. In fact, they made it clear that I was not the object of their scorn. Confronting a cultural taboo requires mutual trust and being accepted by the people.

particularly among the youth. In 2010, Sierra Leone has the fifth highest maternal mortality rate in the world with 890/100,000 live births (CIA 2017a) which rose to 1360/100,000 live births in 2015 (WHO 2015). In 2016, the country ranked 11th among countries with the highest infant mortality rate with 70/1000 live births (CIA 2017b). In 2015, the country's under 5 mortality rate was 120/1000 live births (WHO 2015). The country's total population in 2015 was 7,076,641 with a ratio of 1 doctor per 100,000 people (WHO 2017). In 2009, there were 685 registered nurses, 95 midwives, and 825 health aides (UNICEF 2009).

In 2013, 54.4% of deliveries occurred in healthcare facilities despite the government mandate that all women deliver in healthcare facilities in 2010 (WHO 2015). The study by Dorwie and Pacquiao (2014) found that most women were delivered by traditional birth attendants/TBAs who were valued by mothers, health professionals, and the community because they provided accessible and affordable care to mothers who may otherwise have no access to health services. TBAs needed training, supervision, and resources for effective referral of mothers. Systemic problems in the healthcare system created enormous barriers to effective care for mothers and children independent of TBA practices that may have contributed to high maternal and infant mortality rates (Dorwie and Pacquiao 2014).

37.1 Social Structural Issues

Sierra Leone is a country in West Africa that suffered a civil war in 2002 that lasted 11 years. In addition, the Ebola outbreak has killed close to 4000 of its people between 2014 and 2016 (BBC News 2016). These events had dramatic consequences on its economy and healthcare infrastructure. According to UNDP (2016), Sierra Leone remains among the world's poorest countries, ranking 180th out of 187 countries in the Human Development Index in 2011. Poverty is widespread with more than 60% of the population living on less than US\$ 1.25 a day. Unemployment and illiteracy remain high,

37.2 Cultural Issues

According to Dorwie and Pacquiao (2014), the majority of women belong to the *Mende* tribe and speak *Mende*. Adolescent girls are trained in child care, homemaking, and sexual matters. The value of hard work and respect for husbands, elders, and authorities are emphasized. Most women are active members of the *Sande*, a society that teaches practical knowledge about birthing, healing, and wisdom that evolved over centuries and generations. Adolescent females undergo initiation rites to become members of the *Sande* society marking their transition to womanhood. The *Sande* society is recognized as the guardian and protector of women and influences all aspects of a woman's life. The society forbids women from divulging its secrets such as the birthing process; violations are considered a major infraction (Dorwie and Pacquiao 2014).

Men and nonmembers are not involved in the process of childbirth, and issues surrounding deliveries by TBAs are not discussed with outsiders (Lori and Boyle 2011). Women of childbearing age are the backbone of the community and viewed as capable of becoming leaders or holding political office. High officials in the society are generally skilled in midwifery. The *Sowie* is the leader of the *Sande* society who is accepted as a role model, enforcer of proper social relationships, and protector of women in the community (Dorwie and Pacquiao 2014). *Sowies* and members of the *Sande* society have control over sacred knowledge essential to the success and happiness of *Mende* women and their families. Most TBAs are either *Sande* society members or *Sowies*. *Sowies* are experts in the *Sande* culture and believed to have access to spirits. In the *Mende* culture, childbearing symbolizes a woman's strength and capacity to participate actively in society. Marriage and having a baby are rites of passage to higher status. The more children a woman bears, the higher is her status and influence. A woman's role is primarily devoted to her family's needs, especially among families of low literacy where girls are encouraged to stay at home to work and supplement the family income and care for younger siblings instead of pursuing secondary education (Kallon and Dundes 2010).

37.3 Cross-Cultural Leadership Strategies

37.3.1 Individual Level

1. Develop self-awareness of own strengths and limitations.
2. Develop in-depth awareness of the community's social and cultural characteristics, history, and current health-related issues.

3. Respect valued cultural traditions of the people by:
   - Assuring gender-congruent care services for women
   - Accommodating desired level of privacy and secrecy by pregnant women
   - Promoting confidentiality of information shared by women about their pregnancy
   - Accommodating preference for oral consent
   - Including family in care decisions and encounters
4. Promote trusting relationship by:
   - Demonstrating hospitality and generosity through sharing of food and offering financial support
   - Demonstrating continued commitment and long-term engagement in the community
   - Accommodating established social and family hierarchy
5. Integrate appropriate cultural, linguistic, and literacy factors in communication by:
   - Developing programs and teaching materials using appropriate language and level of literacy
   - Consulting with local community members regarding appropriateness of health education materials and content

37.3.2 Organizational Level

1. Establish a formal structure and systems for goal implementation locally and worldwide.
2. Seek approval and participation in decision making by community stakeholders including village chiefs and elders, government officials, and healthcare administrators.
3. Use culturally appropriate brokers and mediators to negotiate with established community social hierarchy.
4. Develop multisectoral social network in the community through vertical and horizontal collaboration.
5. Demonstrate trustworthiness through long-term engagement and continued commitment to the community.

6. Disseminate programs and initiatives once approved.
7. Collaborate with community members and stakeholders in needs assessment, selection of priorities, program implementation, and evaluation.
8. Maintain close communication with stakeholders regarding progress of initiatives and future plans.

37.3.3 Global Community Levels

1. Develop sustainable multisectoral partnerships in the local community, nationwide and globally.
2. Develop global partnerships and affiliations such as with the UN, healthcare organizations, religious groups/churches, nursing organizations, academic institutions, multidisciplinary health professionals, etc.
3. Seek avenues for funding of initiatives.
4. Engage experts in collaborative implementation and research on outcomes of initiatives.
5. Disseminate program initiatives and outcomes to worldwide audience and stakeholders.

Conclusion

Cross-cultural and global leadership requires in-depth knowledge of the cultural and social context of communities/countries where leadership transpires. In global contexts, leaders should facilitate evidence-based health promotion strategies that are adapted to the local context. Compassionate and culturally competent leadership builds mutual trust and reciprocity and social network supportive of change. Cross-cultural leadership flourishes in a climate of mutual trust and involvement that can foster expansion of local and global connections and networks of support for effective solutions to problems. Sustainable solutions are the outcomes of culturally competent engagement with multisectoral stakeholders and community members in identifying problems, priorities, and solutions.

References

BBC News (2016) Ebola: mapping the outbreak. http://bbc.com/news/world-africa 28755033

CIA (2017a) The world fact book. https://www.cia.gov/library/publications/the-world-factbook/rankorder/2223rank.html

CIA (2017b). The world fact book. https://www.cia.gov/library/publications/the-world-factbook/rankorder/2091rank.html

Dorwie FM, Pacquiao DF (2014) Practices of traditional birth attendants in Sierra Leone and perceptions by mothers and health professionals familiar with their care. J Transcult Nurs 25(1):33–41. https://doi.org/10.1177/1043659613503874

Kallon L, Dundes L (2010) The cultural context of the Sierra Leone Mende women as patients. J Transcult Nurs 21:228–236

Lori JR, Boyle JS (2011) Cultural childbirth practices, beliefs and traditions in post conflict Liberia. Health Care Women Int 32:454–473

UNDP (2016) About Sierra Leone. http://www.sl.undp.org/content/sierraleone/en/home/countryinfo.html

UNICEF (2009) Free healthcare services for pregnant and lactating women and young children in Sierra Leone. Accessed from. https://www.unicef.org/wcaro/wcaro_SL_freehealthcareservices_2010.pdf on 16 March 2018

WHO (2015) Sierra Leone: country health profile. http://www.afro.who.int/en/sierra-leone/country-health-profile.html

WHO (2017) Sierra Leone. http://www.who.int/countrire/sle/en/

Case Study: Nursing Organizational Approaches to Population and Workforce Diversity

38

Lucille A. Joel, Dula Pacquiao, and Victoria Navarro

A group of Filipino internationally educated nurses (IENs), who entered the USA as legal immigrants to join their families, applied to take the registered nurse licensure examination. After evaluation of their school transcripts, the state Board of Nursing rejected their application because the clinical laboratory component of their nursing courses was not taken concurrently with the theory portion of the course. They were deemed ineligible and mandated by the Board of Nursing to retake these nursing courses in an accredited program of nursing. It should be noted that the additional requirement of concurrency of theory and clinical courses was a problem in this state, which is in keeping with states' rights.

In this instance, some of the nurses sought assistance from the state chapter of the Philippine Nurses Association of America (PNAA). PNAA is the national organization representing Filipino nurses in the USA with several statewide chapter

L. A. Joel, Ed.D., R.N., A.P.N., FAAN
School of Nursing, Rutgers University, Newark, NJ, USA
e-mail: ljoel@sn.rutgers.edu

D. Pacquiao, Ed.D., R.N., C.T.N.-A., T.N.S. (✉)
School of Nursing, Rutgers University, Newark, NJ, USA

School of Nursing, University of Hawaii, Hilo, Hilo, HI, USA

V. Navarro, M.S.N., R.N.
Joint Commission International, Oakbrook, IL, USA

affiliates. One of its goals is to foster the positive image and welfare of its constituent members (PNAA 2016). PNAA facilitated a face-to-face meeting between the president of the Philippine Association of Deans of Colleges of Nursing and the state Board of Nursing. According to Dr. Divinagracia (president of the Philippine deans), concurrency between classroom and clinical components is also a standard in the Philippines. However, during the mass recruitment of Filipino IENs by foreign employers, proliferation of hospital-based schools of nursing and large nursing enrollment created overcrowding and shortages of clinical sites. Consequently, some schools allowed students to take the theory portion prior to clinical practice to manage student progression in the curriculum. At the height of the last nursing shortage in the USA and other rich countries, nursing enrollment in the Philippines grew exponentially as entrepreneurs (physicians and hospital owners) established several schools of nursing. Organized nursing leadership was powerless in controlling the growth of these schools due to the support by the Philippine government eager to bolster its dollar reserve from overseas employment of nurses (Jurado 2013).

PNAA collaborated with a local community college to develop a program to remedy the deficits in the nursing curricula of these nurses. It provided initial funding for tuition support of the first cohort of 40 students. This program is continuing as hundreds of Filipino IENs were affected. PNAA developed a position statement on nursing education standards which was shared with the Association of Deans of Colleges of Nursing in the Philippines emphasizing the need for concurrent theory and clinical practice in the nursing curricula. Many of these questionable nursing programs have since closed when foreign demands for nurses dwindled.

Thousands of nurses, the vast majority of them women, migrate each year in search of better pay and working conditions, career mobility, professional development, and sometimes just novelty and adventure (Kingma 2006). Worldwide, nurses comprise the largest group of healthcare workers as well as the largest migrant group among all categories of healthcare workers. About 8% of registered nurses/RNs in the USA are foreign-educated with the Philippines as the major source country accounting for more than 30% of US foreign-educated nurses. Nurse immigration to the USA has tripled since 1994 to about 15,000 annually (Aiken 2007). The USA employs the most international nurses, but foreign-educated nurses comprise only 4% of its nursing workforce, compared to the UK and Ireland (8%) and Canada (6%). The top six countries that export nurses are the Philippines, Canada, India, Nigeria, Russia, and Ukraine (Walker 2010).

The flow of migration of healthcare workforce has consistently followed a pattern from low-income to high-income countries. A paradox exists in the Philippines with as much as 300,000 unemployed nurses while healthcare facilities particularly in rural areas are critically understaffed. Many nurses seek employment outside of nursing, but nursing school enrollment is greatly influenced by employment opportunities abroad. A shortage of highly educated and skilled health workers within the source countries ("brain drain") has had catastrophic effects on the quality of care, disease burden, and mortality in these countries (Allutis et al. 2014; Kingma 2008).

The International Council for Nurses (ICN 2007) recognizes the right of individual nurses to migrate and the benefits of multicultural practice and learning opportunities supported by migration. However, it denounces unethical recruitment practices that exploit and mislead nurses to accept working conditions incompatible with their qualifications and experience. In addition, ICN condemns recruitment of nurses to countries where the authorities have failed to implement sound resource planning and workforce development and retention. It has called for its member national nurses associations to engage in promoting ethical recruitment by guiding informed decision-making and reinforcing sound employment policies on the part of governments, employers, and nurses, as well as supporting fair and cost-effective recruitment and retention practices. According to ICN, governments and nursing leaders of member nations should develop strategic plans for workforce development, employment, and retention in order to build an adequate and sustainable healthcare workforce. In response to the worldwide human and workforce diversity, ICN (2013) has developed a position statement emphasizing the need for culturally competent nursing and healthcare for populations worldwide.

38.1 Social and Cultural Issues

In the USA, the government monitors the safety of consumers and qualifications of individuals seeking to practice as registered nurses through the State Boards of Nursing and a system of licensure, but the development of the profession is chiefly through the private sector. Organized nursing such as the American Nurses Association (ANA), the National League for Nursing (NLN), and the American Association of Colleges of Nursing (AACN) has fought for many years to move entry into practice for nursing to the level of the baccalaureate degree (BSN) with no success. Efforts included requiring the baccalaureate degree for licensure and later requiring, through legislation, that this degree be completed within 10 years of initial entry into practice. It should be noted that ANA's 1965 position statement (Donley and Flaherty 2008) for BSN as entry to practice was the impetus for the implementation of BSN as the sole entry to practice in the Philippines in 1983 (Republic Act 877). This was achieved through leadership by the Philippine Association of Deans of Colleges of Nursing, the Board of Nursing, and the Philippine Nurses Association.

While efforts to push the BSN in the USA as entry to practice failed, the Magnet Program and the Institute for Medicine Report (2011), both private sector initiatives, have revolutionized the workplace and moved the BSN into new prominence through their demands for a more educated nurse, given the growing complexity of healthcare. These demands were evidence-based, drawing directly on research done by Aiken and other scholars (Aiken et al. 2014; Kutney-Lee et al. 2013; Stimpfel et al. 2016). In a partnership referred to as "twinning," Magnet hospitals in the USA have become mentors to institutions in developing countries to enhance care.

Increasing diversity of populations brings a unique challenge in care provision because of cultural and linguistic differences. The Office of Minority Health (2017) has identified the need for culturally competent healthcare services. This directive has been fully adopted by private organizations such as the accrediting bodies for hospitals and other care settings as well as educators in various health professions. Some of the issues that emerged in healthcare have stemmed from cultural differences between patients and health system norms. The need for translation and interpretation has posed conflict between patients and practitioners. While some families may prefer their own family members for language interpretation, this has resulted in some legal problems for practitioners and healthcare organizations. The individual patient's right to confidentiality demands that the patient determines who has access to his/her medical information. Many cultures assume the sick should not be burdened with information about their prognosis or that medical information should only be shared with specific family members such as the oldest son. Care should be taken to reconcile these choices with the legal requirements of a hosting country. Often the expectations of confidentiality and autonomy require educating patients to their rights and then documenting their preference.

IENs need to adapt their clinical practice and communication skills to that of their new environment in order to successfully deliver safe, quality care to patients. They need to be aware of cultural differences between their own home country and that of the USA and negotiate with these differences to enhance care effectiveness. For instance, the individual right of confidentiality and autonomy may be contrary to the ethic of many IENs and doctors. Another example is the alleviation of pain. Pain has long been labeled as the fifth vital sign in the USA. Depending on the preference of the patient, no one needs to suffer pain and pain need not be the natural by-product of illness (Department of Veterans Affairs 2000). As a vital sign, pain should be routinely assessed, and nurses have the responsibility to advocate for the patient's optimal alleviation of pain, sometimes in the face of strident medical or family opposition. These opposing viewpoints can intrude on clinical care. Some of these attributes of caring are guaranteed legally, others are monitored through accreditation, but they all draw from the US culture. Earlier, there was little appreciation that IENs may bring a different philosophy of care. There is much that can be learned from these new colleagues, while remaining vigilant over one's own context of care.

Cultural competence is inextricably linked to linguistic competence. The essence of nursing is communication—the ability to engage patients as true partners in their care and establish the trust relationship that is essential to building that partnership require linguistic competence. Every aspect of nursing practice, from initial assessment to teaching, counseling, and support, depends on linguistic competence. Linguistic competence is the capacity to communicate effectively with persons who have limited language proficiency, who are to some degree illiterate or have a disability inhibiting hearing and/or understanding (National Center for Cultural Competence (NCCC) 2017). This becomes a problem in any culture where the provider or the patient is not proficient in the local language and the appropriate nonverbal communication.

This patient-centric model within the context of nationally established standards and ethics is an expectation of nursing graduates. Respect for multiculturalism is fostered in nursing education and in in-service programs. Private and public sector endorsement of culturally and linguistically competent healthcare services has been promoted by the Office of Minority Health (2017), The Joint Commission, and the Institute of Medicine (2010). The NLN and AACN have developed and promulgated standards for integration of cultural competence in nursing education. Diversity/multiculturalism in education promises to improve the quality of even the best of programs. AACN (2014) has emphasized that diversity among the student body and faculty improves "learning outcomes, thinking and intellectual engagement, motivation, social and civic skills, and empathy…".

Evidence-based practice has become the raison d'etre of nursing which needs to be reinforced in every nurse, regardless of country of origin or date of completion of their entry educational program. Increasing diversity in the US population necessitates evidence-based practices to reflect the demographics of the patient population as well as practitioners. Institutional review board approval should be contingent on this factor. If the major portion of the clinical population is of an immigrant population, risk management, utilization review, quality assurance, and clinical research models should reflect this demographic makeup. Indeed, a review of studies in healthcare by the US Health Resources and Services Administration (HRSA 2006) revealed that patients are more likely to receive quality preventive care and treatment when they share race, ethnicity, language, and/or religious experiences with their providers. This observation holds challenges for both education and practice.

38.2 Approaches by Professional Nursing Organizations

ICN (2017) is a federation of more than 130 national nurses' associations (NNAs), representing more than 20 million nurses worldwide. ANA

is a member of ICN that represents the interests of 3.6 million registered nurses in the USA (ANA 2017). In response to the influx of IENs and other foreign-educated health professionals to the USA, ANA and NLN established the Commission on Graduates of Foreign Nursing Schools (CGFNS) in 1977. CGFNS has evolved to be a federal and national authority for credentials evaluation and verification pertaining to the education, registration, and licensure of nurses and other healthcare professionals across the world (CGFNS 2016).

IENs experienced a high failure rate in the RN licensure exams and were consequently employed in roles below their educational preparation in order to survive in the USA. Many employers and co-workers also noted their difficulty with English communication. CGFNS developed the test of English proficiency and nursing knowledge for IENs that has demonstrated the ability to predict success in the RN licensure exams. These exams were mandated by most states for visa qualification and RN licensure eligibility. Since the RN licensure exams have been offered in countries outside the USA, the requirement for CGFNS exam has been abolished by many states.

Funded by the Kellogg Foundation, CGFNS (2016) has developed coalitions with nursing leaders in Canada and Mexico to identify and examine the challenges and opportunities presented by the North American Free Trade. One of its divisions, the Alliance for International Ethical Recruitment Practices (CGFNS 2016), has recently partnered with the Philippine Labor Organization, the Philippine Overseas Employment Agency, and the Philippine Nurses Association of America to establish standards for employment contracts offered to Filipino IENs by US employers.

As the national organization of Filipino nurses in the USA, the PNAA represents the professional interests of its members. PNAA has strived to align itself with the official position of ANA and has maintained a collaborative relationship with ANA's state affiliates. Filipino nurses comprise the largest group of IENs in the USA. At the height of the nursing recruitment in the 1980s, state chapters of PNAA partnered with local healthcare employers and nursing schools to develop an acculturation program for newly recruited nurses which included hospital educators, managers, and staff. Using feedback from IENs, their employers, and co-workers, these programs have evolved to include cultural differences, communication, critical thinking, decision-making, legal-ethical issues, leadership, teamwork, etc. State chapters of PNAA also partnered with local schools of nursing and healthcare employers in preparing IENs for CGFNS and RN licensure exams.

The Philippine government views labor export especially of healthcare manpower as a big source of dollar revenue. This governmental push has limited the capacity of local nursing leaders to address the nationwide depletion of skilled educators and practitioners and large nursing vacancies in healthcare facilities because of lack of government funding and proliferation of low-quality nursing programs during periods of mass foreign recruitment. PNAA has instituted the annual educational exchange program ("Balik-Turo") to facilitate dissemination of academic and clinical practices to nurses in the Philippines. This annual program is offered in different regions of the Philippines to reach different sectors of practitioners. PNAA has also partnered with the Department of Health in the Philippines to establish the first nurse anesthesia program to address the shortage of anesthesiologists in rural areas.

PNAA has worked with the Philippine Overseas Employment Agency to promote ethical recruitment practices based on the experiences of nurses in the USA. PNAA has referred nurses to the Philippine Human Rights Committee for legal assistance with fraudulent recruitment and contract violations with their employers. The Philippine Commission on Overseas Filipinos has partnered with PNAA to offer a global summit in the Philippines every 2 years to promote understanding of trends and requirements for international nursing employment among local stakeholders, nurses, and students.

38.3 Cross-Cultural Leadership Strategies

38.3.1 Individual Level

- Design mentoring programs for diverse students and nurses to promote academic and professional success.
- Provide consultation to healthcare organizations and professionals on culturally competent leadership strategies.
- Promote development of professional and leadership network for diverse students and nurses.
- Promote active membership of diverse students and nurses in professional nursing organizations.
- Model leadership behaviors for racial and ethnic minority students and professionals.
- Participate in education and training of healthcare professionals in culturally competent care.

38.3.2 Organizational Level

- Design organizational systems and structure to promote delivery of culturally competent healthcare services.
- Promote engagement of organizations and its leaders in vulnerable and underserved communities.
- Implement systems and structure to reward culturally competent practices and prevent discrimination and inequity in healthcare.
- Enhance recruitment, retention, and success of diverse students and nurses.
- Participate in developing position statements and public dissemination of healthcare agenda supportive of culturally competent care and health equity.

38.3.3 Community Level

- Engage in multisectoral and multidisciplinary collaboration to influence laws, policies, and regulations to enhance population health equity.

- Maintain active involvement in professional organizational committees to improve health equity.
- Participate in local, national, and global initiatives to improve workforce development and retention.
- Participate in local, national, and global initiatives to promote healthcare equity worldwide.
- Expand social and professional networks to advance initiatives for health equity.
- Participate in research and evaluation of programs and policies relevant to population health.

Conclusion

Preparation for culturally competent/proficient organizations/communities must start with the individual. Cultural competence requirements should be included in job descriptions, performance appraisals, and promotion criteria. Organizational policies should reflect the characteristics of the workforce and the community served. The healthcare organization is situated in a community and is dependent on the community for its sustenance. The hospital, long-term care facility, home care, or ambulatory care setting should begin to take on the characteristics of the population it serves. It is best to educate healthcare workers to the values and traditions of the people and listen to their community leaders. Know the community, ask their indulgence for one's ignorance, and invite them to speak to staff or provide "friendly" visits to patients. Bring services to the local ethnic population, breaking down barriers and establishing familiarity. Let patient satisfaction data speak for itself and determine the receptiveness of services to diverse populations. Track programs with the volume of services being provided, and determine how this impacts on the organization's bottom line. Be aware that resources cost money, so cultural competence deserves a budget line of its own. The costs of consultation, interpretation, printed material and translation services, and more, deserve to be visible

in the organization's budget (The Joint Commission 2010).

Nursing leaders need to engage with racial and ethnic communities and other stakeholders to implement a strategic plan to build a multicultural student body or the multicultural workforce. This creates a vibrant community for learning and practice, a ready laboratory to advance the science and improve health internationally. This will be one way to provide staff with the resources for culturally competent practice. It is also the way to create a welcoming bridge between the agency and the community it serves.

Engagement with racial and ethnic nursing organizations and communities can promote recruitment of diverse students to nursing and the professions. They serve as a vital social support network for students. These systems and their leaders can provide the link to enhance awareness of culture-specific best practices in education and practice.

Cross-cultural leaders not only transform their organizations toward cultural competence but also engage in regional, national, and international collaborations to promote safe and equitable healthcare globally. Cross-cultural leaders should be mindful of the positions of global experts in healthcare. They can engage their national organizations to collaborate with governmental agencies in their countries to influence policies on workforce development and deployment. Cross-cultural leaders should collaborate with professional nursing organizations globally to create a unified strategy to influence governmental policies to promote local employment and retention of healthcare professionals, allocation of adequate healthcare manpower for local needs, and universal access of local populations to basic care services. International collaboration should promote dissemination of knowledge and best practices in nursing education and care delivery.

Agreements among governments should address ways to compensate for the loss of the financial investment in the education of healthcare professionals and the negative consequences on population health when they decide to leave for more opportunities and better salaries and working conditions. While migration of health professionals might benefit individual families and even countries through their remittances, these gains are rarely used to improve the social agenda of the sending country.

References

AACN (2014) Fact sheet. The need for diversity in healthcare workforce. http://www.aapcho.org/wp/wp-content/uploads/2012/11/NeedForDiversityHealthCareWorkforce.pdf

Aiken LH (2007) U.S. nurse labor market dynamics are key to global nurse sufficiency. Health Serv Res 42(3 Pt 2):1299–1320. https://doi.org/10.1111/j.1475-6773.2007.00714.x

Aiken LH, Sloane DM, Bruyneel L et al (2014) Nurse staffing and education and hospital mortality in nine European countries: a retrospective observational study. Lancet 383:1824–1830. PMCID: PMC4035380

Allutis C, Bishaw T, Frank MW (2014) The workforce for health in a globalized context – global shortages and international migration. Glob Health Action 7:23611. https://doi.org/10.3402/gha.v7.23611

ANA (2017) Members and affiliates. http://www.nursingworld.org/FunctionalMenuCategories/AboutANA/WhoWeAre

CGFNS (2016) Milestones. http://www.cgfns.org/about/history/

Department of Veterans Affairs (2000) Pain as the 5th vital sign toolkit. Geriatrics and Extended Care Strategic Healthcare Group National Pain Management Coordinating Committee Veterans Health Administration, Washington, DC

Donley R, Flaherty J (2008) Revisiting the American Nurses Association's first position on education for nurses. http://www.nursingworld.org/MainMenuCategories/ANAMarketplace/ANAPeriodicals/OJIN/TableofContents/Volume72002/No2May2002/RevisingPostiononEducation.html

HRSA (2006) The rationale for diversity in the health professions: a review of evidence. http://bhpr-hrsa-healthworkforce-reports-diversityreviewevidence

ICN (2007) Position statement: ethical recruitment of nurses. http://www.icn.ch/images/stories/documents/publications/position_statements/C03_Ethical_Nurse_Recruitment.pdf

ICN (2013) Position: cultural and linguistic competence. http://www.icn.ch/images/stories/documents/publications/position_statements/B03_Cultural_Linguistic_Competence.pdf

ICN (2017) Who we are. http://www.icn.ch/who-we-are/who-we-are/

Institute of Medicine (2010) The future of nursing: leading change, advancing health. National Academies Press, Washington, DC

Jurado L (2013) Social construction of Filipino nurses in the Philippines and as foreign-educated nurses in the United States. PhD Dissertation, Rutgers, The State University of New Jersey

Kingma M (2006) Nurses on the move: migration and the global health care economy. Cornell University Press, Ithaca

Kingma M (2008) Nurses on the move: historical perspective and current issues. Online J Nurs 13(2). http://www.nursingworld.org/MainMenuCategories/ANAMarketplace/ANAPeriodicals/OJIN/TableofContents/vol132008/No2May08/NursesontheMove.html

Kutney-Lee AM, Sloane DM, Aiken LH (2013) An increase in the number of nurses with baccalaureate degrees is linked to lower rates of postsurgery mortality. Health Aff 32:579–586. PMCID: PMC3711087

National Center for Cultural Competence (NCCC) (2017) Self-assessment: an essential element of cultural competence. http://nccc.georgetown.edu/foundations/frameworks.html. Accessed 13 May 2017

Office of Minority Health (OMH), US DHHS (2017) The national standards for culturally and linguistically appropriate services in health and health care. minorityhealth.hhs.gov/omh/browse.aspx?lvl=2&lvlid=53. Accessed 10 May 2017

PNAA (2016) Mission. http://mypnaa.org/About-Us

Stimpfel AW, Sloane DM, McHugh MD et al (2016) Hospitals known for nursing excellence associated with better hospital experiences for patients. Health Serv Res 51(3):1120–1134

The Joint Commission (2010) Advancing effective communication, cultural competence, and patient- and family-centered care: a roadmap for hospitals. The Joint Commission, Oakbrook Terrace, IL

Walker J (2010) Migration, brain drain, and going forward. Johns Hopkins Nursing. http://magazine.nursing.jhu.edu/2010/08/the-global-nursing-shortage/

Designing Culturally Competent Interventions Based on Evidence and Research

Marilyn "Marty" Douglas

Guideline: *Nurses shall base their practice on interventions that have been systematically tested and shown to be the most effective for the culturally diverse populations that they serve. In areas where there is a lack of evidence of efficacy, nurse researchers shall investigate and test interventions that may be the most effective in reducing the disparities in health outcomes.*

Douglas et al. (2014: 115)

39.1 Introduction

According to a World Health Organization report of more than a decade ago (WHO 2004), more than half of the world's deaths are preventable with cost-effective interventions that are known and evidence-based. Yet, we neither know how to make these interventions more available to those who need them nor do we adequately direct our efforts and resources toward closing the gap between what is known and what we practice. Consequently, the disparities in healthcare delivery, health inequities, and health outcomes remain a significant challenge worldwide, and one that does not seem to be diminishing even as science makes significant advances in curing human diseases. In an effort to address these challenges, evidence-based practice is now a well-established global priority of nursing, recognizing that nursing practice must be based on findings from the best evidence derived from well-designed research studies (International Council of Nurses 2012; Munten et al. 2010; Saunders and Vehviläinen-Julkunen 2017; Cheng et al. 2017).

39.2 Evidence-Based Practice (EBP)

As the costs of delivering healthcare rise, solutions to aligning quality, improved patient outcomes, and costs have become more urgent. Increasingly, healthcare delivery systems are using standardized practices that are based on the best research findings as a means to improve patient outcomes while at the same time reducing costs. Almost 10 years ago, the US Institute of Medicine set the following goal: "By the year 2020, 90 percent of clinical decisions will be supported by accurate, timely, and up-to-date clinical information, and will reflect the best available evidence (Institute of Medicine 2008: 189)." Furthermore, EBP has been strongly endorsed by several international nursing organizations as a foundation of nursing practice (International Council of Nurses 2013; Sigma Theta Tau International 2017; Royal College of Nursing 2014; American Academy of Nursing 2017; American Nursing Credentialing Center 2015).

M. Douglas, Ph.D., R.N., FAAN
School of Nursing, University of California, San Francisco, San Francisco, CA, USA
e-mail: martydoug@comcast.net;
marilyn.douglas@nursing.ucsf.edu

39.2.1 Definition and Goals

Evidence-based practice is a method used to incorporate the best evidence into the clinical decision-making process. It uses a problem-solving approach to combine three major elements: the best evidence from research, patient's preferences and values, and the clinician's expertise (Melnyk et al. 2014). EBP is a complex process involving clinical nurses, advance practice nurses, and administrative staff. Its goal is to improve patient outcomes as well as staff satisfaction and retention, which ultimately reduces costs in both areas.

39.2.2 Barriers to EBP

Despite the overwhelming support for EBP, many barriers to its implementation remain. In an attempt to identify global barriers to implementing EBP, Ubbink et al. (2013) conducted a systematic review of 31 studies with 10,798 respondents in 17 countries representing all continents. Surprisingly they found that the barriers at both the individual and organizational levels were similar across settings, except for the language barrier in non-English-speaking countries and limited access to electronic databases in some countries. Both nurses and physicians found similar barriers, such as lack of time to access research findings and implement the evidence in their own settings, lack of training in the process of implementation, lack of facility resources, and lack of administrative and staff support for EBP. In addition, nurses cited their lack of authority to change practice, limited understanding of statistics and the research process in general, and their inability to translate the research findings into implications for practice as impeding implementation of EBP.

These findings are consistent with many other studies. Khammarnia et al. (2015) surveyed 280 nurses in Iran to determine barriers to implementing evidence-based practice in six teaching hospitals. Besides the language barriers, they found similar issues related to time, that is, insufficient time to access then read the literature, as well as work overload precluding time to evaluate and change practice. Organizational lack of support, lack of essential knowledge of the EBP process, and unavailability of electronic and library resources were also cited as barriers.

Studies of European nurses have shown similar barriers. Investigators in Spain (Pericas-Beltran et al. 2014) reported nurses' lack of autonomy, perceived lack of inclusion in clinical decision-making, and insufficient leadership support as well as physician resistance as impediments to implementing EBP. Patelarou et al. (2013) confirmed these findings in an investigation of European community settings.

Since standardizing evidence-based practices across large hospital systems is one suggestion for improving patient outcomes and reducing costs, Warren et al. (2016) surveyed 1608 nurses in one large 9-hospital system spread out along the mid-Atlantic area of the USA. These investigators used questionnaires developed by Melnyk et al. (2008) to describe not only the nurses' attitudes, beliefs, and perceptions about EBP (Evidence-Based Practice Belief scale (EBPB)) but also their readiness to implement EBP (Evidence-Based Practice Implementation scale (EBPI)). A third questionnaire used was the Organizational Culture and Readiness for System-Wide Integration of EBP Scale (OCRSIEP) developed by Fineout-Overholt and Melnyk (2006). This questionnaire asked the participants to rate the availability of EBP resources and mentoring staff at their organization, identify key leadership roles in decision-making, and rate the readiness of their organization to implement EBP.

Overall, less than half of the nurses in this study reported having access to resources to implement EBP, while almost 80% had not accessed national guidelines to evaluate a change in their clinical practice within the past 2 months. Almost 2/3 of RNs reported a lack of organizational readiness for EBP, especially in the areas of human and financial resources. And nearly 80% perceived their involvement in clinical decision-making as "None" to "Somewhat." However, notable demographic and educational differences were found. The nurses who were younger, who worked in Magnet® hospitals, and those with less work experience had a much more positive attitude toward EBP, similar to those with graduate nursing degrees. These differences can be attributed to newer curricula in nursing programs and that Magnet® designated hospitals place a strong emphasis on EBP (American Nursing Credentialing Center 2013).

Viewed from a global perspective, the barriers are remarkably similar among nurses around the world. Although more nurses are becoming increasingly aware of the need for EBP, many still report lack of time, resources, and leadership in order to provide care based on the best evidence available.

39.2.3 Facilitators of EBP

Despite the obstacles faced by clinicians to implement evidence-based care, a number of facilitators have been identified. The essential characteristics of an environment that facilitates EBP include nurses with a positive attitude toward EBP and access to the necessary resources to search current research. First and foremost, the healthcare delivery system must embrace a philosophy and culture and mentorship to guide nurses in the interpretation, critical appraisal, and translation of evidence into their practice (Davidson and Brown 2014) that supports EBP and then provide financial, digital, and human resources to support this culture (Melnyk 2017). A belief in the value of EBP to improve patient outcomes, reduce costs, and increase nurse satisfaction is crucial at the executive level. Without this conviction, organizational goals will not be created, and fiscal resources will not be allocated to support EBP.

For nurses to have a positive attitude toward EBP, they need knowledge of its process and benefits. Since younger nurses and those more recently graduated from nursing programs have already been introduced to EBP, more experienced nurses are more critically in need of continuing education programs in these concepts. Integrating EBP and research content into staff orientation, continuing education, and leadership development programs demonstrate one aspect of organizational support and preparation for EBP.

Knowledge alone about EBP does not guarantee its implementation. Mentorship by nurses with advanced EBP training, working side by side with clinical nurses, is essential if the best evidence is going to be integrated into established practice. These EBP mentors are needed to help interpret statistics, select well-designed studies, and identify which findings can be tested in their own settings. Unless organizations allocate funds to hire these EBP mentors, staff nurses will be ill equipped to interpret and integrate EBP.

Nursing leadership at the executive, departmental, and unit levels is required to facilitate the implementation of EBP (Melnyk et al. 2016). Nurse leaders endorse the essential ingredient of *time* to be spent by the nurses to study a problem, gather the necessary evidence, and then evaluate its relevance to their current practice. Nurse leaders foster a positive attitude toward EBP by encouraging staff to partake in EBP classes and projects and by providing the necessary time and resources to accomplish these activities. Nursing leadership legitimizes this commitment by incorporating participation in EBP in job descriptions and clinical ladders and as a competency in the functional statements and performance evaluations of nursing staff at all levels.

Besides time, mentors, and leadership support, material, digital, and human resources also are needed to enable nurses to participate in EBP activities. Access to electronic databases containing relevant research studies is a prerequisite, in whatever form, whether it is at the point of care or accessible through a university. In addition, librarians who can assist the staff with accessing these databases are crucial. These librarians can contribute through instruction in continuing education classes for the staff at the point of care, as well as assisting with identifying and searching the appropriate library resources and databases (Melnyk and Fineout-Overholt 2015).

39.2.4 Strategies for Implementing Evidence-Based Practice

A number of models have been developed to address the barriers to EBP and to emphasize those elements that facilitate the transfer of research findings into clinical practice. Four such models will be discussed: the Iowa model, the Johns Hopkins model, the Advancing Research and Clinical Practice Through Close Collaboration (ARCC ©) model, and the Joanna Briggs Institute (JBI) model of evidence-based healthcare, a model reconsidered.

39.2.4.1 Iowa Model of Research and Practice

The team of Titler et al. (1994, 2001) was a pioneer in developing a coherent framework for infusing nursing research findings into clinical practice. They developed the Iowa Model of Research and Practice©, which was an outgrowth of the Quality Assurance Model Using Research (QAMUR) (Watson et al. 1987). The Iowa model was developed by nursing leaders within the University of Iowa Hospitals and Clinic (UIHC) system, a multi-division healthcare system in the Central USA. The steps in the process of integrating research into practice are illustrated in Fig. 39.1.

Although knowledge of the process is essential, it is insufficient without an adequate structure in which to implement EBP. Nursing administration at UIHC constructed such an environment in the following way:

- *Department of Nursing Research Committee* provides the organizational structure for coordinating all the department's research activities, such as the following:
  - Strategic planning for nursing research, including prioritizing topics to be investigated
  - Consultants to divisional and unit-based nursing research committee*s*
  - Reviewing research protocols
  - Presenting classes and papers on clinical research topics
  - Disseminating research findings to divisional committees
- *Divisional* and *Unit-Based Nursing Research Committees* are composed of front-line care providers such as staff nurses, clinical nurse specialists, and nurse managers. Their activities include as follows:

- Identifying the clinical practice issues in their division or on their units that require exploration of research-based validation
- Critiquing the appropriate research with the help of EBP mentors and support of divisional nursing administrators
- Developing strategies for pilot testing evidence-based practices in their own settings and evaluating the effect of the changes on patient outcomes
- Coordinating any changes needed in practice protocols with the appropriate committees.
- Presenting projects developed at the unit or division level at the Professional Nursing Council, which serves as a platform for sharing and discussing how their experiences and findings have applicability to the work in other divisions and units

In this model, the process of problem identification, evaluation, and implementation is accomplished by point-of-care providers, thus providing some assurance that the research-based changes will be integrated into standard practice.

39.2.4.2 Johns Hopkins Nursing EBP Model

A second model for implementing EBP, the Johns Hopkins Nursing Evidence-Based Practice Model, is one of the easiest to use by the practicing nurse (Dearholt and Dang 2012). It uses a three-step problem-solving approach named PET: (1) practice question, (2) evidence, and (3) translation. A diagram of the model plus nine user-friendly tools is available on the Internet at http://www.hopkinsmedicine.org/evidence-based-practice/jhn.html.

39.2.4.3 Advancing Research and Clinical Practice Through Close Collaboration (ARCC) Model

A third model was designed to be implemented on a system-wide basis. The Advancing Research and Clinical Practice Through Close Collaboration (ARCC©) model was designed and tested by the team of Melnyk et al. (2017). It

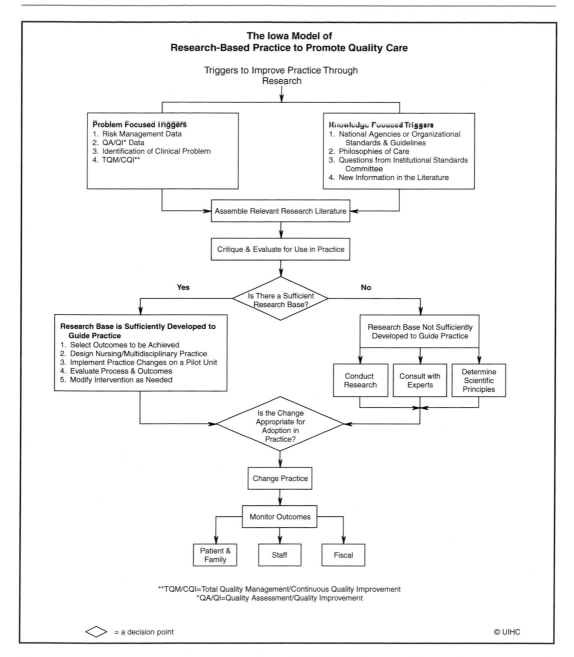

Fig. 39.1 The Iowa model of research-based practice to promote quality. Source: Titler MG, Kleiber C, Steelman VJ, Good C, Rakel B, Barry-Walker J, Small S, Buckwalter K (1994) Infusing research into practice to promote quality care. *Nursing Research*, 43: pg. 309. Reproduced with permission

incorporates an organizational assessment as a first step in identifying the barriers and strengths within the specific healthcare system. Based on the findings from this tool, the Organizational Culture and Readiness for System-Wide Integration of EBP Scale (OCRSIEP) (Fineout-Overholt and Melnyk 2006), system-specific strategies are developed to address the identified strengths and barriers. For example, some potential strengths may be that the organization as a whole places a strong value on EBP, has administrative support, and has potential EBP mentors. Barriers may include inadequate knowledge and skills about EBP among the staff and their perceived lack of value in the benefits of EBP.

After organizational assessment, an evaluation of the point-of-care clinicians is the next step. Findings from two tools administered to staff, the Evidence-Based Practice Belief scale (EBPB) and the Evidence-Based Practice Implementation scale (EBPI) (Melnyk et al. 2008) are used to build a curriculum for orientation and continuing education workshops in EBP and research. Central to these workshops is the seven-step process of EBP outlined in Table 39.1

Table 39.1 The seven steps of evidence-based practice (Melnyk et al. 2014)

Step 0. Cultivate a spirit of inquiry along with an EBP culture and environment
Step 1. Ask the PICO(T)[a] question
Step 2. Search for the best evidence
Step 3. Critically appraise the evidence
Step 4. Integrate the evidence with clinical experience and patient preferences to make the best clinical decision
Step 5. Evaluate the outcome(s) of the EBP practice change
Step 6. Disseminate the outcome(s) (Melnyk and Fineout-Overholt 2015)

[a]PICO(T): P = patient population, I = intervention or issue of interest, C = comparison intervention or issue, O = outcome, T = time for intervention to achieve outcome (if relevant) (Melnyk 2017)
Source: Melnyk BM, Gallager-Ford, L, Long LE, Fineout-Overholt E. (2014). The establishment of evidence-based practice competencies for practicing registered nurses and advanced practice nurses in real-world clinical settings: proficiencies to improve healthcare quality, reliability, patient outcomes, and costs. Worldviews on Evidence-based Nursing. 11: page 6. Reproduced with permission

(Melnyk et al. 2014). Each of these steps can be further expanded into separate courses.

Finally, in order to integrate and sustain EBP within the organizational culture, competencies were developed for both registered nurses and advanced practice nurses, as outlined in Table 39.2 (Melnyk et al. 2014). These competencies provide clear expectations of the staff that EBP is part of the organizational culture.

If the clinical problem of interest involves a racially or ethnically diverse or vulnerable population, then added criteria need to be applied to defining the problem (PICOT question) and evaluating the research for applicability. For example, additional questions to ask are as follows: Was the population of interest included in the study? Were different cultural groups studied and compared? Was the intervention appropriate and feasible for or adapted to the population of interest? Were the outcomes of a culturally specific intervention clinically significant? Was the effectiveness of a particular intervention studied across several cultural groups?

39.2.4.4 The Joanna Briggs Institute Model

This final model, the JBI Model of Evidence-Based Healthcare, a model reconsidered (Jordan et al. 2016), is the most recent revision of the model first published in 2005 by Pearson et al. Evidence-based practice is defined as "clinical decision-making that considers the best evidence; the context in which care is delivered; client preference; and the professional judgement of the health professional" (Pearson et al. 2005: 209). Its major components are broader than the other models in that it includes evidence generation, evidence synthesis, evidence transfer, and evidence utilization, with its newest component of global health.

Its emphasis on the context in which care is delivered and client preferences makes this model particularly relevant and useful with vulnerable populations. At the core of the model are four criteria, which can be applied when evaluating whether the evidence is applicable to diverse populations:

Table 39.2   Evidence-based practice competencies (Melnyk et al. 2014)

Evidence-based practice competencies for practicing registered professional nurses

1. Questions clinical practices for the purpose of improving the quality of care

2. Describes clinical problems using internal evidence (internal evidence=evidence generated internally within a clinical setting, such as patient assessment data, outcomes management, and quality improvement data)

3. Participates in the formulation of clinical questions using PICOT format (P=patient population, I=intervention or area of interest, C=comparison intervention or group, O=outcome, T=time)

4. Searches for external evidence to answer focused clinical questions (external evidence = evidence generated from research)

5. Participates in clinical appraisal of pre-appraised evidence (such as clinical practice guidelines, evidence-based policies and procedures, and evidence synthesis)

6. Participates in the critical appraisal of published research studies to determine the strength and applicability to clinical practice

7. Participates in the evaluation and synthesis of a body of evidence gathered to determine its strength and applicability to clinical practice

8. Collects practice data (e.g., individual patient data, quality improvement data) systematically as internal evidence for clinical decision-making in the care of individuals, groups, or populations

9. Integrates evidence gathered from external and internal sources in order to plan evidence-based practice changes

10. Implements practice changes based on evidence and clinical expertise and patient preferences to improve care processes and patient outcomes

11. Evaluates outcomes of evidence-based decisions and practice changes for individuals, groups, and populations to determine best practices

12. Disseminates best practices supported by evidence to improve quality of care and patient outcomes

13. Participates in strategies to sustain an evidence-based practice culture

Evidence-based practice competencies for practicing advanced practice nurses
All competencies of practicing registered professional nurses plus:

14. Systematically conducts an exhaustive search for external evidence to answer clinical questions (external evidence = evidence generated from research)

15. Critically appraises relevant pre-appraised evidence (i.e., clinical guidelines, summaries, synthesis of relevant external evidence) and primary studies, including evaluation and synthesis

16. Integrates a body of external evidence from nursing and related fields with internal evidence in making decisions about patient care (internal evidence = evidence generated internally within a clinical setting, such as patient assessment data, outcomes management, and quality improvement data)

17. Leads transdisciplinary teams in applying synthesized evidence to initiate clinical decisions and practice changes to improve the health of individuals, groups, and populations

18. Generates internal evidence through outcomes management and EBP implementation projects for the purpose of integrating best practices

19. Measures processes and outcomes of evidence-based clinical decisions

20. Formulates evidence-based policies and procedures

21. Participates in the generation of external evidence with other healthcare professionals

22. Mentors others in evidence-based decision-making and the EBP process

23. Implements strategies to sustain an EBP culture

24. Communicates best evidence to individuals, groups, colleagues, and policy makers

Source: Melnyk BM, Gallager-Ford, L, Long LE, Fineout-Overholt E. (2014). The establishment of evidence-based practice competencies for practicing registered nurses and advanced practice nurses in real-world clinical settings: proficiencies to improve healthcare quality, reliability, patient outcomes, and costs. Worldviews on Evidence-based Nursing. 11:5–15, pg. 11. Reprinted with permission

- *Feasibility*: Would this intervention be workable, practical, and sustainable in the cultural context of interest? Would the population be able to integrate the intervention into their daily life?
- *Appropriateness*: How well does the intervention align with the cultural beliefs and practices of the cultural group?
- *Meaningfulness:* Would the racial, ethnic, or vulnerable population of study respond positively to the intervention? Would they endorse the intervention?
- *Effectiveness*: Does the intervention achieve the desired outcome for this group?

Finally, four overarching principles complete the model: culture, capacity, communication, and collaboration. Further elaboration of the model and the resources provided by the institute can be found at: http://joannabriggs.org.

In summary, knowledge and skills in integrating EBP, human resources in the form of mentors, and a positive attitude within the organization are necessary but insufficient for EBP to be sustainable. Additional administration support is required in the form of clinical release time to participate in research activities, such as library searches, journal clubs, collecting data, funding for attendance at research courses and presentations at research conferences, and mentoring in writing research abstracts and papers. All of these elements are crucial to providing an environment that encourages nurses to seek scientific evidence to underpin their nursing practice.

39.3 Research

Nurse researchers have the opportunity to reduce racial and ethnic disparities in health outcomes by exploring cultural phenomena and testing interventions that have been specifically targeted to the health needs and life ways of specific cultural groups. Both qualitative and quantitative research methodologies are available to those nurse researchers investigating questions related to culturally appropriate care. By providing practitioners with scientifically tested, evidence-based strategies and practices designed for specific groups, nurse researchers play an important role in deceasing global racial and ethnic disparities in health outcomes. An overview of a few, more frequently used research methods are presented below.

39.3.1 Qualitative Methods

Most of the early research in transcultural nursing used a variety of qualitative methodologies to explore cultural phenomenon and culturally specific health beliefs and practices. Qualitative research aims to examine the meanings of a phenomenon and to analyze observations in order to discover patterns of behaviors and relationships. These methods continue to be useful to nurse researchers investigating culturally specific care issues. The choice of the qualitative method used depends heavily on the research question being asked.

39.3.1.1 Ethnography
Ethnography is rooted in techniques developed by anthropologists who spent extended periods of time living among a group of people. Ethnographic research investigates the customs, beliefs, practices, and worldview of a group of people. The researchers using this method construct a comprehensive view of the social framework of the society, not just about health and illness.

Ethnography forms the bases for other research methods as well, such as grounded theory and, more recently, community-based participatory research (CBPR) and mixed-method designs (Morse 2016). Nurse researchers can use some of ethnography's methods to focus on a specific health issue or nursing problem observed in a small group of vulnerable culturally diverse persons. The key elements of ethnographic methods that have proven useful to nurse researchers include the following:

- *Participant observation*. It involves active involvement in activities of the group, study-

Cronbach's alpha of both versions, and (7) factor analysis with varimax rotation for internal consistency. Using this process, the investigators were confident that the cultural self-efficacy tool was valid and adequately adapted to the cultural group that they wish to test in future research.

Another good example of a scale validation study is described by Santos Prudencio et al. (2016: 512). These investigators provide a highly detailed explanation and illustration of the process of cultural and linguistic validation of an instrument into Brazilian Portuguese. In this case, the Patient Expectations and Satisfaction with Prenatal Care scale was analyzed using a homogeneous group of Brazilian women seeking publicly funded prenatal care in one urban area. But because of the sociocultural heterogeneity of the Brazilian population, the investigators recommended further assessment of this instrument with a wider, more diverse sample. This is a poignant observation as caution is warranted when attempting to use a translated instrument for a population different from the one used for the original validation, despite the similarity of languages.

39.3.2.2 Experimental and Quasi-experimental Designs

Experimental designs seek to establish a cause-effect relationship between two or more variables. The major differences between quasi-experimental and true experimental designs are that in quasi-experimental designs the groups being tested are not randomly selected and the independent variable is not manipulated. Common quasi-experimental designs include pre- and posttest designs, posttest-only designs, and interrupted time-series designs.

In true experimental designs, participants are randomly assigned to control and experimental groups, and the researchers attempt to control for all variables except for the one being manipulated, i.e., the independent variable or intervention. The intervention is administered only to the experimental group. Outcome or dependent variables are measured, and comparisons between the two groups are analyzed statistically.

Joseph et al. (2016) describe an intervention study in which a pretest/posttest design was used. The aim of their study was to decrease sedentary behavior and increase moderate activity in a group of young African-American women with a body mass index (BMI) >25 kg/m^2 (overweight and obese). As the intervention, the investigators designed a culturally relevant website that contained exercise demonstration videos; blogs about physical exercise, nutrition, and wellness; online recipes; tools for tracking dietary intake and daily physical exercise (PA); a diary; and a message board. The study participants logged into the website with a username and password. Participants were encouraged to engage in 30–60 min of exercise four times per week for 3 months. Two of the weekly sessions were held at a local indoor track, with research assistants monitoring the participants while they walked. For the other two weekly sessions, participants could choose either to walk alone or join a group exercise class. The dependent variables of BMI, self-efficacy for PA, social support for PA, enjoyment of PA, and weekly amount of physical activity and sedentary screen time (e.g., TV, DVD, computer games) were measured both before the intervention began (pretest) and after 3 months of the intervention (posttest). This study illustrates how complex, resource intensive, and time consuming these designs can be, particularly if the intervention needs to be tailored to cultural sensitivities. However, these efforts are necessary to determine efficacy of our interventions, especially when we are evaluating programs and testing interventions in racial, ethnic, and vulnerable populations.

A major benefit of using quantitative research designs is that the findings may be generalizable to a broader population. These techniques enable the researchers to gather information from a relatively large number of participants, allowing for comparisons. And with the use of numerical rating information, statistical analysis can be used to determine relationships between variables and examine probable cause and effect of this relationship.

39.3.3 Mixed Method Designs

In the past decade, mixed method research designs have become more widely accepted. But as they evolved and gained recognition, their definition became more blurred. Traditionally, mixed methods are characterized by using statistical trends (quantitative data) combined with the stories (qualitative data). A leading expert in mixed methods research has delineated six different strategies to guide the combination and analysis of both types of data. These include sequential explanatory design, sequential exploratory design, sequential transformative design, concurrent triangulation design, concurrent nested (embedded) design, and concurrent transformative design (Creswell 2013). More recently, qualitative researchers such as Morse (2010) and Morse and Cheek (2015) contend that mixed method designs can also apply to the use of two or more methods of the qualitative nature (QUAL-*qual*), such as in-depth interviews as the core component of a research study and participant observation as a second, supplemental data source.

Mixed method research takes advantage of using several ways to explore a research problem and gives a more complete understanding of our research problem than by using just one method. The choice of the appropriate combination of methods cannot be arbitrary. Rather, the researcher selects qualitative and quantitative methods that have complementary strengths and do not have overlapping weaknesses. Data are not just collected and analyzed separately, but, instead, qualitative and quantitative data are integrated and analyzed according to a specific mixed-method design, such as one described by Creswell (2013).

Two studies provide examples of mixed methods designs. De Gagne et al. (2015) explore the healthcare experiences of Asian Indians in the Southeastern United States by using surveys, which provided quantitative data, plus focus groups, which, through content analysis of the transcripts, provided qualitative data. The findings from the combination of qualitative and quantitative data provided both overlapping and different perspectives of the respondents' healthcare experiences. On the other hand, a modified qualitative mixed-method (QUAL-*qual*) design is described by Phillips et al. (2014). To study Australian nurses in small healthcare organizations, these authors used a number of qualitative methods, including semi-structured interviews, structured and unstructured observations, photographs, floor plans, and social scanning data. Their design did not adhere strictly to Morse's requirement for a core method with others being supplemental. Instead, the investigators used two standard qualitative methods as core components, in-depth interviews and structured observations, and the other four methods as supplemental. The combination of these methods rendered a more complete and complex portrayal of the research problem than if only one method was used.

39.4   Evidence-Based Research: Selecting the Most Appropriate Evidence

One of the most crucial stages in the EBP process is searching the literature for the best evidence to address the clinical practice issue and target the individual person or group. But not all evidence is equal. The quality of the evidence is usually described as a hierarchy, with level one producing the greatest degree of current scientific evidence available, as outlined in Table 39.3 (Stillwell et al. 2010).

39.4.1 The "5S" Model

The University of Michigan Library website (2017) provides a wealth of information regarding evidence-based research, including a pyramid further delineating the levels of evidence (Fig. 39.2). This model aligns the hierarchy described in Table 39.3 with a second hierarchy of evidence strength (Haynes 2006; Townsend et al. 2015). For example, *studies*, which most often examine a single aspect of care, are followed by *syntheses*, such as systematic reviews

Table 39.3 Hierarchy of evidence for intervention studies

Type of evidence	Level of evidence	Description
Systematic review or meta-analysis	I	A synthesis of evidence from all relevant randomized, controlled trials
Randomized, controlled trials	II	An experiment in which subjects are randomized to a treatment group or control group
Controlled trials without randomization	III	An experiment in which subjects are nonrandomly assigned to a treatment group
Case-control or cohort study	IV	Case-control study: a comparison of subjects with a condition (case) with those who do not have the condition (control) to determine characteristics that might predict the condition Cohort study: an observation of a group (s) (cohort[s]) to determine the development of an outcome(s) such as a disease
Systematic review of qualitative or descriptive studies	V	A synthesis of evidence from qualitative or descriptive studies to answer a clinical question
Qualitative or descriptive study	VI	Qualitative study: gathers data on human behavior to understand *why* and *how* decisions are made Descriptive study: provides background information on the *what*, *where*, and *when* of a topic of interest
Opinion or consensus	VII	Authoritative opinion of expert committee

Source: Stillwell SB, Fineout-Overholt E, Melnyk BM, Williamson KM. (2010). Searching for the Evidence: Strategies to help you conduct a successful search. *AJN.* 110 (5). p.43. Reprinted with permission

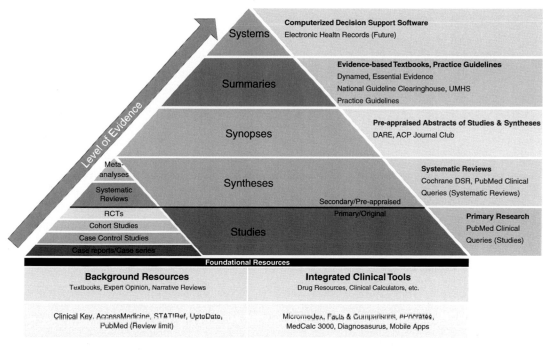

Fig. 39.2 Sources for evidence-based research: integrated "5S" levels of organization of evidence pyramid. Source: Townsend W; Donovan K; Ginier E; MacEachern M; Mani N. "Integrated "5S" Levels of Organization of Evidence Pyramid." September 2015. (http://hdl.handle.net/2027.42/138965). CC BY 4.0 https://creativecommons. org/licenses/by/4.0/. Adapted from: Haynes RB. Of studies, syntheses, synopses, summaries and systems: the "5S" evolution of services for evidence-based health care decisions. ACP J Club. 2006 Nov–Dec;145(3): A8–9. Reprinted with permission

like Cochrane Reviews (Rew 2011). Integrative reviews also fall in the category of syntheses but are the only approach that combines studies using both nonexperimental and experimental research methods to address a research question (Whittemore and Knafl 2005). *Synopses* are concise, abstract-like descriptions of the systematic reviews. *Summaries* compile and integrate the best evidence from the three lower levels in order to extract the full range of evidence for a particular care problem. Finally, *systems*, such as a computerized decision support system (DSS) within the electronic health record, link the individual patient with the best evidence for his or her specific problem. Obviously, this highest *system* level is ideal and would be very useful for racial and culturally diverse populations, specifically in the case of pharmacological efficacy. However, these DSS systems are very expensive and consequently rare; yet they remain the goal. This "5S" pyramid also lists services and resources compiling the evidence at each level.

39.5   Evolution from Evidence-Based to Value-Based Practice

After decades of work dedicated to developing models for implementing evidence-based interventions, there is increasing attention over the past 10 years being given to patient centeredness and the "value" of the treatment as viewed by the patient as well as the healthcare provider and the healthcare system. Brown et al. (2005) first coined the term by defining value-based care as "…incorporating the highest level of evidence-based data with the patient perceived value conferred by health care interventions for the resources expended." Although the original definition of EBP included patient values and preferences, those components were overshadowed by the search for the best evidence. Now the renewed emphasis on patient satisfaction and quality of

life has shifted clinical decision-making toward value-based care (Marzorati and Pravettoni 2017).

But *value* can be defined differently by each of the stakeholders, depending on their perspective. Patients, healthcare providers, healthcare systems, economists, health insurance companies, and employers all can assess value differently. Hence, to date, there is no consensus on what constitutes value. For example, healthcare providers assess value according to clinical effectiveness and evidence-based interventions. On the other hand, health economists define value in terms of clinical benefit achieved for the money spent.

Value, from the individual's perspective, is very personal and incorporates unique preferences and expectations that can be culturally derived. Value encompasses the person's health-related quality of life and goals related to all aspects of life, including levels of functional impairment, pain management, spiritual well-being, and social and cognitive functioning. Mohammed et al. (2016) conducted a systematic review of 36 studies assessing patients' perception of high-quality healthcare. A majority of the studies were published after 2005; the designs included quantitative, qualitative, and combined methods and were conducted in ten countries, although 63% of the studies were in the USA. Most of the study settings were in primary/ambulatory care, but in-patient and emergency services also were studied. Both a longitudinal comprehensive measure of quality of care and a single encounter with the healthcare system were evaluated. Of the ten dimensions of quality care identified, the top three were communication, access, and shared decision-making.

Incorporating cultural competency principles within value-based practice can be easily achieved because of the shared goals of adapting care to the person's unique values, preferences, and aspirations, which in the case of vulnerable and racially and ethnically diverse populations can be culturally defined.

39.6 Implications for Practice, Education, and Research

39.6.1 Individual Level

For healthcare professionals at the point of care, the most important contributions are the identification of researchable care problems and the implementation of evidence-based process and solutions. Unit-based journal clubs to review transcultural health literature can serve as entry points for new nurses and well as those with more work experience but less preparation in EBP and research from their training curricula. Attendance at staff development programs on EBP lays the foundation for participation in the EBP process. Participation on unit-based and system-wide committees that collect data on patient satisfaction, especially from patients of diverse cultural heritages, helps elucidate potential cross-cultural challenges and areas for further exploration. Ultimately, it will be the primary providers of care who will be responsible for implementing any policy changes made as a result of the research process.

Advanced practice nurses (APN) have the additional responsibilities of mentoring staff in the EBP process and conducting continuing education programs on EBP and the research process. In addition, the APNs can serve as leaders of interdisciplinary research teams investigating cross-cultural problems, seeking funding for such projects, and collaborating with professional colleagues and faculties. They can evaluate research tools and services provided for cultural applicability, specifically for the populations they serve. By collaborating with their international colleagues, they can test research instruments with diverse populations around the world, investigate common cross-cultural problems, and consult with and mentor their global colleagues. Finally, the APNs can coordinate and host conferences to disseminate evidence on effective approaches to culturally congruent practice.

For those clinicians working in low to middle income countries, where financial and digital resources are limited, quality assurance projects may be the optimal level achievable. However, the same seven-step process described in Table 39.1 applies. Enlisting the assistance of university librarians and faculty members to aid in the literature searches may be helpful, if such alternatives are feasible.

39.6.2 Organizational Level

As described above, without an organizational climate that supports EBP and research, the financial, digital, and human resources will not be allocated. Staff development programs and time allotted for the staff to attend need to be provided. APNs and medical librarians are needed to guide the staff in searching the literature. Unit-based computers with Internet access to university medical libraries are necessary if an adequate literature search is to be conducted. The job descriptions and performance evaluations of APNs must include EBP mentoring and research to validate those functions as totally integrated into their practice, rather than as "extras" that somehow never are addressed for lack of time.

The organization is also responsible for collection of health data for all its citizens within its "encatchment" or service. This is particularly important where large numbers of vulnerable or racial and ethnically diverse populations reside. These statistics can serve as the basis for investigating cultural applicability and appropriateness of the services for these populations.

39.6.3 Community Level

Collaboration between clinicians and faculty researchers in the community can be mutually beneficial. The clinicians gain from the research expertise of the faculty in designing EBP projects and research studies. And the faculty benefit from the access to clinical settings for data collection for their own research and can identify first-hand clinically relevant and significant researchable problems for their future search.

By expanding this collaboration to include interdisciplinary networks of clinicians and researchers, studies can be designed to include higher proportions of patients from diverse populations than if only conducted in one healthcare system. Findings from these network studies have the potential for greater generalizability of results.

International partnerships between academic and clinical facilities from resource-rich countries and healthcare systems in developing countries can be similarly beneficial to each participant. Collaboration with national and international colleagues provides the structure to share knowledge and expertise about the culture of study. These colleagues can jointly identify culturally relevant clinical problems, collaborate on quality improvement projects, and apply for funding that is often unavailable to and inaccessible by resource-poor countries. Using this shared knowledge and expertise, all members of the international team can work together to design and implement large-scale intervention studies of cultural phenomena. Co-authorship on the publication and dissemination of the results of these studies in professional journals and at transcultural conferences is also a benefit to national and international colleagues alike.

Conclusion

Providing culturally competent care requires that any adaptation or accommodation made to respect the person's cultural beliefs, values, or practices must be grounded in safety and evidence. And this evidence must be based on findings generated from careful study. Optimally, an evidence-based practice approach or a formal research study is the preferred method of identifying culturally competent interventions. However, in situations in which financial and digital resources are limited, quality improvement projects and program evaluations using a similar EBP process can provide useful information. The goal is to provide the most meaningful (valued) intervention based on the best available evidence.

Practice based on evidence has been shown to increase both patient and nurse satisfaction, reduce costs, and improve patient outcomes. Therefore, improving health outcomes, especially among the vulnerable and racially and ethnically diverse populations, may help decrease the racial disparities in health seen today.

References

American Academy of Nursing (2017) Transforming health policy and practice through nursing knowledge: 2017-2020 strategic plan. www.aannet.org/about/strategic-plan-2014-2017. Accessed 25 Apr 2017

American Nursing Credentialing Center (2013) Chapter 4. New knowledge, innovations and improvements. In: 2014 Magnet® application manual. Author, Silver Spring, MD

American Nursing Credentialing Center (2015) Annual report 2015. http://www.nursecredentialing.org/Documents/Annual-Reports-Archive/2015-AnnualReport.pdf. Accessed 26 Apr 2017

Bloomer MJ, Cross W, O'Connor M, Moss C (2012) Qualitative observational in a clinical setting: challenges at end of life. Nurs Health Sci 14:25–31

Boucher LM, Marshall Z, Martin A, Larose-Hébert K, Flynn JV, Lalonde C, Pineau D, Bigelow J, Rose T, Chase R, Boyd R, Tyndall M, Kendall C (2017) Expanding conceptualizations of harm reduction: results from a qualitative community-based participatory research study with people who inject drugs. Harm Reduct J 14:1–18. https://doi.org/10.1186/s12954-017-0145-2

Brown MM, Brown GC, Sharma S (2005) Evidence-based medicine to value-based medicine. AMA Press, Chicago, IL. 5–7, 125–149, 151–181, 193–217, 267–279, 319–324

Carvajal A, Centeno C, Watson R, Martinez M, Rubiales AS (2011) ¿Como validar un instrumento de medida de la salud? [How is an instrument for measuring health to be validated?]. Anales del Sistema Sanitario de Navarra 34(1):63–74

Cheng L, Feng S, Hu Y (2017) Evidence-based nursing implementation in Mainland China: a scoping review. Nurs Outlook 65:27–35

Choi TST, Walker KZ, Palermo C (2017) Culturally tailored diabetes mellitus education for Chinese patients: a qualitative case study. J Transcult Nurs 38:315–323

Creswell JW (2013) What is mixed methods research. https://cirt.gcu.edu/research/developmentresources/research_ready/mixed_methods/choosing_design. Accessed 6 May 2017

Davidson JE, Brown C (2014) Evaluation of nurse engagement in evidence-based practice. AACN Adv Crit Care 25:43–55

De Gagne JC, Oh J, So A, Haidermota M, Lee SY (2015) A mixed method study of health care experiences among Asian Indians in the southeastern United States. J Transcult Nurs 26:354–364

Dearholt SL, Dang D (2012) Johns Hopkins nursing evidence based practice and guidelines, 2nd edn. Sigma Theta Tau International, Indianapolis, IN

Diekelmann N, Allen D, Tanner CA (1989) The NLN criteria for appraisal of baccalaureate programs: a critical hermeneutic analysis. National League for Nursing Press, Washington, DC

Douglas M, Rosenketter M, Pacquiao D, Clark Callister L, Hattar-Pollara M, Lauderdale L, Milsted J, Nardi D, Purnell L (2014) Guidelines for implementing culturally competent nursing care. J Transcult Nurs 25(2):109–221

Fineout-Overholt B, Melnyk BM (2006) Organizational culture & readiness for system-wide integration of EBP. ARCC, IIc, Gilbert, AZ

Ge L, Albin B, Hadziabdic E, Hjelm K, Rask M (2016) Beliefs about health and illness and health-related behavior among urban women with gestational diabetes mellitus in the southeast of China. J Transcult Nurs 27:593–602

Groenewald T (2004) A phenomenological research design illustrated. Int J Qual Methods, 3(1). Article 4. http://www.ualberta.ca/~iiqm/backissues/3_1/html/groenewald.html. Accessed 20 May 2017

Haynes RB (2006) Of studies, syntheses, synopses, summaries and systems: the "5S" evolution of services for evidence-based health care decisions. ACP J Club 145(3):A8–A9. 107326/ACPJC-2006-145-3-A08

Herrero-Hahn R, Rojas JG, Ospina-Diaz JM, Montoya-Juarez R, Restrepo-Medrano JC, Hueso-Montoro C (2017) Cultural adaptation and validation of the cultural self-efficacy scale for Colombian nursing professionals. J Transcult Nurs 28:195–202

Institute of Medicine, McClellan MB, McGinnis M, Nabel EG, Olsen LM (2008) Evidence-based medicine and the changing nature of healthcare: meeting summary (IOM roundtable on evidence-based medicine). National Academies Press, Washington, DC. http://www.nap.edu/catalog/12041.html. p 189. Accessed 5 May 2017

International Council of Nurses (2012) Closing the gap: from evidence to action. International Nurses Day 2012. http://www.icn.ch/images/stories/documents/publications/ind/indkit2012.pdf. Accessed 22 Mar 2017

International Council of Nurses (2013) Position statement: scope of practice. http://www.icn.ch/images/stories/documents/publications/position_statements/B07_Scope_Nsg_Practice.pdf. Accessed 26 Apr 2017

Johns Hopkins Nursing Evidence-Based Practice Model. http://www.hopkinsmedicine.org/evidence-based-practice/jhn.html. Accessed 11 May 2017

Jordan Z, Lockwood C, Aromataris E, Munn Z (2016) The updated JBI model for evidence-based healthcare. The Joanna Briggs Institute. http://joannabriggs.org/assets/docs/approach/The_JBI_Model_of_Evidence_-_Healthcare-A_Model_Reconsidered.pdf. Accessed 15 Aug 2017

Joseph R, Pekmezi D, Dutton GR, Cherrington AL, Kim YI, Allison JJ, Durant NH (2016) Results of a culturally adapted internet-enhanced physical activity pilot intervention for overweight and obese young African American women. J Transcult Nurs 27:136–146

Kara B, Tenekeci EG (2017) Sleep quality and associated factors in older Turkish adults with hypertension: a pilot study. J Transcult Nurs 28:296–305

Khammarnia M, Mohammadi MH, Amani Z, Rezaeian S, Setoodehzadeh F (2015) Barriers to implementation of evidence based practice in Zahedan teaching hospitals, Iran, 2014. Nurs Res Pract. 2015: 1–5. Article ID 357140. https://doi.org/10.1155/2015/357140. Accessed 5 May 2017

Marzorati C, Pravettoni G (2017) Value as the key concept in the health care system: how it has influenced medical practice and clinical decision-making processes. J Multidiscip Healthc 10:101–106

Melnyk BM (2017) The difference between what is known and what is done is lethal: evidence-based practice is a key solution urgently needed. Worldviews Evid Based Nurs 14:3–4

Melnyk BM, Fineout-Overholt E (2015) Evidence-based practice in nursing and healthcare. A guide to best practice, 3rd edn. Wolters Klower, Philadelphia, PA

Melnyk BM, Fineout-Overholt E, May MZ (2008) The evidence-based practice beliefs and implementation scales: psychometric properties of two new instruments. Worldviews Evid Based Nurs 5:208–216

Melnyk BM, Gallager-Ford L, Long LE, Fineout-Overholt E (2014) The establishment of evidence-based practice competencies for practicing registered nurses and advanced practice nurses in real-world clinical settings: proficiencies to improve healthcare quality, reliability, patient outcomes, and costs. Worldviews Evid Based Nurs 11:5–15

Melnyk BM, Gallagher-Ford L, Kosky BK, Troseth M, Wyngarden K, Szalacha L (2016) A study of chief nurse executives indicates low prioritization of evidence-based practice and shortcomings in hospital performance metrics across the United States. Worldviews Evid Based Nurs 13:6–14

Melnyk BM, Fineout-Overholt E, Giggleman M, Choy K (2017) A test of the ARCC© model improves implementation of evidence-based practice. Healthcare culture, and patient outcomes. Worldviews Evid Based Nurs 14:5–9

Miner SM, Liebel D, Wilde MH, Carroll JK, Zicari E, Chalupa S (2017) Meeting the needs of older adult refugee populations with home health services. J Transcult Nurs 28:128–136

Mohammed K, Nolan MB, Rajjo T, Shah ND, Prokop LJ, Varkey P, Murad MH (2016) Creating a patient-centered health care delivery system: a systematic review of health care quality from the patient perspective. Am J Med Qual 31:12–21

Morse JM (2010) Simultaneous and sequential qualitative mixed method designs. Qual Inquiry 16:483–491. https://doi.org/10.1177/1077800410364741

Morse J (2015) Using qualitative methods to assess the pain experience. Br J Pain 9:26–31

Morse J (2016) Underlying ethnography. Qual Health Res 26:875–876

Morse JM, Cheek J (2015) Introducing qualitatively-driven mixed-methods designs. Qual Health Res 25:731–733

Munten G, van den Bogaard J, Cox K, Garretsen H, Bongers I (2010) Implementation of evidence-based practice in nursing using action research: a review. Worldviews Evid Based Nurs 7:135–157

Musa AS, Pevalin DJ, Shahin FJ (2016) Impact of spiritual well-being, spiritual perspective, and religiosity on the self-rated health of Jordanian Arab Christians. J Transcult Nurs 27:550–557

National Institute of Minority Health and Health Disparities (2017) Community-based participatory Research program, program description. https://www.nimhd.nih.gov/programs/extramural/community-based-participatory.html. Accessed 15 May 2017

Nikfarid L, Rassouli M, Borimnejad L, Alavimajd H (2017) Experience of chronic sorrow in mothers of children with cancer: a phenomenological study. Eur J Oncol Nurs 28:98–106

Nypaver CF, Shambley-Ebron D (2016) Using community-based participatory research to investigate meaningful prenatal care among African American Women. J Transcult Nurs 27:558–566

Patelarou A, Patelarou E, Brokalaki H, Dafermos V, Thiel L, Melas C, Koukia E (2013) Current evidence on the attitudes, knowledge and perceptions of nurses regarding evidence-based practice implementation in European community settings: a systematic review. J Commun Health Nurs 30:230–244. https://doi.org/10.1080/07370016.2013.838501

Pearson A, Wiechula R, Court A, Lockwood C (2005) The JBI model of evidence-based healthcare. Int J Evid Based Healthc 3:207–215

Pericas-Beltran J, Gonzalez-Torrente S, Pedro-Gomez J, Morales-Asencio J, Bennasar-Veny M (2014) Perception of Spanish primary healthcare nurses about evidence-based clinical practice. A qualitative study. Int Nurs Rev 61:230–244. https://doi.org/10.1080/07370016.2013.83851

Phillips CB, Dwan K, Hepworth J, Pearce C, Hall S (2014) Using qualitative mixed methods to study small health care organizations while maximizing trustworthiness and authenticity. BMC Health Serv Res 14:559–571. https://doi.org/10.1186/s12913-014-0559-4

Rew L (2011) The systematic review of literature: Synthesizing evidence for practice. J Spec Pediatr Nurs 16:64–69

Royal College of Nursing (2014) Defining nursing 2014. ISBN: 9781910672020. https://www.rcn.org.uk/professional-development/publications/pub-004768. Accessed 4 May 2017

Santos Prudencio P, Hilfinger Messias DK, Villela Mamede F, Spadoti Dantas RA, de Souza L, Villela Mamede M (2016) The cultural and linguistic adaptation to Brazilian Portuguese and content validity of the patient expectations and satisfaction with prenatal care instrument. J Transcult Nurs 27:509–517

Saunders H, Vehviläinen-Julkunen K (2017) Nurses evidence-based practice beliefs and the role of evidence-based practice mentors at university hospitals in Finland. Worldviews Evid Based Nurs 14:35–45

Sigma Theta Tau International (2017) Evidence-base nursing position statement. http://www.nursingsociety.org/why-stti/about-stti/position-statements-and-resource-papers/evidence-based-nursing-position-statement. Accessed 4 May 2017

Speziale HJS, Carpernter DR (2007) Qualitative research in nursing. Advancing the humanistic imperative, 4th edn. Lippincott Williams & Wilkins, Philadelphia

Squires A, Aiken LH, van den Heede K, Sermeus W, Bruyneel L, Lindqvist R, Schoonhoven L, Stromseng I, Busse R, Brzostek T, Ensio A, Moreno-Casbas M, Rafferty AM, Schubert M, Zikos D, Matthews A (2013) A systematic survey instrument translation process for multi-country, comparative health workforce studies. Int J Nurs Stud 50:264–273

Stillwell SB, Fineout-Overholt E, Melnyk BM, Williamson KM (2010) Searching for the evidence: strategies to help you conduct a successful search. AJN 110:41–47

Teshuva K, Borowski A, Wells Y (2017) The lived experience of providing care and support services for Holocaust survivors in Australia. Qual Health Res 27:1104–1114

Titler MG, Kleiber C, Steelman VJ, Goode C, Rakel B, Barry-Walker J, Small S, Buckwalter K (1994) Infusing research into practice to promote quality care. Nurs Res 43:307–313

Titler MG, Kleiber C, Steelman VJ, Rakel BA, Budreau G, Everett LQ, Buckwalter KC, Tripp-Reimer T, Goode CJ (2001) The Iowa model of evidence-based practice to promote quality care. Crit Care Nurs Clin North Am 13:497–509

Townsend W, Donovan K, Ginier E, MacEachern M, Mani N (2015) Integrated "5S" levels of organization of evidence pyramid. September 2015. (http://hdl.handle.net/2027.42/138965). CCBY 4.0 https://creativecommons.org/licenses/by/4.0/. Adapted from: Haynes RB. Of studies, syntheses, synopses, summaries and systems: the "5S" evolution of services for evidence-based health care decisions. ACP J Club 145(3):A8–A9

Ubbink DT, Guyatt GH, Vermeulen H (2013) Framework of policy recommendations for implementation of evidence-based practice: a systematic scoping review.

BMJ Open 3(1): e001881. https://doi.org/10.1136/bmjopen-2012-001881. https://www-ncbi-nlm-nih-gov.ucsf.idm.oclc.org/pmc/articles/PMC3563143/. Accessed 25 Apr 2017

University of Michigan Library (2017) Research guides/nursing/hierarchy of evidence resources. http://guides.lib.umich.edu/c.php?g=282802&p=1888245. Accessed 2 Aug 2017

Warren JI, McLaughlin M, Bardsley J, Eich J, Esche CA, Kropkowski L, Risch S (2016) The strengths and challenges of EBP in healthcare systems. Worldviews Evid Based Nurs 13:15–24

Watson CA, Bulechek GM, McCloskey JC (1987) QAMUR: a quality assurance model using research. J Nurs Qual Assur 2:21–27

Whittemore R, Knafl K (2005) The integrative review: updated methodology. J Adv Nurs 52:546–553

World Health Organisation (2004) World report on knowledge for better health: strengthening health systems. WHO, Geneva

Yost KJ, Bauer MC, Buki LP, Austin-Garrison M, Garcia LV, Hughes CA, Patten CA (2017) Adapting a cancer literacy measure for use among Navajo women. J Transcult Nurs 28:278–285

Case Study: Domestic Violence of an Elderly Migrant Woman in Turkey

40

Gülbu Tanriverdi

Fatma is a 67-year-old Kurdish Muslim woman who practices in the Shafi'i Muslim sect. She is married with three children and literate and works as a housewife. Fatma's husband is 70 years old, Kurdish, and also practices in the Shafi'i Muslim sect. He completed his primary school education. Fatma and her husband were both born and raised in a village located in the easternmost part of Turkey. This is also where they married and had their children. Forty-five years ago, Fatma and her husband and children migrated to an urban area in western Turkey due to financial reasons. Fatma's husband was a construction foreman. Because the weather in eastern Turkey is cold and snowy in winters, it was impossible for construction workers to find a permanent job year-round. However, the climate conditions were appropriate for construction in almost every season when they moved to their new location in western Turkey.

When they moved, their children were 1, 2, and 3 years of age. Fatma and her husband encountered a culture that was very different from their own when they first migrated to the city in western Turkey. They did not have any social support. Fatma had 6 siblings, and her husband had 17 siblings, but none of them was living in or near them in their new location. They did not adapt well to this different culture, but the working conditions compelled them to stay. Fatma's husband was spending long days working in construction with other workers, who came from a culture that was similar to his. Fatma, on the other hand, was spending time alone at home with the children.

She did not like this city at first. Residents of the city were not friendly. She thought they did not like her and looked down on her. No one who lived close by had more than two children, and she felt that everybody was avoiding her and her children. Fatma remembered an elderly woman who said hello to her once, and this woman was the first person she talked to. When she saw the elderly woman again, she became happy and felt as if she had seen a member of her own family.

Fatma and her husband were worried about their children. They thought that they could not raise their children in this city according to their own cultural values. In their opinion, young people in this big city were too free. Their clothing and lifestyles did not conform to the standards of the culture of Fatma and her husband. They did not approve of the relationships between young women and men. This was not in accordance with the culture of Fatma and her family. They feared that their children could grow up to be like these young people, and this was unacceptable in their culture. There were some migrant families

G. Tanriverdi, Ph.D.
Canakkale School of Health, Terzioglu Campus,
Canakkale Onsekiz Mart University,
Canakkale, Turkey
e-mail: gulbu@comu.edu.tr

that went back to their hometown for these reasons alone.

On the one hand, Fatma and her husband were making efforts to raise their children in accordance with their own cultural beliefs. On the other hand, they did not make any effort to accommodate themselves to this new culture to which they had migrated. They socialized with other migrant families whose culture was similar to their own. One study found that families who migrated to another city in Turkey created various solidarity networks with other migrants living in their city. Through these social networks, they coped with the difficulties of living in a city that was strange to them (Canatan and Yıldırım 2009).

In her new life in western Turkey, Fatma was conducting herself and behaving in ways that were specific to her own culture. She tried to solve the problems she faced within these patterns because she was aware of the consequences she would face if she did not behave in accordance with her culture.

However, 6 months ago, Fatma behaved unintentionally in a way that was inappropriate to her culture. It occurred when Fatma went to see a doctor. She had entered the examination room of a male doctor, unaccompanied by her husband, even though she knew this would make her husband angry. Her husband had brought her to the hospital, but he left to do a short errand just before Fatma's turn came to see the doctor. Fatma did not know how to behave when her turn came to see the doctor, because her husband was not there to accompany her to the examination room. She felt uncomfortable with the strange looks the others in the waiting room gave her, but she nevertheless entered the examination room with the male doctor, without her husband. When her husband returned, he could not find Fatma where he had left her.

After she had seen the doctor, Fatma told her husband that she was not alone in the examination room. She told him that she had merely showed her medical analysis results to the doctor and was not examined, but she could not convince him of this explanation. Fatma swore on the Qur'an and suggested to her husband that he view the surveillance tape recorded by the hospital cameras. However, her husband told her that he could not accept her explanation.

Thus, Fatma began having horrible days, with her husband becoming violent toward her almost every day. At first, she believed that she deserved this. Her husband insulted her and used physical violence against her, and they had sexual intercourse rarely, only when he wished. But there was no emotional expression of fondness or love. Sexual violence then was added to what first began as physical and emotional violence. She continued to believe that she deserved this violence. Fatma could not say no to the sexual desire of her husband despite everything she experienced. Eventually she experienced a psychological breakdown, for which she blamed herself. She felt ashamed, desperate, scared, and worried because she was subjected to violence. She prayed for this violence to stop and awaited God's help.

Fatma did not tell anyone about these episodes of violence, but instead she remained silent. While her husband was committing physical violence against her, she tried to protect her face, and she did not make a sound. She did not want anyone outside to hear her screams. Fatma believed that no one should know about the violence that she was subjected to by her husband. She should resist this violence by herself as much as she could. In this way, she would stay married, and her husband would not be punished. She wanted to prevent any damage to the reputation of her family. She believed that if their neighbors reported the violent acts to a government agency, such as the police, gendarmerie, health institutions, or prosecutor's office, there would be irreversible negative consequences. Although their home was only a few minutes from the Family Health Center, Fatma did not report the violence to her family doctor or nurse. With the continuing violence, Fatma felt desperate at times. She even thought of committing suicide, but this was against her religious beliefs. She believed that if she committed suicide, she would go to hell. Another way to stop the violence would be to get a divorce, but she felt ashamed to even consider this. In her culture, it is unacceptable for a woman, particularly an elderly one, to get divorced. The same belief statements were observed in a qualitative research conducted in Turkey (Yalcin Gursoy and Tanriverdi 2017).

40.1 Cultural Issues

According to Fatma's beliefs, when a woman needs to visit a male doctor, a man or a woman must accompany her. Their culture requires this. A study found that, in some cultures in Turkey, it is important that the doctor who examines a woman is female and that if the doctor is not female, the woman does not get examined (Özçelik Adak 2002; Tanriverdi et al. 2011; Yalcin Gursoy and Tanriverdi 2017).

Defining violence is difficult in Turkish culture. Because the family is regarded as sacred and private, it is not acceptable for other people to interfere in one's family life. This issue comes into question more in traditional societies. Elderly people may not accept that their families have a problem regarding violence. The elderly may feel ashamed of their family members' behaviors. They may be worried about how their relatives would react and believe that their relatives might mistreat them when they report the violence. Many of the older generations think that they have caused the problems they face, and they may not want to tell anyone else about their problems (Yeşil et al. 2016).

The cultural structure forces women to give into difficulties, to continue their marriages in all circumstances, and to question what they have done to deserve the violence. Moreover, women accept violence for reasons such as fear of being lonely, feeling ashamed, fear of having to appear in court, fear of losing financial support, and worrying about their children (Ibiloglu 2012). Many elderly people in Turkey do not want to disclose to anyone out side of their families that they are experiencing violence. They prefer to remain silent about who is committing violent acts, believing that their relatives will be punished if the violence is reported to governmental agencies (Kalaycı and Şenkaynağı 2015). In Turkish

culture, proverbs such as "men both love and beat," "no one can come between husband and wife," and "beating is heaven-sent" are used to normalize violence, while other proverbs such as "you can leave the house where you have come with your wedding dress only with your shroud" are used to make divorce seem impossible (Yüksek Oktay 2015).

A nationwide study conducted in Turkey reported that among women, 14% think that it is acceptable, in some cases, for men to commit physical violence against them, while 48.5% do not talk about the physical and emotional violence they experience. Also, 92% do not seek help from any institution because of violence; and of the women who are exposed to physical and sexual violence, 55% do not want to receive any kind of support, and 91.8% do not want to receive support from government agencies (The General Directorate on the Status of Women 2009). Another study conducted in Turkey reported that 39.3% of the women surveyed approved of this type of violence. In the same study, approximately one in five women stated that the cause of violence is cultural (Kocacık and Çağlayandereli 2009).

40.2 Social Structural Factors

In Turkey, life expectancy at birth is 75.3 years for males, 80.7 years for females, and 78 years on average. There are approximately 6.6 million persons 65 years or older, comprising 8.3% of the Turkish population. A higher percentage of elderly (13.5%) live in the city to which Fatma migrated. Nearly half of the elderly people in Turkey only have a primary school education of five grades.

One of the common social problems in Turkey is violence against women (Guvenc et al. 2014; Lök 2015). Studies conducted on the elderly in Turkey found that the incidence of physical violence varies between 2 and 10% (Artan 2016) and the people who commit violent acts are generally the relatives of the victims (Artan 1996). Studies found that being female and having a low educational level are the factors that increase violence (Kissal and Beşer 2011; Tanriverdi and Şipkin 2008; Fadıloğlu and Şenuzun 2012). Moreover, not being submissive was regarded as a risk factor for violence directed against women (Ali et al. 2015).

For several decades violence against women in Turkey was interpreted and understood to be a domestic issue. This viewpoint changed because of the influence of the women's movement in the 1980s, which upheld that domestic violence is a crime and therefore local law enforcement should protect women against such violence based on enforceability of the law. As a result, it became a matter of public discussion in the society as opposed to being a private personal matter. The first legal dictate preventing violence against women under Turkish law was the Family Protection Law No. 4320, known as the Act No. 4320, which came into effect on January 17, 1998. Subsequently, Act No. 4320 was inadequate, and it became evident that either the law needed to be enforced or amendments were required to the existing Act. Finally, two new laws were passed: the Act of Family Protection and Prevention of Violence Against Women was passed on March 8, 2012, and then on January 18, 2013, the Regulation on the Act of Family Protection and Prevention of Violence Against Women was approved and enforced (Ozturk 2017).

Furthermore, international treaties were signed, such as the Convention on the Elimination of all Forms of Discrimination Against Women (CEDAW) and the Council of Europe Convention (2011) on preventing and combating violence against women and domestic violence (Istanbul Convention https://rm.coe.int/168046031c). The Istanbul Convention brings several obligations to signatory states, from prevention of all kinds of discriminations related to gender, sexual orientation, and gender identity and prevention of male violence to taking necessary measures against violence, providing compensations for women who were victims of violence, and inflicting penalties for perpetrators that are commensurate with the severity of the violent act. The treaty, which Turkey was one of the first to sign in 2011, is the first international Convention for European

Council that is binding and which has a monitoring mechanism.

On the other hand, the Act of Family Protection and Prevention of Violence Against Women of March 8, 2012 was passed after long meetings and spirited debates between members of the Ministry of Family and Social Policies and the Stop Violence Platform, which consisted of more than 250 women organizations. This law aims to protect women who are married, divorced, and engaged and whether in a relationship or single. It also protects children and family members who have already been victims of violence or who live under the threat of violence as well as all individuals who are victims of "persistent pursuit." According to the Stop Violence Platform, the law was based on the Istanbul Convention, and despite the Act's shortcomings when compared to the Convention itself, it has been a significant achievement in terms of advocacy. It provides two main measure injunctions as protective measures and preventive measures. Protective measures cover injunctions for the woman who is the victim of violence, such as access to shelter, legal assistance, and psychological support. Preventive measures cover injunctions for the author of the violent act, such as suspension. Those injunctions can be handed down by family court judges and in urgent cases enforced by the police (Ayhan 2017).

However, the rights acquired may not always be put into practice and used to protect women because of cultural reasons. Discussions about the fact that this topic is a specific problem that needs to be solved within the family are still ongoing (Salacin 2016).

40.3 Culturally Competent Strategies Recommended

40.3.1 Individual-/Family-Level Interventions

- In the cases of migrants, the reasons for migration, the migration process of the family, and their post-migration experiences should be examined. Some of these issues include cultural conflict, cultural shock, cultural pain, and cultural lag that Fatma and her husband have experienced.

- The cultural differences of the family should be examined. For example, the native language of the family was Kurdish, and the sect of the family was Shafi'i. Because women do not actively take part in the decision-making process, they could not make individual decisions.
- The family's perception of violence and the cultural reasons for violence should be examined. Explore how Fatma and her husband perceive violence against women or domestic violence. Do women deserve violence? Should the occurrence of violence be kept secret within the family? Is committing violence against women a right granted to men? etc.
- Employ culturally preferred means to combat domestic violence. These may include remaining silent, not revealing anything about the violence, denying the violence, consulting a traditional healer, etc.
- The cultural obstacles to combating domestic violence should be examined, such as wishing to remain in the marriage and worrying that reporting violence can damage the reputation of the family.
- Women who are victims of violence should be evaluated within the framework of their own cultures, and they should not be forced to exhibit any behavior that is deemed inappropriate within their cultures. The ways to combat domestic violence should be explained to women with patience. Strategies appropriate to their culture should be developed, and women should be persuaded to adopt these strategies. Female victims of violence should be assured that the violent acts are not reported to any government agencies such as police or gendarmerie without their consent.
- The cultural obstacles that hinder victims of violence and/or perpetrators of violence from seeking help from institutions, such as stigmatization and fear of exclusion, should be explored.

40.3.2 Organizational-Level Interventions

- Strategies should be developed for combating domestic violence that are in accordance with the various cultures. Pamphlets and leaflets in the language and literary level of the patients should be prepared and educational programs arranged. Concerns about privacy and fear of stigmatization related to domestic violence should be eliminated. Awareness among the staff and the patients should be raised about ways to combat domestic violence.
- Long-term solutions that do not ignore the cultural consequences of violence should be planned in combating domestic violence. Women should not be encouraged to get divorced before the consequences of divorce in their cultures are clearly identified.
- The support of religious leaders should be sought for combating domestic violence.

40.3.3 Community- and Societal-Level Interventions

- Strategies and interventions should be planned that prevent victims of violence and perpetrators of violence from being socially stigmatized.
- Community events should be planned to help remove the cultural obstacles to combating domestic violence. For example, women who come to a new region through migration could be invited to participate in social activities that are not contrary to their own cultures; this can help to raise their awareness.
- Support mechanisms should be developed that are appropriate to the cultures of women who are victims of violence. Communication lines organized and advisory hotlines appropriate to the various cultures can be established for victims of domestic violence.
- Public awareness of ways to combat domestic violence in a way that is appropriate to the various cultures should be raised, and help and

support should be provided by governmental as well as nongovernmental organizations. Such assistance can be obtained from foundations, social life centers, or violence prevention centers that are founded in accordance with the various cultures.

40.4 Conclusions: Case Study Follow-Up

40.4.1 Culture Care Preservation/ Maintenance

Although Fatma was a victim of violence, she did not reveal this situation to anyone and did not seek a way of combating it because of cultural reasons. On follow-up visits, Fatma was not marginalized or judged by her healthcare providers because of her decision, and her decision to maintain privacy was accepted with respect. Assurance was given in helping her feel culturally safe.

40.4.2 Culture Care Accommodation/ Negotiation

At first, Fatma was interviewed without her husband present. During these interviews, her healthcare provider spoke with Fatma using a nonjudgemental tone and with cultural sensitivity. She was asked how she perceives violence, why she did not use effective ways of combating violence, why she preferred to remain silent, and why she did not report the violence to anyone. Fatma was assured that she would not be forced to do anything against her will. The negative health effects of violence and ways of combating violence were explained to Fatma. She stated that she would not accept any approach that would harm her husband. It was suggested to Fatma that she share this situation with her family doctor and her children. It was also recommended that she consult a psychiatrist along with her husband, without telling anyone outside of the family.

40.4.3 Culture Care Repatterning/ Restructuring

Fatma agreed to tell her doctor and son about the episodes of domestic violence. Her family doctor spoke with Fatma's husband and told him that she needed to see a psychiatrist. Fatma went to a private psychiatric clinic with her son and husband. Her husband was also included in the process of the treatment, and after the second interview he began to receive treatment. Fatma's husband had difficulty in accepting treatment. At times, her husband did not want to take his medication. Fatma took her doctor's advice and gave her husband his medication by dissolving it in fruit juice. Except for their children, no one else knew about the episodes of violence or about their visits to a psychiatric clinic. The violence ended after a course of 4 weeks of treatment. Fatma's son began to visit his parents with his wife and children more often. Their grandchildren sometimes spent weekends with them. Fatma's husband began to work at his son's workplace during the day. All these changes were good for Fatma. Fatma was invited to a neighborhood social life center in order to mix with her peers and have an enjoyable time. However, her husband did not allow her to go. Fatma continued to spend most of her day performing domestic chores associated with her role as a woman, according to her culture and religious practices. A life without violence became the major source of happiness for Fatma.

Except for her children, no one was told that Fatma had been a victim of violence. She was not forced to do anything against her will or her desires. She was sent to the psychiatrist in strict confidence through the referral of her family doctor, and the response to treatment was positive.

References

Ali PA, Naylor PB, Croot E, O'Cathain A (2015) Intimate partner violence in Pakistan: a systematic review. Trauma Violence Abuse 16(3):299–315
Artan T (1996) Domestic physical Elder Abuse. Unpublished Master Thesis. Istanbul University

Department of Social Sciences Institute of Forensic Medicine, Istanbul

Artan T (2016) Financial abuse as a type of elderly abuse among elderly people residing in senior centers. HSP 3(1):48–56

Ayhan T (2017) Protecting the woman or the family? Contradiction between the law and its practice in violence against woman cases in Turkey. Marmara Univ J Polit Sci 5(1):137–162

Canatan K, Yıldırım E (2009) Family sociology. Acilim Book. 1st edn. İstanbul

Fadıloğlu Ç, Şenuzun AF (2012) Approach to abuse and neglect in the elderly. Ege J Med 51(Suppl):69–77

Guvenc G, Akyuz A, Cesario SK (2014) Intimate partner violence against women in Turkey: a synthesis of the literature. J Fam Violence 29(3):333–341

Ibiloglu AO (2012) Domestic violence. Curr Approaches Psychiatry 4(2):204–222

Kalaycı I, Şenkaynağı A (2015) Violence perception of the old people's attendants: sample of Suleyman Demirel University Hospital. Elderly Issues Res J 8(1):22–33

Kissal A, Beşer A (2011) Elder abuse and neglect in a population offering care by a primary health care center in Izmir, Turkey. Soc Work Health Care 50(2): 158–175

Kocacık F, Çağlayandereli M (2009) Domestic violence towards women: Denizli case study. Int J Hum Sci 6(2):25–43

Lök N (2015) Elder abuse and neglect in turkey: a systematic review. Curr Approach Psychiatry 7(29):149–156

Özçelik Adak N (2002) Health sociology women and urbanization, 1st edn. Birey Publishing, İstanbul, p 319

Ozturk N (2017) Ailenin korunması ve kadına karşi şiddetin önlenmesine dair kanunun getirdiği bazi yenilikler ve öneriler. Inonu Univ Law Revew 8(1):1–32

Salacin S (2016) Hollistic approches to the combating violence against women and expectations from İstanbul convention. Turkiye Klinikleri J Foren Med-Special Topics 2(2):6–18

Tanriverdi G, Şipkin S (2008) Effect of educational level of women on the domestic violence at Primary Health Care Unities in Canakkale. Fırat Med J 13(3):183–187

Tanriverdi G, Bayat M, Seviğ Ü, Birkök C (2011) Evaluation of the effect of cultural characteristics on use of health care services using the Giger And Davidhizar's Transcultural Assessment Model: a sample from a village in Eastern Turkey. Dokuz Eylül Univ School Nurs Electron J 4:19–24

The General Directorate on the Status of Women (2009) Domestic violence against women in Turkey. Elma Technical Printing, Ankara, Turkey

Yalcin Gursoy M, Tanriverdi G (2017) Comparison of violence against the elderly in different cultures living in Canakkale: a qualitative research. In: 3nd international congress on violence and gender, 21–22 April 2017, Kocaeli-Turkey

Yeşil P, Taşci S, Öztunç G (2016) Elder abuse and neglect. J DU Health Sci Inst 6(2):128–134

Yüksek Oktay E (2015) The common problem of Turkey and the world: violence against women. J Acad Stud 16(64):57–118

Case Study: Sources of Psychological Stress for a Japanese Immigrant Wife

Noriko Kuwano

Miho is a 32-year-old married Japanese woman who accompanied her husband on his posting overseas, together with their 2-year-old child. Before marriage, Miho worked for 2 years as a contract employee at a trading company after graduating from junior college. Six months ago, they relocated from a large metropolitan area in Japan to a suburban area near a big city on the east coast of the USA. In Japan, she had been a full-time homemaker who provided support for her busy husband and cared for their child. By contrast, moving with a young child to another country in which she was not fluent in the language meant that she started her life in the USA with a great deal of anxiety.

Last month, her menstruation persisted for 3 weeks. At first, she thought this was due to the stress of the move and thus just decided to monitor the situation. However, the bleeding continued for several more days, so she decided to visit the hospital. Although she had health insurance that could be used in the USA, finding a hospital that actually accepted it took longer than she had expected, leading to further increases in stress before her appointment. Moreover, her child was still small and needed constant attention. Her busy husband could not provide much support, and she did not know anyone in the neighborhood

to ask advice. As a result, she was very anxious at the time of her examination.

After the initial examination, she made several more appointments to undergo all of the necessary tests. Finally, she received a diagnosis of uterine fibroids. To complicate matters even further, she was also looking for a pediatrician who could administer the necessary vaccinations to her child. In addition, even though she wanted to properly support her husband, who continued to be busy after the move, she was unable to do so because of her illness, causing more stress. Owing to the time it took her to receive a diagnosis, the unfamiliar American healthcare system and lifestyle, and the stress of parenting, her stress began to accumulate. With no one to turn to for advice, she became depressed.

In order to visit hospitals and grocery stores, she needed to visit an area of the city that was not very safe. Crime rates, especially for robberies, were above the national average, and there had previously been shootings in that area. Because she lacked confidence in being able to communicate with taxi drivers, she relied on the subway to get around when she was not with her husband. Taking her child with her on the subway in a dangerous part of town was another substantial source of stress for Miho.

In Japan, her husband had led a work-centered lifestyle, leaving all domestic matters to Miho. These responsibilities had not changed after they came to the USA. If anything, she carried more of the domestic duties because her husband was

N. Kuwano, Ph.D., R.N., M.W., P.H.N.
International Nursing Department, Oita University of Nursing and Health Sciences, Oita, Japan
e-mail: kuwano@oita-nhs.ac.jp

© Springer International Publishing AG, part of Springer Nature 2018
M. Douglas et al. (eds.), *Global Applications of Culturally Competent Health Care: Guidelines for Practice*, https://doi.org/10.1007/978-3-319-69332-3_41

working even harder every day to adapt to the new environment. Although he had noticed that Miho was becoming depressed, he felt helpless because he did not know how to support her. Miho also felt very guilty about the burden she was putting on her husband.

After receiving her diagnosis, Miho was given several options regarding further treatment and was provided explanations about the effects and side effects of each. However, her English was not adequate to understand most of what she was told, so she just kept saying, "yes, yes" repeatedly. It soon became apparent to the nurse that she did not understand what was being said, so halfway through the explanations, the nurse hurriedly arranged for a volunteer medical interpreter to attend. With the assistance of the medical interpreter, Miho was able to grasp the essential content of the conversation. But when she was asked to decide between either continuing to monitor her condition or to begin treatment immediately, she became confused and was silent. She only managed to say, "Let me talk to my husband." The nurse recommended that for her next visit, Miho should be accompanied by her husband. Miho then scheduled her next appointment and went home.

The nurse subsequently arranged for a professional Japanese-American medical interpreter to attend Miho's next appointment. In addition, because Miho appeared to be emotionally distressed, Miho's healthcare team decided that it would be beneficial to introduce her to a therapist. Therefore, a list of mental health clinics in her area was prepared for her next visit.

On the day of the next appointment, Miho came with her husband. With the assistance of the interpreter, they were able to discuss the treatment options and make a decision. She and her husband agreed that she would first undergo drug treatment under continued observation. Thereafter, her physician would evaluate the situation to determine whether she would need to temporarily return to Japan for an operation. They received information on mental health clinics in her area but politely declined after offering their thanks. They seemed reluctant to have Miho undergo a psychological evaluation at a clinic.

41.1 Cultural Issues

Although traditional Japanese culture and values have been influenced greatly by the West, personal perspectives and communication styles remain the basis of Japanese behavior and thought (Takemura 2005). In Japanese culture, a strong emphasis is placed on family bonds, harmonious interpersonal relationships between group members, emotional restraint, and the avoidance of stigma or shame (Cheung et al. 2013).

Some studies have found that traditional gender roles—males working outside the home to provide for the family while females manage the household—remain dominant in Japan (Kozuki et al. 2006; Gunderman and Hua 2014). A central role of married Japanese women, one that takes precedence even over their own needs, is to maintain harmony within the family (Makabe and Hull 2000). Excessive self-sacrifice sometimes adversely affects the mental and physical health of married women, especially in new immigrants or those who are socially isolated.

Communication among Japanese people is known to be more indirect than that among Westerners. Effective nonverbal communication, including subtle gestures such as pausing between words, nodding the head, and silently smiling, is very important to the Japanese because it conveys the important content of a message (Makabe and Hull 2000). In terms of interaction, Japanese people rely on context, shared experience, and nonverbal clues (Gunderman and Hua 2014). In contrast to communication in Western culture, which is based on the spontaneous feelings and thoughts of the parties involved, communication in Japan is based on how accurately the person who initiates communication responds to the recipient's nonverbal needs and thoughts, which are defined by numerous social roles and norms (Kozuki et al. 2006). In Japan, people tend to regard tacit understanding as being a natural form of communication and might demand others understand what they have in mind without being told (Masaki et al. 2014). Furthermore, asking others about their feelings or disclosing one's feelings to another without being asked are both considered impolite (Kozuki et al. 2006).

In Japanese culture, non-verbalization and guessing (tacit understanding) in interpersonal relationships can sometimes lead to excessive hypersensitivity and in turn, psychological distress (Kozuki and Kennedy 2004). In addition, Japanese people rarely touch each other or maintain eye contact in communication (Yamashita and Doutrich 2013). One exception would be Japanese nurses, who sometimes utilize touching and eye contact to demonstrate special concern for their patients (Takada and Nagae 2012).

Some reports in the literature note that Japanese people prefer to seek informal rather than formal help when they have psychological distress because of the shame and social stigma associated with such mental illnesses as depression (Cheung et al. 2013). Whether deliberate or instinctual, patients sometimes present their depressive symptoms as a physical health issue, since expressing emotional distress as a manifestation of physical illness may be seen as more appropriate in Japanese culture. For Japanese persons, physical symptoms are understood to be a possible indication of emotional distress (Makabe and Hull 2000).

41.2 Social Structure Factors

The healthcare delivery system in the USA is different from that in Japan. Consequently, Japanese patients may find it confusing and considerably stressful when attempting to access it. Japan has a universal "free access" health insurance system through which anyone can receive a medical examination at any institution (Ministry of Health, Labor and Welfare 2013), and no scheduled appointment is required for the first visit.

In the healthcare setting, Japanese patients often prefer to wait rather than decide on a treatment plan on their own, even though healthcare providers try to provide sufficient information to patients and encourage them to make decisions with respect to their rights and quality of life. Japanese patients, especially those of the older generations, tend to trust healthcare providers as the authority and often consider it impolite to ask questions. Furthermore, Japanese patients typi-

cally share decision-making with their relatives (Takemura 2005).

Although historically, Japan is a homogeneous society, it has been progressively transitioning into one that is more culturally diverse. However, as of 2016, foreign residents only accounted for 1.82% of the population (Statistics Japan 2016), indicating that Japanese people still have few chances to communicate with culturally and linguistically diverse residents in daily life. Some Japanese therefore remain unaware of their unique communication style and underlying cultural values, as well as those of other countries.

41.3 Culturally Competent Strategies Recommended

In 2015, a total of 419,610 Japanese citizens resided in the USA, an increase of 5.4% within the last 5 years and with more females than males (Ministry of Foreign Affairs of Japan 2015). Even though the Japanese population in the USA is a very small proportion of the entire population, because of the uniqueness of Japanese culture, the following recommendations might be useful to improving culturally appropriate care for this population.

41.3.1 Individual-/Family-Level Intervention

- Listen carefully to clients' somatic complaints because the disclosure of physical symptoms can sometimes serve as a means for reporting psychological distress.
- Provide educational information about psychological distress, and reframe the negative concept of seeking mental help.
- Respect clients' help-seeking behavior, and suggest finding support to release tension.
- Maintain constant openness to cultural differences in the caring process.
- Contact family members and try to involve them in the individual's treatment plan.
- Consider differences in communication patterns, and be aware of the reliance on nonverbal

communication patterns; for example, saying "yes" does not mean affirmation or that I understand but rather "Yes, I hear you."

- Show strong interest in the person, and encourage them to talk about his or her feelings in a place where their privacy is protected.

41.3.2 Organizational-Level Intervention

- Establish organization-wide committees to address the promotion of culturally competent care delivery to all individuals.
- Provide printed materials on multiple conditions in the major languages of the population served.
- Provide a certified interpreter when the patient has limited language proficiency in the language that is different from the healthcare providers.
- Provide easy-to-express environment for patients when they have difficulty in expressing opposition to the decision made by the physician and/or family (Takemura 2005)
- Collaborate with the mental health therapist and psychologists/psychiatrists who understand Japanese culture and the unique characteristics of the Japanese to foster effective care.

41.3.3 Community-Level Intervention

- Establish a partnership with the Japanese community in your area or coalitions, such as an association of people from the same prefecture of Japan, to foster mutual support for healthy lifestyles both physically and mentally.
- Collaborate with the Japanese community in your area or coalitions such as an association of people from the same prefecture of Japan to bring isolated Japanese persons together within the community.

- Establish a partnership with the Japanese community coalition to assist with mental health education, such as during health fairs.

Conclusion

Various forms of cultural issues and social structural factors influenced Miho's physical and mental health status. Because of the traditional gender roles, Miho assumed that she should devote herself to her family, focusing on her function as full-time homemaker even under the pressures of moving to another country. As a consequence of limited exposure to the new environment, her acculturation process may have been delayed, and she was becoming socially isolated. The cumulative stressors, such as the disturbing symptoms, problems dealing with a health delivery system different from her original country, and her limited English proficiency, all led to her depressive symptoms. Furthermore, because of the stigma of mental illness in her culture, she may have failed to share her emotions and thus gain advice about and assistance with mental health problems.

In order to improve her health, an approach involving families and community is needed in order to be effective. It is important to try to reframe the negative concept of help-seeking for mental health problems through providing educational information both for clients and their families. A constant openness to cultural differences and challenges and efforts to understand a person's ways of preserving health and coping behavior in the care setting are indispensable.

References

Cheung M, Leung P, Tsui V (2013) Japanese Americans' health concerns and depressive symptoms: implications for disaster counseling. Soc Work 58(3):201–211

Gunderman R, Hua C (2014) Education in cultural competency in Japan. Acad Radiol 21(5):691–693

Kozuki Y, Kennedy MG, Tsai JH (2006) Relational experiences of partnered Japanese immigrant women with affect disorders. J Adv Nurs 53(5):513–523. https://doi.org/10.1111/j.1365-2648.2006.03753.x

Kozuki Y, Kennedy MG (2004) Cultural incommensurability in psychodynamic psychotherapy in Western and Japanese traditions. J Nurs Scholarsh 36(1):30–38. http://dx.doi.org/10.1111/j.1547-5069.2004.04008.x

Makabe R, Hull MM (2000) Components of social support among Japanese women with breast cancer. Oncol Nurs Forum 27(9):1381–1390

Masaki S, Ishimoto I, Asai A (2014) Contemporary issues concerning informed consent in Japan based on a review of court decisions and characteristics of Japanese culture. BMC Med Ethics 15:8. https://doi.org/10.1186/1472-6939-15-8

Ministry of Foreign Affairs of Japan (2015) Annual Report of Statistics on Japanese Nationals Overseas. http://www.mofa.go.jp/mofaj/files/000162700.pdf

Ministry of Health, Labor, and Welfare (2013) Health insurance: general overview. http://www.mhlw.go.jp/english/policy/healthmedical/healthinsurance/dl/health_insurance_bureau.pdf

Statistics Japan (2016) The number of registered foreign nationals in Japan. http://www.moj.go.jp/nyuukoku-kanri/kouhou/Nyuukokukanri04_00060.html

Takada M, Nagae M (2012) Hisesshokubunka dearu nihon no kango rinsho genba ni oite touching ga yuko ni hataraku yoin: togoteki bunkenkenkyu (Factors for effectiveness of touching in clinical ward in Japan where has contactless culture: literature review) (in Japanese). Bull Jpn Red Cross Toyota Coll Nurs 7(1):121–131

Takemura Y (2005) Cultural traits and nursing care particular to Japan. In: de Chesnay M (ed) Caring for the vulnerable: perspectives in nursing theory, practice, and research. Jones and Bartlett Publishers, Sudbury, MA, pp 235–243

Yamashita CY, Doutrich DL (2013) Japanese Americans. In: Giger JN (ed) Transcultural nursing: assessment & intervention, 6th edn. Elsevier, St. Louis, MO, pp 309–339

Case Study: Early Childbearing and Contraceptive Use Among Rural Egyptian Teens

42

Azza H. Ahmed

Hala is a 19-year-old Egyptian immigrant woman who came to the emergency room (ER) with heavy bleeding after miscarriage. Hala was 8 weeks pregnant with her second baby. The obstetrician performed a D&C, and blood testing revealed that her hemoglobin was 9.5. Iron supplements were ordered for her.

Hala did not have any prenatal visits for this recent pregnancy. She and her husband had looked for a prenatal care clinic in their area, and when they ultimately found such a clinic, they scheduled an appointment. However, the miscarriage occurred before the appointment. Hala's older baby is an 11-month-old boy who was born in Egypt. Hala mentioned that she had made two visits to the health center during this pregnancy in Egypt, but she gave birth at home with the assistance of a traditional birth attendant (daya) despite the risk of having premature birth.

Hala and her 26-year-old husband Othman were born and raised in a rural county in northern Egypt. When Hala was 17 1/2 years old, they married in an Egyptian traditional marriage arranged through their families. Hala became pregnant immediately after the wedding, and her first child was born at 35 weeks gestational age. After the birth of their son, Othman was permitted to immigrate to the USA with the lottery

A. H. Ahmed, DNSc, RN, IBCLC, CPNP
School of Nursing, Purdue University,
West Lafayette, IN, USA
e-mail: ahmedah@purdue.edu

green card he received because of an application submitted 2 years earlier, in which he cited financial limitations. He traveled alone to the east coast of the USA and found minimum wage work as an accountant and worker in a small business company. Hala joined her husband about 7 months ago.

Hala is a member of a large Muslim family with ten household members, including seven siblings who are younger than herself. She did not complete her high school education because she was always busy helping her mother with raising her younger siblings. When she married, she dropped out of school completely. Her father is a religious conservative man who does not believe in contraceptive use. Hala's husband Othman has four siblings. He received his bachelor's degree in commerce from a state university in northern Egypt. After serving his 1-year requirement of military service, he worked for the Egyptian government as an accountant for 2 years before immigrating to the USA.

Hala and her husband are currently living in a small apartment in a predominantly Arab community. They have very few fiends as Othman is working most of the time and Hala just recently arrived from Egypt. They visit their local mosque for prayer during the month of Ramadan and whenever there is a special event or celebration. Because of her limited English language ability, Hala does not like to interact with non-Arab neighbors. Consequently, she only shops when accompanied by her husband and only on the weekends when he is free of work responsibilities. She does not have a driving license. Since she did not drive in Egypt, she first needs to learn driving skills as well as learn enough English to obtain a driver's license in her new country of residence.

In the emergency department, during post-miscarriage counseling, the couple was asked about contraceptive use. Othman said that they never discussed this topic before or after getting married and they were not aware of the different options or types of contraception that they could use. Hala said that she and her mother never talked about using any contraceptive methods and that her mother-in-law told her that she would not get pregnant while she is breastfeeding.

Although the recent pregnancy was not planned, Hala and her husband were very sad about the loss of their baby. They started to discuss the need to visit a health provider and ask about contraceptive alternatives they could use. Othman said that he would love to have another baby, but not until Hala's condition stabilizes and their son gets older, as she doesn't have family to help her in the USA. In the Egyptian tradition, the women who had had a miscarriage stay home with family, and friends visit her to provide support and cook for the family until the mother's condition is improved. Family and friends also provide help with taking care of the children during this time. Based on Islamic ruling, if the fetus of the miscarriage is around 12 weeks of gestation or the body of the fetus is complete, the family should ask that the fetus be named. In addition, they need to follow the rules for any dead child, such washing the body in the Islamic way, laying it in a coffin (three layers of fabric), praying for the deceased person in the Mosque, and, finally, burying the body. In Hala's case, this process was not required as she was 8 weeks pregnant and the body of the fetus was not complete.

42.1 Cultural Issues

In the Egyptian culture sex education and intimate sexual relationships, including contraceptive use, are not topics that parents discuss with their chil-

dren, mostly out of shyness. Therefore, as part of their prenuptial counseling, mothers do not teach their daughters and sons about the need to use contraception during marriage. Not only do the parents avoid this topic, but schools in Egypt also do not provide needed information about successful use of contraceptive methods. Studies by Eltomy et al. (2013) and Awadalla (2012) found that lack of knowledge and cultural issues were the main barriers to contraceptive use and family planning among Egyptian women. This phenomenon is more common and predominant in rural areas where families consider discussing sex education and contraceptive use to be totally inappropriate and shameful. This phenomenon in rural areas is also combined with marriage at an early age, which leads to high rates of pregnancy, contraception nonuse, abortions, and other consequences, such as prematurity and maternal and infants' mortality and morbidities (WHO 2014; Awadalla 2012). In addition, married couples rarely discuss contraceptive use and family planning before marriage out of shyness and may discuss it only with precaution after getting married.

A qualitative study was conducted by Farrag and Hayter (2014) to examine Egyptian school nurses' knowledge and perception about sex education. The study highlighted several barriers to sex education: these include parents' concerns about discussing this topic with their children, saying that it a Western topic that is not appropriate for their children; cultural and religious issues that do not allow discussing the topic with children; and the nurses' concerns about their ability, skills and self-confidence to teach sex education. Therefore, the main source of information about intimate relations and contraceptive use is from the women's peers who often provide inaccurate information. Women even feel shy to discuss this topic if they have male healthcare providers.

Some aspects of sex education have been described in Islamic oral teachings. It is documented by the companions of Prophet Muhammad (peace be upon him) that He practiced coitus disruption as a method to prevent pregnancy. The following Hadiths (the Prophet's Sunnah) explains: "As Jaabir ibn Abdullah (may Allah be pleased with) said: 'We used to practice *azl* (coitus interruptus) while our Qur'an was being revealed. Jabir added 'We used to practice coitus interruptus during the lifetime of Allah's messenger (blessings and peace of Allah be upon him)'" (al-Bukhari, 5208) Imam Muslim al Naysaburi (1440) added: "This (the news of this practice) reached Allah's Apostle (blessings and peace of Allah be upon him) and he did not forbid it. Currently in Egypt, IUDs are the most commonly used contraceptive method (36%), followed by the pill (12%) (Family Planning 2020 2016; The world Bank 2016).

A study by *Darmstadt* et al. (2008) found that mothers usually received antenatal care from physicians in healthcare centers but traditional birth attendants (*dayas*) conducted most deliveries. They found that *dayas* attended roughly half of deliveries and were more common birth attendants than physicians, nurses, or relatives. More recent statistics found that slightly more than 9% of total births in rural areas in Egypt are done by traditional birth attendants, as compared to 3% in the urban areas (Egypt 2014). Despite the efforts of the Ministry of Health and WHO projects to ensure facility delivery and decrease maternal morbidity and mortality, traditional birth attendance still exist in rural and urban areas in Egypt, and *dayas* are still prominent and widely accepted care providers for the large share of births at home in rural Egypt, suggesting that expanding their skills to provide intrapartum care and antenatal and postnatal advice to recognize and encourage care-seeking for complications could improve neonatal outcome.

Another cultural aspect in Hala's case relates to the fact that in Egyptian culture, the oldest daughter has the responsibility of helping her mother and family in taking care of younger siblings. This cultural aspect combined with early marriage played a role in Hala's case of not being able to complete her high school education.

42.2   Social Structural Factors

Several sociodemographic factors are associated with the early childbearing and contraceptive use, including age, education, employment status, and income. In addition, adolescent fertility adversely affects not only young women's health, education, and employment prospects but also that of their children. Births to women aged 15–19 years old have the highest risk of infant and child mortality as well as a higher risk of morbidity and mortality for the young mother (WHO 2014).

According to WHO (2014), in the Arab Republic of Egypt, there are over 15.6 million adolescents aged 10–19 years, which is 18.4% of the country's total population. More than 50% of adolescents live in rural areas, 55.8% of adolescent girls and 47.8% of adolescent boys. By age 19, the mean number of years of school attended by married adolescent girls is 9.2. Among married adolescent girls who become parents before age 20, the average age at which they have their first baby is 17.9 years.

The WHO report also reported that most women who reported using contraceptive methods were 30–39 years old, were employed, were rich, were educated, and lived in urban governorates. According to the Egypt Demographic and Health Survey (EDHS) conducted by the Ministry of Health and Population (MOHP 2015), 79.5% of married adolescent girls aged 15–19 are not using a method of contraception. However, while 38.3% of married adolescent girls reported that they did not want a child in the next 2 years, only 23.4% of these are currently using any method to prevent pregnancy. The main reasons these adolescents report for not using a contraceptive method include menses has not returned after giving birth (41.8%), infrequent sex (28.5%), and breastfeeding (10.0%). When contraceptives are used, IUDs, one of the most effective methods, and pills are the most common modern methods used (9.8% and 7.1% of these adolescent girls, respectively). Injectable contraceptives are used by 0.9%, and lactational amenorrhea (LAM) is used by 1.6% (WHO 2016).

In Egypt, while early childbearing is more prevalent among the poor compared to rich counterparts, the rich-poor gap in prevalence of early childbearing is similar across cohorts. Findings from a study conducted in a rural area in northern

Egypt by El-Shazly et al. (2015) found that most of the women in the study were not aware of physiological, surgical, and emergency contraceptive methods. The most common contraceptive method used by this cohort of women was contraceptive pills.

In Egypt, the literacy rate among females aged 15 and above is 58%. Fewer girls are enrolled in primary schools compared to boys, with a ratio of female to male primary enrollment of 95%. The World Bank Report (2011) acknowledged that economic progress and greater investment in human capital of women will not translate into better reproductive outcomes if women lack access to reproductive health services. It is thus important to ensure that health systems provide a basic package of reproductive health education and services, including family planning (The World Bank 2016).

In order to improve maternal health including positive pregnancy outcomes, mothers should have access to prenatal care and family planning services. In Egypt, only about one quarter of pregnant women receive antenatal care from skilled medical personnel (physician, nurse, or midwife) with merely 66% of these having the recommended four or more antenatal visits. Nationally, 79% of pregnant women deliver their babies with the assistance of skilled medical personnel. But while 97% of women in the wealthiest quintile delivered with skilled health personnel, only 55% of women in the poorest quintile obtained such assistance. Furthermore, 86% of urban women as compared to 59% of rural women delivered their babies with assistance from skilled health personnel. Moreover, 45% of all pregnant women are anemic (defined as hemoglobin <110 g/L), increasing their risk of preterm delivery, low birth weight babies, stillbirth, and newborn death. Among all women aged 15–49 years who had given birth, 34% had no postnatal care within 6 weeks of delivery, while only 0.1% received postnatal checkup from a traditional birth attendant (Ministry of Health and Population (MOHP) 2015). These data are highly related to Hala's situation in terms of being a young mother who came from rural Egypt and experienced early childbearing with

preterm birth, anemia, inadequate prenatal care, and ultimate miscarriage.

42.3 Culturally Competent Strategies Recommended

Gender equality and women's empowerment are important for improving reproductive health, especially in developing countries. Higher levels of women's autonomy, education, wages, and labor market participation are associated with improved reproductive health outcomes (Shaikh et al. 2013).

42.3.1 Individual-/Family-Level Interventions

- Consider cultural assessment in all aspects including language, care preferences, religious beliefs, education, and socioeconomic status.
- Consider asking about parents and parents' in-law involvement in the family's decision-making.
- Be sensitive when addressing intimate partner relationships.
- Consider privacy and discuss the topic with each partner separately and then both together.
- Encourage sexual awareness and early introduction of contraceptive use and its benefits for families and their children.
- Provide premarital information sessions for couples about important topics for marriage, including contraceptive use in collaboration with the local Egyptian community.
- Teach the couples decision-making skills, including family planning. Awadalla (2012) reported that whatever the level of education, the majority of women thought that family planning decisions should be made by both partners. It is better to discuss contraceptive use with both partners together and help them to take an informed decision by educating them about different types of contraception available.

- Introduce Hala to the Special Supplemental Nutrition Program for Women, Infants, and Children (WIC) for her child and herself. WIC provides healthy nutrition that could help with her low hemoglobin level and breastfeeding, and she could receive correct information about lactation amenorrhea.
- Introduce Hala to community resources to learn life skills and be an active member in her community.

42.3.2 Organizational-Level Interventions

- Provide a licensed, culturally competent, and proficient interpreter to assist with communication between healthcare providers and Hala and her husband, especially with the discussion of types of contraceptives and selecting the appropriate method.
- Provide translated information in Arabic about the different types of contraception and written in educationally appropriate terminology. Partner with the local Egyptian community to raise awareness about the availability of contraceptive service available in the community and their correct uses.
- Provide English conversation classes to empower women like Hala to improve her English so she could be able to engage in more social relationships and understand her right to information and education.

42.3.3 Community-/Societal-Level Interventions

- Collaborate with local community mosques, and involve religious leaders in family planning programs. Shaikh et al. (2013) reported that the involvement of religious leaders in family planning programs had a positive influence on rural women.
- Discuss the importance of school nurses' and teachers' training sessions on how to discuss contraceptive use with middle and high school students in Muslim community schools if they have private Islamic schools. Farrag and Hayter (2014) reported that school nurses had concerns about their ability and self-confidence to discuss the topic with middle and high school students.
- Connect Hala with community resources to complete her education.

Conclusion

Hala is a typical case of an Egyptian teenager in rural Egypt who did not complete her high school education because of family and marriage responsibilities, got married early, and did not use any contraceptive methods to plan her family. Several factors played a role in Hala's case. Lack of knowledge, low educational level, and cultural and family issues all contributed to Hala's situation. Hala married when she was 17 1/2 years old, did not complete her basic education, had no information about contraceptive use and its benefits, and experienced a preterm birth with her first baby and a miscarriage with heavy bleeding in her second pregnancy. All these factors not only affect Hala's health but also her whole family and their future. Strategies to address Hala's situation should be discussed by culturally competent providers who should consider all social, cultural, religious, and familial aspects.

References

al-Bukhari M. The Sunnah of Muhammad. Book 67 Wedlock and Marriage, Hadith 142, hadith # 5208–5209. https://sunnah.com/bukhari/67

Awadalla HI (2012) Contraception use among Egyptian women: results from egypt demographic and health survey in 2005. J Reprod Infertil 13(3):167–173

Darmstadt G et al (2008) Practices of rural Egyptian birth attendants during the antenatal, intrapartum and early neonatal periods. J Health Popul Nutr 26(1):36–45

El-Shazly H, Elkilani O, Nashat N, Elshishiny R (2015) Evaluation of family planning services in a rural area in Al-Shohdaa district, Menoufiya governorate. Menoufia Med J 28(3):650–656. http://www.mmj.eg.net/article.asp?issn=1110-2098;year=2015;volume=28;issue=3;spage=650;epage=656;aulast=Anwar

Eltomy EM, Saboula NE, Hussein AA (2013) Barriers affecting utilization of family planning services among rural Egyptian women. Eastern Mediterr Health J 19(4):400–408

Family Planning 2020 (2016) Egypt: Family Planning 2020 Core Indicator Summary Sheet 2016. http://www.track20.org/download/pdf/2016%20FP2020%20CI%20Handouts/english/Egypt%202016%20FP2020%20CoreIndicators.pdf. Accessed August 2017

Farrag S, Hayter M (2014) A qualitative study of Egyptian school nurses' attitudes and experiences toward sex and relationship education. J School Nurs 30(1):49–56

Ministry of Health and Population (MOHP) [Egypt], El-Zanaty and Associates [Egypt], and ICF International (2015) Egypt demographic and health survey 2014. Ministry of Health and Population and ICF International, Cairo, Egypt. https://dhsprogram.com/pubs/pdf/fr302

Imam Muslim. The Sunnah of Muhammad. Book 16. The book of marriage. Hadith 164, hadith # 1440. https://sunna.com/muslim/16

Shaikh B, Azmat S, Mazhar A (2013) Family planning and contraception in Islamic countries: a critical review of the literature. J Pak Med Assoc 63(4 Suppl 3):S67–S72

The World Bank (2016) Reproductive health at a GLANCE, Egypt. http://documents.worldbank.org/curated/en/575751468233940262/pdf/629610BRIEF0Eg0BOX0361514B00PUBLIC0.pdf. Accessed June 2017

World Health Organization (2014) Arab Republic of Egypt: adolescent contraceptive use. WHO Publications. http://apps.who.int/iris/bitstream/10665/252445/1/WHO-RHR-16.69-eng.pdf?ua=1

World Health Organization (WHO) (2016) Adolescent contraceptive use: data from the Egypt demographic and health survey 2014 (EDHS). http://apps.who.int/iris/bitstream/10665/252445/1/WHO-RHR-16.69-eng.pdf. Accessed 24 July 2017

Case Study: A Chinese Immigrant Seeks Health Care in Australia

43

Patricia M. Davidson, Adam Beaman, and Michelle DiGiacomo

The forces of globalization and migration have enriched diversity across the globe as well as intensified certain migration corridors (Czaika and Haas 2014). Australia is a diverse and culturally pluralistic society with people from a range of cultural, ethnic, linguistic, and religious backgrounds (Radermacher and Feldman 2017). Aboriginal and Torres Strait Islander people have inhabited Australia for tens of thousands of years and are the traditional owners of the land (Brown 2009). Most Australians are immigrants or the descendants of immigrants who arrived over the last two centuries from more than 200 countries. Mainland China continues to remain the biggest country from which immigrants come to Australia, and in recent years, it has overtaken the United Kingdom to become its largest source of immigrants.

Differences between the Australian and Chinese health-care systems are evident and beyond language. Many factors, including differences in knowledge, values, and beliefs

P. M. Davidson, Ph.D., MEd., R.N., FAAN (✉)
A. Beaman, M.P.H.
School of Nursing, Johns Hopkins University, Baltimore, MD, USA
e-mail: pdavidson@jhu.edu; pdavids3@jhu.edu; abcaman1@jhu.edu

M. DiGiacomo, Ph.D.
University of Technology Sydney, Faculty of Health, Sydney, NSW, Australia
e-mail: michelle.digiacomo@uts.edu.au

about health, challenge Chinese Australians' access to health care. It is also impossible to deny that many Australians are not accepting of the rising Chinese influence (Grigg and Manderson 2016). Living in this environment can be challenging for individuals experiencing such discrimination and may affect their level of trust when interacting with their health team. Therefore, it compels health-care professionals to explore their own knowledge, attitudes, and beliefs about other cultural groups. Every day, millions of individuals fail to receive optimal care and are either exposed to medical errors or lack access to care. Ethnicity, culture, and sociodemographic factors are important considerations influencing these challenges (Vincent and Amalberti 2016). The antecedent and moderating factors for this situation are complex and multifaceted and require innovative and collaborative solutions. The story provided below is not an unusual one. It underscores the importance of ensuring there is both understanding of the health information provided to the client and its follow-up, particularly in individuals with limited English language proficiency and health literacy.

It is a busy Wednesday in the cardiology clinic when the clinical trial nurse looks up at Mr. Wang's face. She sees a 54-year-old Chinese man who migrated to Australia from Mainland China 3 years ago. He was recently admitted to the hospital with a diagnosis of chronic heart failure and was eager to engage in conversation with the nurse. He is smiling, and the nurse and Mr. Wang are engaging in social chatter before the interpreter arrives to explain a clinical trial that Mr. Wang has agreed to consider. Mr. Wang has working knowledge of English, and he is employed as a painter in a local company. He confesses that he is very tired, and it is harder to do his job.

While assessing eligibility to participate in the clinical trial, the nurse is perplexed to see that Mr. Wang had been scheduled for coronary bypass surgery 3 months earlier, but it appeared that the surgery was not done—at least not at this hospital. She makes a note that this is an important issue to explore when the health-care interpreter arrives. During a discussion with the health-care interpreter, it was clear that the surgery was not performed and that Mr. Wang was not aware of the severity of his condition. In addition, he had not followed up with his primary care provider following the hospitalization. What evolved was this serendipitous visit to consider a clinical trial that might save Mr. Wang's life. Through the direct intervention of the clinical trial nurse, who worked with the interpreter to assure that Mr. Wang understood his condition and the need for surgery and follow-up medications, treatment for his chronic heart failure, finally started. The surgery for his triple-vessel coronary artery disease was scheduled, and therapy for his chronic heart failure was initiated.

Mr. Wang also told the nurse and interpreter that he goes to the traditional Chinese medicine doctor in Chinatown for his health problems and does not see the primary care physician listed in his medical record. This is an important observation in ensuring adherence with recommended medications and avoiding drug interactions. The nurse and interpreter emphasized to Mr. Wang the importance of engaging in regular contact with his primary care physician and carefully disclosing all of his medications, including herbal preparations.

It was evident from this encounter that Mr. Wang had "slipped through the cracks" in the system. His "working" English had led to many assumptions by the health-care providers regarding his literacy. Plus, his agreeable and non-confronting attitude had likely led the clinical staff to assume he could both read and understand the written discharge instructions. A lack of systematic follow-up as well as exploring the reasons for not presenting for his surgical procedures was a missed opportunity. Mr. Wang seemed to still hold onto many of his traditional beliefs about health and wellness, and it did not appear that he understood the seriousness of receiving a diagnosis of chronic heart failure, nor the importance of managing his coronary artery disease and engaging in secondary prevention strategies. These factors should have been considered in his discharge planning and in developing a follow-up plan. His belief and faith in traditional Chinese medicine was also an important flag to ensure that drug interactions are explored (Daly et al. 2002; Davidson et al. 2003). It is important for health-care professionals to promote a culture that enables individuals and their families to discuss their traditional beliefs and explore how they align with recommended treatment strategies. By openly discussing and asking about home remedies used, health-care providers can project a receptive attitude toward traditional health-care beliefs and practices.

43.1 Social and Structural Factors Underling the Vulnerability of This Population and Influencing the Problem

Although migrants often have a "healthy immigrant effect," this effect diminishes over time (Gushulak 2007). The process of migration, whether forced or voluntary, is a stressful event. Immigrants are commonly identified as vulnerable populations. But there is, in fact, heterogeneity in the exposure to these susceptibilities, which are largely moderated by social determinants of health and access to resources. Derose et al. (2007) consider factors such as socioeconomic circumstances, immigration status, language proficiency, access to publicly funded health care, residential location, stigma, and marginalization that can have an impact on health-care outcomes. Sadly, global nationalistic forces can amplify the alienation and marginalization of many migrant groups, particularly those who visibly appear different from the mainstream population or hold specific religious and cultural beliefs (Gostin and Friedman 2017).

It is difficult for health-care professionals to address issues such as residential location and stigma. Yet, with thought, preparation, and training, health-care professionals can address health literacy and improve communication and coordination of care through tailored and targeted strategies. Nurses are in an excellent position to activate these important strategies, including addressing health literacy. Health literacy is the degree to which individuals have the capacity to obtain, process, and understand basic health information and services needed to make appropriate health decisions. Health literacy can often be a stronger predictor of health outcomes than social and economic status, education, gender, and age (DeWalt et al. 2004; Nutbeam 2008). Providing health information and addressing language, literacy, and numeracy are important to addressing the needs of individuals and populations (Batterham et al. 2016).

43.2 Culturally Competent Strategies Recommended

43.2.1 Individual-/Family-Level Interventions

Achieving familiarity with a cultural and environmental context is essential for nurses to provide culturally competent communication. Culturally relevant guidelines provide a useful backdrop and contextual information. However, it is always important to avoid stereotyping of cultural issues and take steps to identify and discuss each individual's own knowledge, attitudes, and beliefs about their health situation (Davidson et al. 2007). The following factors should be considered within a comprehensive clinical, cultural, and social assessment to

ensure individuals like Mr. Wang obtain optimal care:

- Effective cultural communication demonstrates respect, dignity, and appreciation of differences and, like any other skill, requires training and practice.
- As part of the admission process, there should be an assessment of the person's cultural self-identity, health-seeking behaviors, home remedies used, language preferences, and environmental, occupational, socioeconomic, and educational status.
- Engagement with certified health-care interpreters is crucial in ensuring that individuals understand their condition and treatment strategies.
- Translation deals with written communication, while interpretation involves the spoken word, both of which are important in achieving a level of shared understanding.
- Understanding traditional health beliefs is important in developing plans of care. Mr. Wang's use of traditional medicines may cause interactions with other medications.
- Promotion of a culture that enables the individual to feel comfortable with disclosure is important.
- There are many websites and resources available to assist in providing culturally appropriate and translated material. Reliable sources are provided by the Centers for Disease Control and Prevention (National Center for Health Statistics 2016).
- Many lesbian, gay, bisexual, transsexual, and queer persons may have great difficulty in obtaining high-quality health care, and this experience is often amplified for those persons if they are members of minority populations (Wilson and Yoshikawa 2007).

43.2.2 Organizational Level

Ideally, our health-care institutions should be seen as part of our communities, and the staff working in these institutions should reflect the sociodemographic and cultural profile of the local community. The following factors are useful in promoting cultural competence and optimal patient outcomes at the level of the organization and community:

- Engagement with core community organizations is crucial in increasing alignment of institutional programs and resources with the community's goals.
- The use of community health workers and liaison staff can be useful additions to the health-care team within the organization.
- Implementation of system-wide interdisciplinary programs for cultural competence development should be a priority of the organization.
- The health-care system should ensure that its budget includes human and financial resources for both health-care interpreters and translation of materials.
- Interpreters via telephone and video-based conferencing can be useful in emergency situations.
- Health-care interpreters must ensure confidentiality, be knowledgeable about health-care language, and conduct all sessions in an ethical manner.
- Policies and systems should be available to monitor health outcomes and ensure quality improvement and progress in addressing the care needs of diverse patients and communities.

43.2.3 Societal Level

Programs and policies that address social determinants of health are crucial. For societies to be engaging and welcoming to migrants, policies should be enabling and appreciative of differences. The Australian Bureau of Statistics (2016) estimated that as of 30 June 2016, 28.5% of the Australian population was born overseas, equal to 6.9 million people, underscoring the importance of this issue.

Immigrants often face disproportionate barriers to accessing health coverage and care (Artiga et al. 2016). Challenges can be the lack of knowledge in how to enter the health-care system as well as discrimination and stigmatization. It is particularly challenging for those with nonoffi-

cial status and no health insurance. Many immigrants to Australia are not covered by reciprocal health-care agreements, and the cost of private health insurance can be prohibitive. Just and civil societies provide a safety net for all individuals regardless of immigration status. Globally, more and more individuals are displaced by geopolitical instability, climate change, and environmental disasters. A study from the United Nations Refugee Agency found a total of 65.3 million people were displaced at the end of 2015, and this number continues to grow, challenging health-care systems across the globe (Langlois et al. 2016). It is critical that health-care providers are prepared for the associated changes and challenges that lie ahead, particularly in relation to patient populations.

Conclusion

Achieving cultural competency requires a multilevel approach. Realizing equity, social justice, and optimal outcomes requires interventions at the level of the individual, organization, and society. Social ecological frameworks have been widely adopted, recognizing that no single factor can explain or predict a particular phenomenon (Baron et al. 2014; Fleury and Lee 2006). Given the complexity of the environments in which nurses serve the health of others, an understanding of the dynamic interplay between the dimensions influencing culture, work environments, and practice is necessary. Addressing health disparities at the local, national, and global level requires making fundamental changes in health-care delivery. Much of this can be achieved by interventions at the policy level and requires data-driven approaches to advocacy. Viewing health care within a social ecological context is important for considering this complex interaction (Davidson et al. 2016). Policies have the power to have an impact on changing systems and the health of populations. We can see the impact of the Affordable Care Act in the United States on improving access to care and, as a consequence, health outcomes (McManus et al. 2016).

Optimal health outcomes, especially for vulnerable groups, are intimately linked with socioeconomic and ecological factors and political situations, with cumulative risks to health. Health-care professionals should understand the sociopolitical structures and processes for policy making. Nurses should have the ability to work with different political and community groups and organizations to establish policies addressing social and environmental inequities and disparities in health care. Understanding broad social issues affecting the health of populations and developing the skills in building effective coalitions at local, national, and global levels are important for addressing health disparities.

Across the globe, professional nursing organizations are galvanizing to promote a culture of health and advancing equity and social justice (Hanks et al. 2017). From the International Council on Nursing advocating for universal health coverage to the *Future of Nursing: Campaign for Action in the United States* to improve America's health through nursing advocacy for the people we serve, professional advocacy is increasing in importance. An important part of this advocacy is promoting respect, tolerance, and recognition of the cultural diversity and pluralism of contemporary society and their implications for health care.

References

Artiga S, Damico A, Young K, Cornachione E, Garfield R (2016) Health coverage and care for immigrants. Kaiser Family Foundation, Washington, DC

Australian Bureau of Statistics (2016) 3412.0—migration, Australia, 2015–16. http://www.abs.gov.au/ausstats/abs@.nsf/Latestproducts/3412.0Main%20Features32015-16?opendocument&tabname=Summary&prodno=3412.0&issue=2015-16&num=&view=. Accessed 12 June 2017

Baron SL, Beard S, Davis LK, Delp L, Forst L, Kidd-Taylor A et al (2014) Promoting integrated approaches to reducing health inequities among low-income workers: applying a social ecological framework. Am J Ind Med 57(5):539–556

Batterham R, Hawkins M, Collins P, Buchbinder R, Osborne R (2016) Health literacy: applying current concepts to improve health services and reduce health inequalities. Public Health 132:3–12

Brown A (2009) Bridging the survival gap between Indigenous and non-Indigenous Australians: priorities for the road ahead. Heart Lung Circul 18(2):96–100

Czaika M, Haas H (2014) The globalization of migration: has the world become more migratory? Int Migr Rev 48(2):283–323

Daly J, Davidson P, Chang E, Hancock K, Rees D, Thompson DR (2002) Cultural aspects of adjustment to coronary heart disease in Chinese-Australians: a review of the literature. J Adv Nurs 39(4):391–399

Davidson P, Hancock K, Leung D, Ang E, Chang E, Thompson DR, Daly J (2003) Traditional Chinese Medicine and heart disease: what does Western medicine and nursing science know about it? Eur J Cardiovasc Nurs 2(3):171–181

Davidson PM, Macdonald P, Moser DK, Ang E, Paull G, Choucair S et al (2007) Cultural diversity in heart failure management: findings from the DISCOVER study (Part 2). Contemp Nurse 25(1–2):50–62

Davidson P, Phillips JL, Dennison-Himmelfarb C, Thompson S, Luckett T, Currow D (2016) Providing palliative care for cardiovascular disease from a perspective of sociocultural diversity: a global view. Curr Opin Support Palliat Care 10(1):11–17

Derose KP, Escarce JJ, Lurie N (2007) Immigrants and health care: sources of vulnerability. Health Aff 26(5):1258–1268

DeWalt DA, Berkman ND, Sheridan S, Lohr KN, Pignone MP (2004) Literacy and health outcomes. J Gen Intern Med 19(12):1228–1239

Fleury J, Lee SM (2006) The social ecological model and physical activity in African American women. Am J Commun Psychol 37(1–2):129–140

Gostin LO, Friedman EA (2017) Reimagining WHO: leadership and action for a new Director-General. Lancet 389(10070):755–759

Grigg K, Manderson L (2016) The Australian Racism, Acceptance, and Cultural-Ethnocentrism Scale (RACES): item response theory findings. Int J Equity Health 15(1):49

Gushulak B (2007) Healthier on arrival? Further insight into the "healthy immigrant effect". Can Med Assoc J 176(10):1439–1440

Hanks RG, Starnes-Ott K, Stafford L (2017) Patient advocacy at the APRN level: a direction for the future. Paper presented at the Nursing Forum

Langlois EV, Haines A, Tomson G, Ghaffar A (2016) Refugees: towards better access to health-care services. Lancet 387(10016):319–321

McManus KA, Rhodes A, Bailey S, Yerkes L, Engelhard CL, Ingersoll KS et al (2016) Affordable care act qualified health plan coverage: association with improved HIV viral suppression for AIDS drug assistance program clients in a medicaid nonexpansion state. Clin Infect Dis 63(3):396–403

National Center for Health Statistics (2016) Health, United States, 2015. with special feature on racial and ethnic health disparities

Nutbeam D (2008) The evolving concept of health literacy. Soc Sci Med 67(12):2072–2078

Radermacher H, Feldman S (2017) Cultural diversity, health and ageing. In: O'Loughlin K, Browning C, Kendig H (eds) Ageing in Australia. Springer, New York, pp 83–101

Vincent C, Amalberti R (2016) Safer healthcare. Springer, Cham

Wilson PA, Yoshikawa H (2007) Improving access to health care among African-American, Asian and Pacific Islander, and Latino lesbian, gay, and bisexual populations. In: Meyer IH, Northridge ME (eds) The health of sexual minorities. Springer, Boston, MA, pp 607–637